T0362521

Current Controversies in Diagnostic and Interventional Radiology

Editors

DOUGLAS S. KATZ
JOHN J. HINES JR

RADIOLOGIC CLINICS
OF NORTH AMERICA

www.radiologic.theclinics.com

Consulting Editor
FRANK H. MILLER

November 2024 • Volume 62 • Number 6

ELSEVIER

1600 John F. Kennedy Boulevard • Suite 1800 • Philadelphia, Pennsylvania, 19103-2899

http://www.theclinics.com

RADIOLOGIC CLINICS OF NORTH AMERICA Volume 62, Number 6
November 2024 ISSN 0033-8389, ISBN 13: 978-0-443-24626-5

Editor: John Vassallo (j.vassallo@elsevier.com)
Developmental Editor: Malvika Shah

Radiologic Clinics of North America (ISSN 0033-8389) is published bimonthly by Elsevier Inc., 360 Park Avenue South, New York, NY 10010-1710. Months of issue are January, March, May, July, September, and November. Periodicals postage paid at New York, NY and additional mailing offices. Subscription prices are USD 561 per year for US individuals, USD 100 per year for US students and residents, USD 643 per year for Canadian individuals, USD 754 per year for international individuals, USD 100 per year for Canadian students/residents, and USD 315 per year for international students/residents. For institutional access pricing please contact Customer Service via the contact information below. To receive student and resident rate, orders must be accompanied by name of affiliated institution, date of term and the signature of program/residency coordinatior on institution letterhead. Orders will be billed at individual rate until proof of status is received. Foreign air speed delivery is included in all *Clinics* subscription prices. All prices are subject to change without notice. Orders, claims, and journal inquiries: Please visit our Support Hub page https://service.elsevier.com for assistance.

Reprints. For copies of 100 or more of articles in this publication, please contact the Commercial Reprints Department, Elsevier Inc., 360 Park Avenue South, New York, New York 10010-1710. Tel.: +1-212-633-3874; Fax: +1-212-633-3820; E-mail: reprints@elsevier.com.

Radiologic Clinics of North America also published in Greek Paschalidis Medical Publications, Athens, Greece.

Radiologic Clinics of North America is covered in *MEDLINE/PubMed (Index Medicus), EMBASE/Excerpta Medica, Current Contents/Life Sciences, Current Contents/Clinical Medicine, RSNA Index to Imaging Literature, BIOSIS, Science Citation Index,* and *ISI/BIOMED.*

Contributors

CONSULTING EDITOR

FRANK H. MILLER, MD, FACR, FSAR, FSABI
Lee F. Rogers, MD, Professor of Medical Education; Chief, Body Imaging Section; Medical Director, MRI; Professor, Department of Radiology, Northwestern Memorial Hospital, Northwestern University, Feinberg School of Medicine, Chicago, Illinois, USA

EDITORS

DOUGLAS S. KATZ, MD, FACR, FSAR, FASER
Vice Chair for Research, Professor of Radiology (Scholar Track - Clinical), Department of Radiology, NYU Grossman Long Island School of Medicine, NYU Langone Hospital - Long Island, Mineola, New York, USA

JOHN J. HINES Jr, MD, FACR
Associate Professor, Department of Radiology, Zucker School of Medicine at Hofstra/ Northwell, Huntington, New York, USA

AUTHORS

GREGG BLUMBERG, DO
Resident Physician, NYU Grossman Long Island School of Medicine, NYU Langone Hospital – Long Island, Mineola, New York, USA

THIAGO A. BRAGA, MD
Assistant Professor, Department of Radiology, Jackson Memorial Hospital, University of Miami-Miller School of Medicine, Miami, Florida, USA

KIM M. CABAN, MD
Assistant Professor, Department of Radiology, Jackson Memorial Hospital, University of Miami-Miller School of Medicine, Miami, Florida, USA

HERSH CHANDARANA, MD
Professor, Department of Radiology, NYU Langone Health, New York, New York, USA

LUIS COLON-FLORES, MD
Resident Physician, NYU Grossman Long Island School of Medicine, NYU Langone Hospital – Long Island, Mineola, New York, USA

BARI DANE, MD
Director of Computerized Tomography, Associate Professor, Department of Radiology, NYU Grossman School of Medicine, Director of Quality and Safety Main Campus Outpatient Imaging, NYU Langone Health, New York, New York, USA

KUSH R. DESAI, MD
Associate Professor, Division of Vascular and Interventional Radiology, Department of Radiology, Northwestern University Feinberg School of Medicine, Chicago, Illinois, USA

DANIELA GALAN, MD
Assistant Professor, Department of Radiology, Jackson Memorial Hospital, University of Miami-Miller School of Medicine, Miami, Florida, USA

ELENA GHOTBI, MD
Post-Doctoral Research Fellow, Johns Hopkins University School of Medicine, Baltimore, Maryland, USA

TARIK GOZEL, MD
Resident, Department of Radiology, Albert
Einstein College of Medicine, Jacobi Medical
Center, Bronx, New York, USA

JASON C. HOFFMANN, MD, FSIR
Attending Physician, NYU Langone
Hospital – Long Island, Associate Professor
of Radiology, NYU Grossman Long Island
School of Medicine, Mineola, New York,
USA

JULIE HONG, MD
Resident Physician, Department of Surgery,
New York-Presbyterian Queens Hospital,
Flushing, New York, USA

SHAYAN CHASHM JAHAN, BS
PhD Student, Department of Computer
Science, University of Maryland, College Park,
Maryland, USA

STELLA K. KANG, MD, MSc
Associate Professor of Radiology and
Population Health, Associate Chair, Population
Health Imaging and Outcomes, NYU
Grossman School of Medicine, New York,
New York, USA

**DOUGLAS S. KATZ, MD, FACR, FSAR,
FASER**
Vice Chair for Research, Professor of
Radiology (Scholar Track - Clinical),
Department of Radiology, NYU Grossman
Long Island School of Medicine, NYU Langone
Hospital - Long Island, Mineola, New York,
USA

FOAD KAZEMI, MD
Post-Doctoral Research Fellow, Johns
Hopkins University School of Medicine,
Baltimore, Maryland, USA

JESI KIM, MD
Chief Resident, Department of Diagnostic
Radiology, NYU Grossman School of
Medicine, Department of Radiology, NYU
Langone Health, New York, New York,
USA

DANIEL B. KOPANS, MD, FACR, FSBI
Professor, Department of Radiology, Harvard
Medical School, Boston, Massachusetts,
USA

ROCÍO G. MÁRQUEZ, MD
Resident, Division of Vascular and
Interventional Radiology, Department of
Radiology, Northwestern University Feinberg
School of Medicine, Chicago, Illinois,
USA

JENNIFER S. McDONALD, PhD
Associate Professor, Department of Radiology,
Mayo Clinic, Rochester, Minnesota,
USA

ROBERT J. McDONALD, MD, PhD
Assistant Professor, Department of Radiology,
Mayo Clinic, Rochester, Minnesota, USA

BENJAMIN M. MERVAK, MD
Associate Professor, Department of Radiology,
Michigan Medicine, Ann Arbor, Michigan,
USA

ALIREZA MOHSENI, MD
Post-Doctoral Research Fellow, Johns
Hopkins University School of Medicine,
Baltimore, Maryland, USA

ANITA MOHSENI, BS
Graduate Student, Azad University Tehran
Medical Branch, Tehran, Iran

KRISHNA MUNDADA, MD
Medical Officer, Department of Nuclear
Medicine, Seth G.S. Medical College and
K.E.M Hospital, Mumbai, India

FELIPE MUNERA, MD
Professor, Department of Radiology,
Jackson Memorial Hospital, University of
Miami-Miller School of Medicine, Miami,
Florida, USA

A. ORLANDO ORTIZ, MD, MBA, FACR
Professor, Department of Radiology, Albert
Einstein College of Medicine, Jacobi Medical
Center, Bronx, New York, USA

FABIO M. PAES, MD, MBA
Associate Professor, Department of Radiology,
Jackson Memorial Hospital, University of
Miami-Miller School of Medicine, Miami,
Florida, USA

PARI V. PANDHARIPANDE, MD, MPH
Professor and Chair of Radiology, The Ohio
State University College of Medicine,
Columbus, Ohio, USA

JOHN S. PELLERITO, MD, FSRU, FAIUM
Vice Chair of Clinical Affairs and Residency
Program Director, Department of Radiology,
Division of US, CT and MRI, Peripheral
Vascular Laboratory, North Shore - Long Island
Jewish Health System, New Hyde Park,
New York, USA

**MARGARITA V. REVZIN, MD, MS, FAIUM,
FSRU, FACR, FSAR**
Associate Professor, Department of Radiology
and Biomedical Imaging, Yale School of
Medicine, New Haven, Connecticut, USA

AMIRALI SHABABI, BS
Medical Student, School of Medicine, Iran
University of Medical Sciences, Tehran, Iran

NILOUFAR SHABABI, MD
Post-Doctoral Research Fellow, Johns
Hopkins University School of Medicine,
Baltimore, Maryland, USA

KRISHNA SHANBHOGUE, MD
Professor, Department of Radiology,
NYU Langone Health, New York, New York,
USA

LEANDRO SINGERMAN, MD
Department of Radiology, Jackson
Memorial Hospital, University of Miami-Miller
School of Medicine, Miami, Florida,
USA

BENJAMIN SRIVASTAVA
Wilton Public High School, Wilton,
Connecticut, USA

MILTIADIS TEMBELIS, MD
Resident Physician, Department of Radiology
NYU Grossman Long Island School of
Medicine, NYU Langone Hospital – Long Island,
Mineola, New York, USA

Contents

At its best, the practice of medicine involves careful integration of experience and evidence. Generating evidence to address controversies in radiology – and translating such evidence to practice – requires appropriate selection of methods, and an understanding of the strengths, shortcomings, and biases inherent to different research designs and analyses. Equipped with such knowledge, the radiologic community can ensure that both research and clinical practice in our discipline excels, and that those questions that will be the most critical to answer will be formulated for successful investigation in the years to come.

The integration of artificial intelligence (AI) in radiology has brought about substantial advancements and transformative potential in diagnostic imaging practices. This article presents an overview of the current research on the application of AI in radiology, highlighting key insights from recent studies and surveys. These recent studies have explored the expected impact of AI, encompassing machine learning and deep learning, on the work volume of diagnostic radiologists. The present and future role of AI in radiology holds great promise for enhancing diagnostic capabilities, improving workflow efficiency, and ultimately, advancing patient care.

Immediate hypersensitivity reactions to iodinated contrast media and gadolinium-based contrast media can be life-threatening. While corticosteroid premedication or agent-switching may mitigate risk, evidence is largely indirect and based on historical studies; recent literature refutes the efficacy. Guidance on premedication varies between organizations worldwide. No strategy eliminates reactions, and indirect consequences of premedication are substantial. Accelerated regimens are often used for emergencies, but are of questionable efficacy. Identifying "high-risk" patients is complex, but a history of reactions (to the same contrast class) is the biggest risk factor.

Iodinated contrast material (ICM) is a critical component for many radiologic examinations and procedures. However, ICM has often been withheld in the past out of concern for its potential nephrotoxicity and increased risk of morbidity and mortality, often at the expense of diagnostic accuracy and timely diagnosis. Evidence from controlled studies now suggest that most cases of acute kidney injury (AKI) caused by ICM were instead due to contrast-independent causes of AKI or normal variation in renal function. This article will discuss current knowledge of contrast-induced AKI, including the incidence, sequelae, risk factors, and prevention strategies of this potential complication.

There are many misconceptions related to the usage of intravenous contrast agents for medical imaging. These misconceptions can affect patient care, as they can lead to nonoptimal examination usage. Knowledge of the current contrast-related misconceptions can help radiologists provide higher quality care to their patients.

Osteoporotic vertebral compression fractures can be quite challenging to treat, especially since they often occur in older adults and can be associated with significant morbidity and mortality. The standard treatment for these fractures has been medical management, as many of these patients are not candidates for open surgery. Vertebral augmentation procedures have emerged as another treatment option. Though initially accepted by clinicians, the benefit of these procedures has been questioned by several clinical trials. Safety concerns related to adjacent level fractures and cement extravasation have also been raised. We review these controversies in the context of the current literature.

The following is an overview of the numerous efforts to reduce access for women to breast cancer screening. Misinformation has been promoted over the many years to suggest that screening only works for women aged 50 years and over. In fact, there are no scientifically derived data to support the use of the age of 50 years as a threshold for screening. The randomized, controlled trials have proved that screening saves lives for women aged 40 to 74 years (the age of the women who participated).

Lower extremity deep venous thrombosis (DVT) is estimated to occur in 1 in 1000 persons annually in adult populations, with prevalence predicted to double by the year 2050. While acute DVT and pulmonary embolism are a major cause of cardiovascular morbidity and mortality, the long-term prognosis for patients with venous thromboembolism is in part determined by the development of post-thrombotic syndrome (PTS), which occurs in up to 50% of patients. PTS refers to a chronic syndrome complex, invariably characterized by intractable edema, pain, stasis dermatitis, and venous stasis ulceration when severe.

Hepatocellular carcinoma (HCC) is a leading cause of cancer-related deaths worldwide. Early detection of HCC is a key factor in enabling curative therapies and improving overall survival. Worldwide, several guidelines are available for surveillance of at-risk populations and diagnosis of HCC. This article provides a current comprehensive update on screening and diagnosis of HCC.

Jesi Kim and Bari Dane

CT and MR enterography are cross-sectional imaging examinations used in the assessment of inflammatory bowel disease. Consistent reporting and standardized nomenclature are important for clear communication with referring clinicians. Enterography has not only been used to depict inflammation in the small bowel, but it has also been used to quantify disease activity, assess distribution of disease, and detect complications including penetrating disease. This article reviews cross-sectional imaging findings in inflammatory bowel disease, including the current literature focusing on small bowel Crohn's disease and ulcerative colitis, with evidence-based guidelines on appropriate protocols and imaging procedures.

Krishna Mundada, John S. Pellerito, Benjamin Srivastava, and Margarita V. Revzin

Intravenous contrast-enhanced ultrasound (CEUS) is a rapidly evolving imaging technique that uses a microbubble contrast agent to enhance ultrasonographic images by augmenting characterization of blood vessels and organ perfusion. CEUS is considered as a useful problem-solving tool and as an indicated first-line imaging modality in select settings. CEUS technique has an inherent advantage over its predecessor B-mode and Doppler imaging. This article reviews different approved and off-label use of CEUS in the pediatric and adult population and also discusses Food and Drug Administration-approved contrast agents in the United States, their reported side effects, and ongoing efforts in the field.

Daniela Galan, Kim M. Caban, Leandro Singerman, Thiago A. Braga, Fabio M. Paes, Douglas S. Katz, and Felipe Munera

Imaging plays a crucial role in the immediate evaluation of the trauma patient, particularly using multi-detector computed tomography (CT), and especially in moderately to severely injured trauma patients. There are specific areas of relative consensus, while other aspects of whole-body computed tomography (WB-CT) use remain controversial and are subject to opinion/debate based on the current literature. Even a few hours of a delayed diagnosis may result in a detrimental outcome for the patient. One must utilize all the tools available to enhance the interpretation of images. It is also important to recognize imaging pitfalls and artifacts to avoid unnecessary intervention.

JOURNAL TITLE: Radiologic Clinics

ISSUE: 62.6

PROGRAM OBJECTIVE

The objective of the *Radiologic Clinics of North America* is to keep practicing radiologists and radiology residents up to date with current clinical practice in radiology by providing timely articles reviewing the state of the art in patient care.

TARGET AUDIENCE

Practicing radiologists, radiology residents, and other healthcare professionals who provide patient care utilizing radiologic findings.

LEARNING OBJECTIVES

Upon completion of this activity, participants will be able to:

1. Describe improvements in radiologists' performance when aided by AI as a diagnostic support tool.
2. Discuss the misconceptions about using intravenous contrast agents for medical imaging.
3. Recognize collaboration between physicians and scientists will likely yield the highest-quality research and optimize the implementation of research results.

ACCREDITATION

The Elsevier Office of Continuing Medical Education (EOCME) is accredited by the Accreditation Council for Continuing Medical Education (ACCME) to provide continuing medical education for physicians.

The EOCME designates this journal-based CME activity for a maximum of 12 *AMA PRA Category 1 Credit*(s)™. Physicians should claim only the credit commensurate with the extent of their participation in the activity.

All other healthcare professionals requesting continuing education credit for this enduring material will be issued a certificate of participation.

DISCLOSURE OF RELEVANT FINANCIAL RELATIONSHIPS

The EOCME assesses conflict of interest with its instructors, faculty, planners, and other individuals who are in a position to control the content of CME activities. All relevant conflicts of interest that are identified are thoroughly vetted by EOCME for fair balance, scientific objectivity, and patient care recommendations. EOCME is committed to providing its learners with CME activities that promote improvements or quality in healthcare and not a specific proprietary business or a commercial interest.

The authors and editors listed below have identified no financial relationships or relationships to products or devices they have with ineligible companies related to the content of this CME activity:
Gregg Blumberg, DO; Thiago A. Braga, MD; Kim M. Caban, MD; Hersh Chandarana, MD; Luis Colon-Flores, MD; Daniela Galan, MD; Elena Ghotbi, MD; Tarik Gozel, MD; John J. Hines Jr, MD; Jason C. Hoffmann, MD, FSIR; Julie Hong, MD; Shayan Chashm Jahan; Stella Kang, MD, MSc; Douglas S. Katz, MD, FACR, FSAR, FASER; Foad Kazemi, MD; Jesi Kim, MD; Rocío G. Márquez, MD; Benjamin M. Mervak, MD; Alireza Mohseni, MD; Anita Mohseni; Krishna Mundada, MBBS; Felipe Munera, MD; A. Orlando Ortiz, MD, MBA, FACR; Fabio M. Paes, MD, MBA; Pari V. Pandharipande, MD, MPH; John Stephen Pellerito, MD, FACR, FAIUM, FSRU; Margarita V. Revzin, MD, MS, FACR, FSAR, FAIUM, FSRU; Amirali Shababi; Niloufar Shababi, MD; Krishna Shanbhogue, MD; Leandro Singerman, MD; Benjamin S. Srivastava; Miltiadis Tembelis, MD

The authors and editors listed below have identified financial relationships or relationships to products or devices they have with ineligible companies related to the content of this CME activity:
Bari Dane, MD: Speaker/Researcher: Siemens Healthineers

Kush R. Desai, MD: Consultant: Boston Scientific, Cook Medical; Advisor: BD, Medtronic, W.L. Gore & Associates, Penumbra, Inc., Philips

Daniel B. Kopans, MD, FACR, FSBI: Royalties: IZI Medical Products; Advisor: DART Imaging Technology Co., Ltd., Malcova

Jennifer S. McDonald, PhD: Advisor/Consultant/Researcher: GE Healthcare

Robert J. McDonald, MD, PhD: Advisor/Consultant/Researcher: GE Healthcare

The Clinics staff listed below have identified no financial relationships or relationships to products or devices they have with ineligible companies related to the content of this CME activity:
Kothainayaki Kulanthaivelu; Michelle Littlejohn; Patrick J. Manley; Malvika Shah; John Vassallo

UNAPPROVED/OFF-LABEL USE DISCLOSURE

The EOCME requires CME faculty to disclose to the participants:

1. When products or procedures being discussed are off-label, unlabelled, experimental, and/or investigational (not US Food and Drug Administration [FDA] approved); and

2. Any limitations on the information presented, such as data that are preliminary or that represent ongoing research, interim analyses, and/or unsupported opinions. Faculty may discuss information about pharmaceutical agents that is outside of FDA-approved labelling. This information is intended solely for CME and is not intended to promote off-label use of these medications. If you have any questions, contact the medical affairs department of the manufacturer for the most recent prescribing information.

TO ENROLL

To enroll in the *Radiologic Clinics of North America* Continuing Medical Education program, call customer service at 1-800-654-2452 or sign up online at http://www.theclinics.com/home/cme. The CME program is available to subscribers for an additional annual fee of USD 340.00.

METHOD OF PARTICIPATION

In order to claim credit, participants must complete the following:
1. Complete enrolment as indicated above.
2. Read the activity.
3. Complete the CME Test and Evaluation. Participants must achieve a score of 70% on the test. All CME Tests and Evaluations must be completed online.

CME INQUIRIES/SPECIAL NEEDS

For all CME inquiries or special needs, please contact elsevierCME@elsevier.com.

RADIOLOGIC CLINICS OF NORTH AMERICA

SERIES OF RELATED INTEREST

Advances in Clinical Radiology
Available at: https://www.advancesinclinicalradiology.com/
Magnetic Resonance Imaging Clinics
Available at: https://www.mri.theclinics.com/
Neuroimaging Clinics
Available at: www.neuroimaging.theclinics.com
PET Clinics
Available at: www.pet.theclinics.com

THE CLINICS ARE AVAILABLE ONLINE!
Access your subscription at:
www.theclinics.com

Preface

Controversial Topics in Radiology—Where Is the Current Evidence?

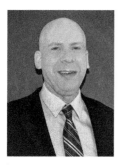

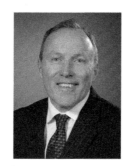

Douglas S. Katz, MD, FACR, FSAR, FASER   John J. Hines Jr, MD, FACR

Editors

In a controversy the instant we feel anger we have already ceased striving for the truth and have begun striving for ourselves.
    —Attributed to Buddha (and to others)

Some years ago, we approached Dr Frank Miller and the Elsevier Editorial Staff to do a "controversies in radiology" issue for the *Radiologic Clinics of North America*. The response was rapid, terse, and negative. "We don't do controversies. *The Clinics* are education journals." Really? There's no debate or controversy in medicine, or in radiology in particular? Everything is known and fixed in stone? Since when is that the case? One of us had been told that 25 to 30 years later, nearly half of what you learn in medical school will be wrong; you just don't know which half that will be. Perhaps an exaggeration, but not that far off.

More recently, we pitched the concept again, and the response was more positive, and more poised. OK, so long as it is evidence-based. So here it is. We aren't aware of a similar past issue of a *Radiologic Clinics of North America* or a purely general radiology education journal—and perhaps that's why the previous hesitancy—although we might have missed it. Hopefully different, but still

educational, useful to those in various practice settings, and possibly inspirational as well. We hope to spark further debate, and interest, in the selected potpourri of topics.

We greatly appreciate the contributions of our scholarly authors to this issue. The authors range from very senior attendings, to more junior attendings, to fellows and even senior radiology residents, and even high school students. We have carefully chosen the more senior authors, who have international-level expertise in the topics they discuss.

We could have done a multi-volume issue on "controversial issues in medical imaging," but we had to "zoom in" on only a few choice topics. The level of controversy varies substantially in the issue—think heat level in hot peppers—ranging from "mild" (eg, imaging of inflammatory bowel disease, with much established in the literature, and with some continuing areas of research and debate), to "incendiary"/off-the-charts hot (breast imaging controversies). The latter, covered by probably the most skilled gladiator in the breast imaging controversies arena, Dr Daniel Kopans, cites over 100 references, skewers his critics (along with, well, some peppers), using tons of evidence. I'm told this is just the tip of the iceberg,

Radiol Clin N Am 62 (2024) xv–xvi
https://doi.org/10.1016/j.rcl.2024.05.001
0033-8389/24/© 2024 Published by Elsevier Inc.

with an entire book now planned on breast imaging controversies. Other topics vary along the "controversy severity hotness scale/spectrum," from "relatively mild" (eg, whole-body trauma CT), to "moderate" (eg, the use of IV contrast in ultrasound, contrast nephropathy), to "relatively marked" (eg, vertebral augmentation).

Of course, everyone has their own point of view, within and outside of radiology. If you are a hammer, everything looks like a nail, or you want everything to be a nail. Any topic can be made into a controversy if you want it to be. Established criteria, the "RADS," consensus documents, prior literature, can all be dissected, debated, and rebuffed with statistics, reanalysis, and the latest literature.

As with our last guest issue, which was plagued with delays due to the COVID-19 pandemic, getting a series of authors to contribute articles to an evidence-based controversies issue, with increasing clinical and other demands, is no easier than herding cats, or like Rocky Balboa in *Rocky II*, no easier than catching a chicken when training to take on Apollo Creed again, especially a chicken that is greased.

We thank Dr Miller and John Vassallo and his excellent staff at Elsevier for their assistance, their guidance, and their patience. We hope this issue spurs debate, subsequent similar issues in the future, and further research into these controversial topics.

Douglas S. Katz, MD, FACR, FSAR, FASER
Department of Radiology
NYU Grossman Long Island School of Medicine
NYU Langone Hospital - Long Island
259 First Street, Mineola, NY 11501, USA

John J. Hines Jr, MD, FACR
Department of Radiology
Zucker School of Medicine at Hofstra/Northwell
Huntington, NY, USA

E-mail addresses:
douglasscottkatzmd@gmail.com (D.S. Katz)
jhinesmd@gmail.com (J.J. Hines)

How Do We Assess Controversies Using Evidence-Based Radiology?

Pari V. Pandharipande, MD, MPH[a],[*], Stella K. Kang, MD, MSc[b]

KEYWORDS

• Evidence • Test performance • Study design • Bias

KEY POINTS

- Knowledge of common study designs and analytical methods is critically important for conducting research and for providing the best possible imaging care.
- While randomized controlled trials are often considered to be the strongest form of evidence, they are rare in radiology due to extensive resource requirements; moreover, they address only limited populations who are eligible for participation.
- Each research study design has strengths and shortcomings, and each is susceptible to various forms of bias, for example, selection bias, verification bias, and confounding bias, among several others.
- Collaboration between physicians and scientists will likely yield the highest-quality research and optimize the implementation of research results, while also generating new ideas to advance our field in the coming years.

INTRODUCTION

Many argue that the practice of medicine must be fully grounded in published evidence. For physicians who practice medicine, it is clear that much of what they do still relies on their personal "database" and intuition from years of experience. Even when interpreting just 1 computed tomography (CT) scan, radiologists must make 100 or more decisions based on their own mind's inventory of thousands of organ contours and textures, liver abnormalities, adrenal nodules, adnexal cysts, compression fractures, injection granulomas, and other findings. Nevertheless, there is too much complexity in human conditions, and too many biases that physicians invoke as human beings, to believe that a practice based on instinct alone is optimal, even when considering the most experienced and talented physicians.[1] The importance

of grounding radiologists' practice in an external evidence base, whenever possible, and of understanding how to conduct evidence-based practice, is paramount to providing the best possible patient care, particularly in areas of controversy, where providers' baseline practice and experience varies. In this article, the authors briefly review and provide an overview of study designs and concepts, which are commonly used in clinical research, and they also highlight their strengths and shortcomings when relied upon to inform everyday medical decision-making.[1,2]

DIAGNOSTIC TEST PERFORMANCE

Historically, a dominant focus of research in radiology has involved the determination of performance characteristics of imaging examinations for the detection of disease. These characteristics

[a] The Ohio State University College of Medicine, 450 Faculty Tower, 395 West 12th Street, 4th Floor, Columbus, OH 43210, USA; [b] Population Health Imaging and Outcomes, NYU Department of Radiology, 660 First Avenue, Room 333, New York, NY 10016, USA

[*] Corresponding author.

E-mail address: Pari.Pandharipande@osumc.edu

Radiol Clin N Am 62 (2024) 929–934

https://doi.org/10.1016/j.rcl.2024.05.002

are as follows: sensitivity (true positive/true positive + false negative result); specificity (true negative/true negative + false positive result); positive predictive value (PPV, true positive/true positive + false positive result); and negative predictive value (NPV, true negative/true negative + false-negative result) (**Fig. 1**).

To provide an example of imaging research in which these test performance characteristics are reported, a recent body of work advances an MRI-based scoring algorithm for renal masses.[3–5] The algorithm includes multiple MRI features (eg, T2 signal intensity, enhancement) to ascertain whether an indeterminate renal mass is likely to represent a clear cell carcinoma.[3–5] Such a determination can help to inform management – that is, biopsy, surgery, or active surveillance – given that clear cell carcinoma is a more aggressive cancer subtype relative to other forms of primary renal tumors.[6] In a recent, multi-center study, Schieda and colleagues[3] reported sensitivity, specificity, and PPV of 75%, 78%, and 76%, respectively, for the detection of clear cell carcinoma when leveraging the MRI-based imaging algorithm using a relatively higher score threshold. Using a lower score threshold, they reported an NPV of 88%.[3] They concluded that the overall test performance of the algorithm was moderate; the strongest attribute of the examination was to identify those who

do not have the clear cell subtype among those who tested negative (NPV).[3]

THE EFFECT OF DISEASE PREVALENCE ON SENSITIVITY AND SPECIFICITY

Mathematically, PPV and NPV depend on the pre-test probability of disease, that is, the disease prevalence, whereas sensitivity and specificity do not.[7] This is important to recognize when evaluating the potential benefit of a given imaging examination for a population. For example, when considering the value of imaging-based screening for cancer or cardiovascular disease detection, the PPV of a given examination when applied to the population of interest, and not only the sensitivity, is critically important to consider.[6] As demonstrated in **Fig. 1**, when a population is at high risk for a disease, this is by definition associated with a greater number of true-positive test results compared to an average-risk population; the PPV of the test is increased relative to an average-risk population. This means that for a given level of sensitivity for disease detection, in a setting where patients are at elevated risk, more patients who test positive will have the disease, thereby increasing the likelihood of benefit at the population level.[7] This principle underlies the promise of some imaging-based examinations for screening in patients with a genetic predisposition for pancreatic cancer – when such examinations (MRI, endoscopic ultrasound) may not be of benefit in average-risk patients.[8]

RANDOMIZED CONTROLLED TRIALS

The "reference or gold standard" research method for comparing diagnostic imaging examinations or imaging-guided interventions is the randomized controlled trial (RCT). In an RCT, eligible patients are randomized to one form of examination (or intervention) versus another, and the results are compared to determine if there is a statistically significant difference in outcomes. Importantly, this methodology minimizes the risk of various biases – if patients are appropriately randomized and the research study is correctly powered, it should be possible to ascertain whether or not the test or intervention leads to a difference in outcomes. In general, in radiology, RCTs are rare because even the most effective imaging examinations and interventions are typically associated with relatively small, directly attributable outcomes improvements; therefore, the resources needed to conduct an appropriately powered trial can be prohibitively high. Two examples of well-known RCTs in radiology include the National Lung Screening Trial

	Disease +	**Disease -**
Test +	TP	FP
Test -	FN	TN

TP – True Positive   Sensitivity = TP/TP+FN
FN – False Negative   Specificity = TN/TN+FP
FP – False Positive   PPV   = TP/TP+FP
TN – True Negative   NPV   = TN/TN+FN

Fig. 1. Sensitivity, Specificity, Positive Predictive Value (PPV), Negative Predictive Value (PPV), and Implications of Pre-Test Probability on Test Performance. By definition, pre-test probability (or disease prevalence) is reflected by all disease-positive cases (*light blue*). Sensitivity and specificity are generally prevalence-independent metrics, whereas PPV and NPV depend on disease prevalence. In high-risk populations, where disease prevalence is high, PPV (TP/TP + FP) increases.

(NLST)[9] and a randomized trial of vertebroplasty for spinal fractures, an interventional trial.[10]

The NLST was a landmark RCT that was conducted to determine whether low-dose CT for lung cancer screening in high-risk individuals results in a reduction of mortality attributable to lung cancer.[9] Eligible participants were aged 55 to 74 years and had a 30-pack per year or greater smoking history.[9] In the CT study arm (n = 26,722), patients underwent low-dose CT, while in the comparator study arm (n = 26,732), patients underwent chest radiography.[9] A 20% relative reduction in lung cancer mortality was identified, when comparing patients who received CT versus radiography screening – notably, the trial was discontinued early as criteria for stopping were met early.[9] Through the application of an RCT design, this study has definitively changed practice recommendations for many patients who are current or previous smokers.

Kallmes and colleagues conducted a multi-center RCT to evaluate outcomes of vertebroplasty (n = 68), compared to a simulated procedure (n = 63), when performed for osteoporotic fractures.[10] The study was designed to identify differences in measures of pain and associated disability.[10] When comparing results, there was no statistically significant difference in primary study measures.[10] This study ultimately raised substantial controversy about the benefits and value of vertebroplasty for osteoporotic fractures at the population level,[10] a topic that will be further covered in a subsequent article.

SYSTEMATIC REVIEW AND META-ANALYSIS IN RADIOLOGY

Systematic review and meta-analysis refers to methods used to synthesize the data from multiple published studies on a given topic – and ideally, through meta-analysis, combining the data to increase the available sample and the validity of a given result or conclusion. Meta-analysis methodology can be applied to study RCT results or observational diagnostic studies. However, as described, RCTs are rare in imaging. Therefore, most related analyses in imaging are conducted to aggregate reported test performance or other observational characteristics from multiple studies, in order to determine more robust estimates. Two examples of systematic review and meta-analysis in radiology are shared here.[11,12]

Smith-Bindman and colleagues published a meta-analysis that has been used for decades to inform the threshold for distinguishing normal from abnormal endometrial thickness, on endovaginal ultrasound, in post-menopausal patients with vaginal bleeding.[11] The authors analyzed related, published studies from 1966 to 1996.[11] They exposed study heterogeneity using the following test: if the 95% confidence interval of a given study did not include the pooled estimate, the study was considered heterogeneous.[11] The authors determined that at a threshold of 5 mm, the sensitivity of ultrasound to detect cancer was 96% (95% confidence interval = 94–98%)[11] – to date, 5 mm remains the threshold used to refer patients to endometrial biopsy in the setting of abnormal vaginal bleeding.

In a second example, Rosenkrantz and colleagues published a systematic review and meta-analysis estimating discrepant rates of imaging interpretations in second-opinion settings.[12] They evaluated studies encompassing 12,676 second-opinion interpretations (n = 29). They utilized the Quality Assessment of Diagnostic Accuracy Studies-2 (QUADAS-2) standard, adapted to the study question, to help inform and expose measures of study quality, as quality assessment is a recommended component of all systematic reviews.[12,13] They also used a random effects model to develop reported, pooled estimates, thereby analytically accounting for heterogeneity across studies when deriving such estimates.[12,14] Comparing primary and secondary interpretations, the overall discrepancy rate was 32%, while for major findings it was 20%, a substantial and clinically important rate of discrepancy.[12]

DECISION-ANALYTIC AND SIMULATION MODELING

Decision-analytic and simulation modeling methods are used to synthesize existing published data, or data from national registries or other population sources, in order to project or estimate patient outcomes.[15,16] In each, disease processes, as well as patients' experiences of different "health states" are simulated. Hypothetical cohorts or individual patients pass through a decision-analytic or simulation model based on probabilities of incurring specific events, including cancer progression or recurrence, and the cumulative experience of the population is analyzed to determine relevant outcomes, for example, life expectancy, quality-adjusted life expectancy, or costs. Such methods are ideally suited for evaluating the effectiveness of diagnostic interventions in settings where RCTs are prohibitively resource intensive – for example, in cancer screening scenarios, where the duration of precancerous focal abnormalities is long. Another advantage of using modeling techniques to evaluate interventions is that more patient populations can be readily evaluated, for example, patients with varied levels of co-morbidities. While modeling cannot replace RCTs or observational studies, it can provide a complementary approach to evaluate health outcomes at the population level in ways that are not possible using other research methods.[15,16]

A widely recognized example of the use of decision analysis in diagnostic testing is a study by members of the National Cancer Institute- sponsored Cancer Intervention and Surveillance Modeling Network that informed the United States Preventative Services Task Force (USPSTF) of the differential value of various colorectal cancer screening strategies.[17] Using modeling techniques, the authors estimated life-years gained and the burden of colonoscopy across a wide spectrum of colorectal cancer screening strategies when implemented at the population level.[17] They concluded that beginning screening at the age of 45 provided an optimal balance of life-years gained and colonoscopy burden, when employing optical colonoscopy, CT colonoscopy, or stool tests for screening.[17] This analysis ultimately informed the USPSTF's decision to lower the recommended age of colorectal cancer screening initiation in the US to 45 in 2021.[18]

REGRESSION ANALYSIS, PROPENSITY SCORE METHODS, AND ARTIFICIAL INTELLIGENCE

Regression analysis and propensity score methods are 2 techniques commonly used, in analyses of observational data, to evaluate associations between exposures and outcomes. Linear and logistic regression analysis involves identifying an outcome of interest (dependent variable), and factors that may predict that outcome, or which may control for the relationship between an exposure and that outcome (independent variables). For example, in a survey study examining barriers to diversity in radiology and radiation oncology workforces, multiple logistic regression analysis was used to evaluate responses.[19] In one such analysis, the item response was the dependent variable (yes/no to the question: "have you personally felt you were treated unfairly or with disrespect because of your gender…"); gender was a hypothesized predictor variable (independent variable), and training status was a control variable (independent variable).[19] Women were found to be much more likely – with statistical significance – to respond that they had experienced unfair or disrespectful treatment in the workplace, attributable to their gender (51% [women] and 5% [men], odds ratio = 18 [95% confidence = 9–35]).[19]

Propensity score methods are techniques that can be used to simulate an RCT using retrospective observational data. Using regression analysis, the probability of exposure ("propensity score") for a given patient is first determined. This score can then be used in different ways – for example, in one method, exposed and unexposed individuals can then be matched based on the propensity score, ultimately allowing, to a degree, discernment of the independent effect of the exposure in the population.[20] Among the most well-recognized studies in imaging that have used propensity score methods are those that have sought to identify the association between intravenous contrast and acute kidney injury.[20–22] From a methodologic standpoint, these studies used propensity score methods to test the hypothesis that iodinated contrast material is causally associated with acute kidney injury and associated downstream outcomes.[20–22] Related work will be discussed in a subsequent article.

While controversies related to artificial intelligence (AI) will be discussed in a subsequent article as well, it should be noted that AI applications draw from regression analysis and other related techniques to identify associations.[23] Importantly, the scale of such analysis is substantially larger than typical regression analysis, and the researcher's (software engineer's) knowledge of specific associations tested may be comparatively much more limited.[23]

In all methods, utilizing retrospective observational data—to test for associations or causality—the risk of residual bias remains. Risks of confounding and selection bias are particularly important to consider.[24] Confounding occurs when both the exposure and outcome variables are associated with an external variable that is not included in the analysis. For example, in a study in which multiple imaging characteristics are being evaluated for their association with malignancy, if age is a primary driver of both a given imaging characteristic and malignancy, but is not controlled for in the regression analysis, then a statistically significant but false association between the imaging characteristic and malignancy may be reported. Selection bias is further discussed as follows.

BIAS IN IMAGING RESEARCH

Several forms of bias are important to consider when evaluating studies that compare different imaging interventions.[2,24] Confounding has already been described, in the setting of regression analysis. Here, the authors highlight 2 additional potential sources of bias that are common in the imaging literature and critically important to consider when designing studies or adapting published imaging results into practice.

Selection bias occurs when the cohort of study patients (or findings) under evaluation is not representative of the population to which the results are ascribed or used.[2,24] For example, consider a hypothetical study in which the performance of a new MRI imaging protocol is being evaluated for its ability to characterize focal liver abnormalities in cirrhosis. In a single-institution study, if the study population is part of a successful screening program, the abnormalities of interest may be smaller than if such findings are primarily detected later, by symptoms. This difference in population could affect reported test performance, making the study results subject to selection bias, most pronounced when applied to a broader population.

In AI applications, the introduction of selection bias – particularly related to gender, race, and ethnicity – is a recognized and growing concern.[23] If the training data are restricted to a specific race, gender, or ethnicity, then the corresponding algorithm or application for disease detection may be invalid when applied to other populations. Moreover, given that algorithms are built in ways that allow for them to continuously learn and update their performance; they are vulnerable to circumstances in which they can be prospectively degraded by selection bias. For these reasons, there is growing recognition about the critical need for transparency in the development of AI algorithms, and the need for robust standards for the development and maintenance of such algorithms.

Verification bias is a type of selection bias that is very common in diagnostic imaging research.[2,25] It can occur, for example, when diagnostic test performance (or other) results are reported from a population in which close follow-up or pathologic correlation are required as inclusion criteria. If only the most suspicious abnormalities – based on either imaging or patient-level characteristics – are closely followed or surgically resected, then bias is introduced when the results of corresponding studies are generalized to broader populations, in whom follow-up or surgery may not be pursued. Reported malignancy rates for incidentally detected findings are particularly subject to verification bias, for example, in the setting of pancreatic cysts, where the likelihood of such bias has been substantiated through analyses of existing, population-level data.[25,26]

DISCUSSION

An evidence-based approach to imaging care is critically important for ensuring that radiologists provide the best possible service to our patients. As a medical specialty, the radiology community has an imperative to generate evidence that addresses primary controversies and issues of high impact in our field, and to implement corresponding practices responsibly. Such evidence may pertain to the practice of imaging itself – for example, renal tumor classification at MRI – or to other aspects of imaging care delivery, such as the effects of contrast on kidney function, second-opinion interpretations, or our workforce. In this article, the authors reviewed the strengths and drawbacks of several study designs, as well as important biases to consider. However, this article only begins to breach the depth of methodologies and biases that are important to consider in our field. For physicians and scientists alike, whether seeking to conduct research or implement published findings, the benefits of collaboration between providers and methodologists cannot be overstated. With such collaboration, not only do the specific projects gain benefit, but new and unforeseen ideas for addressing controversies are born, creating invaluable opportunities for advancing our field in the years to come.

CLINICS CARE POINTS

- Controversies in imaging – and more broadly, in the field of radiology – can be addressed with a variety of research methods, ranging from analyses of test performance, to RCTs, meta-analysis, decision analysis, regression analysis, propensity score methods, and AI techniques, among several others.

- Each clinical research method has strengths and shortcomings, and each is susceptible to various biases; as such, a basic understanding of study designs and attendant biases, when conducting research or implementing published results, is critically important.

- Close collaboration between physicians and scientists can help to guide research design and the translation of results to practice, and also fosters a singular environment for the advancement of new ideas and their successful execution in the years to come.

DISCLOSURE

P.V. Pandharipande was a member of the Association of University Radiologists – General Electric Radiology Research Academic Fellowship Board of Review (2022–2023); she has ended this responsibility. SKK receives royalties from Wolters Kluwer for unrelated work.

REFERENCES

1. Busby LP, Courtier JL, Glastonbury CM. Bias in radiology: the how and why of misses and misinterpretations. Radiographics 2018;38:236–47.
2. Lijmer JG, Mol BW, Heisterkamp S, et al. Empirical evidence of design-related bias in studies of diagnostic tests. JAMA 1999;282(11):1061–6.
3. Schieda N, Davenport MS, Silverman SG, et al. Multicenter evaluation of multiparametric MRI clear cell likelihood scores in solid indeterminate small renal masses. Radiology 2022;303(3):590–9.
4. Pedrosa I, Cadeddu JA. How we do it: managing the indeterminate renal mass with the MRI clear cell likelihood score. Radiology 2022;302(2):256–69.
5. Pedrosa I. Invited commentary: MRI clear cell likelihood score for indeterminate solid renal masses: is there a path for broad clinical adoption? Radiographics 2023;43(7):e230042.
6. Kang SK, Huang WC, Elkin EB, et al. Personalized treatment for small renal tumors: decision analysis of competing causes of mortality. Radiology 2019; 290(3):732–43.
7. Marcus PM. Assessment of cancer screening: a primer [Internet]. Bethesda (MD): National Cancer Institute (US); 2019. Chapter 3, Performance measures. . [Accessed 5 May 2024].
8. Goggins M, Overbeek KA, Brand R, et al, International Cancer of the Pancreas Screening (CAPS) consortium. Management of patients with increased risk for familial pancreatic cancer: updated recommendations from the International Cancer of the Pancreas Screening (CAPS) consortium. Gut 2020; 69(1):7–17.
9. National Lung Screening Trial Research Team, Aberle DR, Adams AM, Berg CD, et al. Reduced lung-cancer mortality with low-dose computed tomographic screening. N Engl J Med 2011;365(5): 395–409.
10. Kallmes DF, Comstock BA, Heagerty PJ, et al. A randomized trial of vertebroplasty for osteoporotic spinal fractures. N Engl J Med 2009;361(6):569–79.
11. Smith-Bindman R, Kerlikowske K, Feldstein VA, et al. Endovaginal ultrasound to exclude endometrial cancer and other endometrial abnormalities. JAMA 1998;280(17):1510–7.
12. Rosenkrantz AB, Duszak R Jr, Babb JS, et al. Discrepancy rates and clinical impact of imaging secondary interpretations: a systematic review and meta-analysis. J Am Coll Radiol 2018;15(9): 1222–31.
13. Whiting PF, Rutjes AW, Westwood ME, et al, QUADAS-2 Group. QUADAS-2: a revised tool for the quality assessment of diagnostic accuracy studies. Ann Intern Med 2011;155:529–36.
14. DerSimonian R, Laird N. Meta-analysis in clinical trials. Control Clin Trials 1986;7:177–88.
15. Plevritis SK. Decision analysis and simulation modeling for evaluating diagnostic tests on the basis of patient outcomes. AJR 2005;185:581–90.
16. Rutter CM, Knudsen AB, Pandharipande PV. Computer disease simulation models: integrating evidence for health policy. Acad Radiol 2011;18(9): 1077–86.
17. Knudsen AB, Rutter CM, Peterse EFP, et al. Colorectal cancer screening: an updated modeling study for the US Preventive Services Task Force. JAMA 2021;325(19):1998–2011.
18. United States Preventive Services Task Force. Final recommendation statement: screening for colorectal cancer. 2021. Available at: https://www.uspreventive servicestaskforce.org/uspstf/announcements/final-recommendation-statement-screening-colorectal-cancer-0. [Accessed 4 May 2024].
19. Pandharipande PV, Mercaldo ND, Lietz AP, et al. Identifying barriers to building a diverse physician workforce: a national survey of the ACR membership. J Am Coll Radiol 2019;16(8):1091–101.
20. McDonald RJ, McDonald JS, Bida JP, et al. Intravenous contrast material-induced nephropathy: causal or coincident phenomenon? Radiology 2013;267(1): 106–18.
21. McDonald JS, McDonald RJ, Carter RE, et al. Risk of intravenous contrast material-mediated acute kidney injury: a propensity score-matched study stratified by baseline-estimated glomerular filtration rate. Radiology 2014;271(1):65–73.
22. McDonald JS, McDonald RJ, Williamson EE, et al. Is intravenous administration of iodixanol associated with increased risk of acute kidney injury, dialysis, or mortality? A propensity score-adjusted Study. Radiology 2017;285(2):414–24.
23. Lee MD, Elsayed M, Chopra S, et al. A no-math primer on the principles of machine learning for radiologists. Semin Ultrasound CT MR 2022;43(2): 133–41.
24. Haneuse S. Distinguishing selection bias and confounding bias in comparative effectiveness research. Med Care 2016;54(4):e23–9.
25. Weaver DT, Lietz AP, Mercaldo SF, et al. Testing for verification bias in reported malignancy risks for side-branch intraductal papillary mucinous neoplasms: a simulation modeling approach. AJR Am J Roentgenol 2019;212(3):596–601.
26. Gardner TB, Glass LM, Smith KD, et al. Pancreatic cyst prevalence and the risk of mucin-producing adenocarcinoma in US adults. Am J Gastroenterol 2013;108(10):1546–50.

Artificial Intelligence in Radiology

What Is Its True Role at Present, and Where Is the Evidence?

Check for updates

Alireza Mohseni, MD[a],[*], Elena Ghotbi, MD[a], Foad Kazemi, MD[a],
Amirali Shababi, BS[b], Shayan Chashm Jahan, BS[c], Anita Mohseni, BS[d],
Niloufar Shababi, MD[a]

KEYWORDS

- Artificial intelligence • Radiology • Medical imaging • Machine learning • Deep learning
- Radiomics

KEY POINTS

- Recent studies show artificial intelligence (AI) improves radiologists' accuracy and efficiency.
- Machine learning in AI streamlines diagnostic processes, improving workflow efficiency.
- Challenges like data quality and regulatory concerns require careful navigation for successful integration into clinical practice.

INTRODUCTION

The integration of artificial intelligence (AI) into radiology has brought about major advancements and transformative potential in diagnostic imaging practices. Recent studies have explored the impact of AI on the expected future workload of radiologists, simultaneously questioning whether radiologists could potentially be replaced by AI in domains such as breast imaging, given promising results.[1,2] However, multiple studies now show that radiologists' diagnostic performance is significantly improved when aided by AI tools for detection and decision support, affirming the useful role of AI as an assistive technology rather than as a replacement.[3] For example, retrospective simulation studies have examined how AI triaging could decrease radiologists' workloads for evaluating screening mammograms, while still maintaining or boosting cancer detection rates.[4]

Beyond such potential workflow and efficiency optimizations, rapid advances are being made in applying AI approaches across radiology subspecialties including neuroradiology, facilitated by the digitalization of medical imaging data.[5] Musculoskeletal imaging similarly exhibits transformative potential throughout its imaging workflow using AI techniques for analysis and interpretation tasks.[6] Initial evidence also indicates that AI elevates diagnostic accuracy over human radiologists alone when analyzing complex imaging, such as liver tumor evaluation on ultrasound.[7] However, a review of commercially available radiology-focused AI highlights that large gaps are still present in their underlying evidence base and calls for more rigorous validation.[8] Therefore,

[a] Johns Hopkins University School of Medicine, 600 N. Wolfe Street / Phipps 446, Baltimore, MD 21287, USA;
[b] School of Medicine, Iran University of Medical Sciences, Hemat Highway next to Milad Tower 14535, Tehran, Iran; [c] Department of Computer Science, University of Maryland, 8125 Paint Branch Drive College Park, MD 20742, USA; [d] Azad University Tehran Medical Branch, Danesh, Shariati Street, Tehran, Iran 19395/1495
* Corresponding author. 600 N. Wolfe Street / Phipps 446, Baltimore, MD 21287.
E-mail address: amohsen4@jhmi.edu
Twitter: @Alireza_Mhsn1 (A.M.)

Radiol Clin N Am 62 (2024) 935–947
https://doi.org/10.1016/j.rcl.2024.03.008

while perspectives vary on how AI may reshape and integrate into radiology, addressing these research gaps and guiding careful implementation remains critical.[9]

ARTIFICIAL INTELLIGENCE IN RADIOLOGY: TRANSFORMING IMAGING TECHNIQUES AND PROTOCOLS

AI has transformed imaging protocols across modalities including MR imaging and computed tomography (CT) to facilitate quantitative analyses.[10] It has also enhanced protocols for AI-based applications through standardization and optimization.[11] AI has additionally enhanced hanging protocols, guiding the presentation of current and previous examinations, including outcomes generated by AI, to radiologists for their interpretation.[12]

ARTIFICIAL INTELLIGENCE AND IMAGING FINDINGS/PATHOLOGY

AI has transitioned into clinical use, helping radiologists identify and interpret findings.[13] Applications are being customized for subspecialties including pediatric radiology to address specific needs such as differences in anatomy, physiology, and pathology compared to adults.[14] Moreover, the application of AI in radiologic evaluation and interpretation is perceived as a transformative avenue for learning, with the capability to revolutionize the entire field of radiology.[15]

CLINICAL APPLICATIONS

Integrating AI into radiology can improve diagnostic precision, workflow efficiency, and patient outcomes. AI has shown efficacy in expediting disease diagnosis and treatment, including coronavirus disease 2019 (COVID-19).[16] It can be used to optimize workflows and to aid radiologists in detection and monitoring to elevate care.[17] However, structured frameworks and validation are vital for successful clinical integration.[18]

REDEFINING DIAGNOSTIC CRITERIA

By accurately analyzing imaging, AI could influence diagnostic criteria for conditions including neoplasms, lung pathologies, and other abnormalities.[17] Moreover, advances in diagnostic radiology with AI have increased radiological investigations globally, potentially transforming diagnostic landscapes.[19] Additionally, AI introduces the prospect of a transformative educational opportunity, reshaping the realm of radiology and potentially impacting the establishment of diagnostic criteria for different diseases.[20]

CURRENT LANDSCAPE OF ARTIFICIAL INTELLIGENCE IN RADIOLOGY
Overview of Artificial Intelligence Applications

AI applications in radiology encompass image interpretation and decision support, bringing transformative changes to radiologists' workflow.[18,21]

Rates of Artificial Intelligence Integration in Radiology Practices

Based on available data, it is estimated that roughly 30% of radiologists in the United States are currently utilizing AI within their practice.[22] Additionally, only 30% of current radiology practices reportedly employ AI tools.[23] Despite the relatively modest current adoption rate, there is a growing expectation for AI to become significantly involved in radiology practice in the future.[24] The slow implementation of AI in clinical radiology practice is attributed to the complexity of integration and the necessity for further validation of its efficacy.[18]

Research focuses on the frequency and challenges of AI integration in radiology practices, driven by cost control and innovation strategies, although obstacles such as technical proficiency and unclear additional value persist.[25]

Key Players and Technologies

The incorporation of AI into radiology involves multiple components and technologies. Radiologists, leveraging their extensive expertise, play a pivotal role in this domain, and AI technologies function as supportive tools aimed at improving diagnostic precision.[26] The impact of the COVID-19 pandemic has influenced the perceived integration of AI with digital radiology, leading to suggestions for electronic interaction mechanisms to gather the perspectives of medical radiology technologists.[27] For the advancement of AI-based imaging research and application, it is crucial to establish supportive infrastructure and operational standards, ensuring the compatibility of AI applications with existing clinical radiology workflows.[11] Moreover, the effective integration of AI into radiology departments necessitates training programs, transparent policies, and motivation for radiographers.[28]

PROMISES OF ARTIFICIAL INTELLIGENCE IN RADIOLOGY
Improved Accuracy, Efficiency, and Diagnostic Capabilities

AI statistically significantly enhances diagnostic accuracy and efficiency, promising transformative changes in radiology.[10,28–30]

Potential Cost Savings

While AI holds significant promise for enhancing radiologist efficiency, its full potential and effectiveness in clinical settings are still being realized. While there is growing evidence and numerous studies showcasing the benefits of AI in radiology, including improved efficiency, accuracy, and workflow optimization,[5,13,18,22,31] further research and validation in real-world clinical settings are necessary to conclusively establish its impact.

The integration of AI in radiology offers the prospect of potential cost savings, as the heightened efficiency provided by AI enables radiologists to engage in more value-added tasks, increasing their visibility to patients and playing a crucial role in multidisciplinary clinical teams. The anticipated implementation of AI in radiology over the coming decade is expected to notably enhance the quality, value, and depth of radiology's contributions to patient care and population health, leading to a transformation in the workflows of radiologists. AI implementation in radiology offers potential cost savings, but concerns about adoption hesitancy need further exploration.[18,32]

TYPES OF ARTIFICIAL INTELLIGENCE IN RADIOLOGY
Machine Learning and Deep Learning

The integration of machine learning (ML) and deep learning (DL) in radiology has transformed the field, offering applications in order scheduling, triage, decision support, image analysis, and interpretation[33] (**Table 1**). ML, as a data analysis technique, empowers computers to learn from experience and make intelligent decisions.[34] DL, utilizing artificial neural networks, excels in handling complex tasks, particularly in medical image analysis.[35] Despite the potential, effective deployment of DL in radiology requires addressing challenges in data curation and model training.[36,37] ML and DL hold the promise to revolutionize diverse fields, including medicine, by automating processes and making intelligent decisions.

Natural Language Processing

Natural language processing (NLP) has become invaluable in radiology, leveraging techniques to extract information from unstructured medical texts.[45] Its application shows promise in medical education, diagnostic imaging, and clinical documentation.[46] NLP facilitates the extraction of valuable medical information, contributing to improved health care delivery and patient outcomes.[47–49] NLP has also facilitated the extraction of imaging observations, automated outcome classification from medical reports, and longitudinal analysis of pain in patients, demonstrating its potential to enhance diagnostic precision and patient care in radiology and beyond.[50–55] As NLP evolves, it holds the promise of transforming the processing of medical information, ultimately contributing to improved health care delivery and patient outcomes.

Computer-Aided Detection and Computer-Aided Diagnosis

CAD and CADx have, for years now, substantially influenced radiology, providing tools to aid radiologists in detecting abnormalities in medical images.[46] These systems enhance diagnostic accuracy across various modalities, including CT, MR imaging, and mammography.[56,57] The combined use of CAD and CADx has proven effective in enhancing sensitivity, contributing to improved diagnostic accuracy and patient care.[58,59]

Several research studies have investigated the effects of CAD or CADx systems on diagnostic accuracy across various radiological domains. In the realm of mammography, there is a divergence of findings regarding the impact of CAD on diagnostic accuracy. While certain studies suggest that CAD systems do not substantially enhance radiologists' diagnostic performance in mammography interpretation,[60–62] others propose that CAD may improve diagnostic accuracy, particularly when integrated with digital mammography or breast tomosynthesis.[63–65] Additionally, CAD systems have shown utility in characterizing suspicious microcalcifications on mammograms, potentially aiding in clinical decision-making.[65]

Furthermore, CAD systems have undergone evaluation in other radiological domains such as bone fracture detection and brain lesion recognition. Studies indicate that CAD systems, especially those utilizing DL algorithms, can enhance clinicians' abilities in detecting fractures and brain abnormality recognition and focal brain findings.[66,67]

Computer Vision

Computer vision, integrated with DL, promises to reshape traditional paradigms of medical image analysis.[68] This technology automates the analysis of imaging modalities, offering support for radiologists in identifying structures and abnormalities.[69] Computer vision algorithms, particularly those rooted in DL, exhibit promise in improving the safety and efficiency of procedures, advancing patient care through sophisticated image analysis.[70] Collaboration between radiologists and computer vision experts is crucial for unlocking the full potential of AI and DL in radiology.[71]

Table 1
Different types of artificial intelligence in radiology

AI Type	First Establishment	Foundation	Potential Applications in Radiology and Medicine
Natural language processing	1950[38]	Used for processing and understanding human language	Extraction of structured information from radiology reports[39]; analyzing radiology reports for clinical inquiries[40]
ML[41]	1952	Pattern and complex relationship recognition; learning from datasets	Image segmentation; image registration; computer-aided detection (CAD); and diagnosis systems from CT and MR imaging
CAD and computer-aided diagnosis (CADx)	1980	Automated tools aiding radiologists in detecting and characterizing abnormalities	Enhancing diagnostic performance in tasks such as tuberculosis screening, lung nodule assessment, and breast abnormality identification
DL[42]	2000	Multilayer neural networks for autonomous learning and decision-making	Analysis of high volumes of data, including radiograph, MR imaging, CT scans, for various diagnostic and predictive applications
Computer vision[43]	Evolved in past decade	Acquiring information and comprehension from sequences of images or videos	Object classification; object detection; image segmentation; and assisting in medical image analysis and interpretation
Radiomics[44]	Ongoing research	Extraction and analysis of quantitative features from medical images	Enhancing diagnostic precision, predictive modeling, and treatment planning based on quantitative image features

Radiomics: Transforming Quantitative Imaging

Radiomics, focused on extracting quantitative features from medical images, contributes to personalized medicine by capturing the heterogeneity of phenotypes.[72] Despite being distinct from AI, radiomics is closely linked to it, and the integration of radiomics with DL features enhances predictive capacities in radiology.[73] Radiomics outperforms traditional models in predicting clinical outcomes, offering supplementary guidance in clinical decision-making.[74] Its integration into nomograms demonstrates excellent discrimination in predicting various pathologic and clinical features.[75]

CHALLENGES AND LIMITATIONS
Data Quality and Quantity

One of the principal hurdles in AI in radiology pertains to the quality and quantity of data. The precision of data-driven AI systems is inherently tied to the quality of the data, and the restricted generalizability of AI systems frequently necessitates substantial customization by local experts to address regional intricacies in reporting syntax for enhanced performance. Consequently, the presence of high-quality, diverse, and well-annotated datasets is essential for the effective creation and implementation of AI applications in radiology.[76]

Collaborative efforts are underway to develop AI systems that are more generalizable. These initiatives bring together various stakeholders, including radiologists, other specialist clinicians, and researchers, to advance the implementation of AI in radiology.

One notable study by Kaviani and colleagues[77] showcases the application of AI to reduce missed findings on chest radiographs in an international, multicenter study. The AI model developed in this study demonstrated generalizability across different sites, geographic locations, patient genders, and age groups. This underscores the effectiveness of a collaborative approach involving multiple centers in developing AI solutions that can be applied effectively in diverse settings.

Regulatory and Ethical Concerns

The use of AI in radiology comes with concerns related to regulations and ethics, creating significant obstacles for its widespread use. While regulatory approval is more common, the scientific validation of AI products is not as extensive. Additionally, the limited adaptability of NLP systems often means they need a lot of customization by local experts to work well in specific areas. It is crucial to ensure ethical governance, explainability, interpretability, and ethical auditing to address concerns of fairness, accountability, and transparency in the use of AI in radiology.[78]

Integration with Existing Systems

Incorporating AI into current radiology systems poses difficulties regarding how well it works with them, including issues particularly interoperability, data security, and optimizing how tasks are done. The expected implementation of AI in radiology over the next 10 years is likely to greatly enhance the quality, value, and scope of radiology's impact on patient care and overall public health, transforming the way radiologists work. However, the idea of completely replacing current systems has sparked strong reactions within the radiology profession, underscoring the importance of carefully integrating and adjusting AI technologies within the existing radiological setups.[18]

Efforts by major commercial medical imaging vendors to incorporate AI algorithms into their equipment and software have been a prominent focus within the health care technology sector. Companies operating in the medical technology industry, particularly in fields like radiology, have actively integrated AI, including ML algorithms, into their offerings.[79] The integration of AI into medical imaging has garnered significant attention due to its potential to improve diagnostic precision and efficiency. AI and ML have hastened the development of robust processing tools in medical imaging, facilitating advancements in tasks such as region delineation, image denoising, reconstruction, and tissue characterization.[80] Despite the growing interest in AI among established imaging vendors, the market remains fragmented, and comprehensive AI solutions spanning different modalities are still in the developmental stages.[81]

Impact on Radiologist–Patient Relationship

The introduction of AI in radiology sparks concerns about how it might affect the relationship between radiologists and patients. The radiology community needs training on how to carefully assess the possibilities, risks, and threats linked to the implementation of new AI tools. Moreover, the real challenge is not to resist the inclusion of AI in professional practices but to embrace the inevitable shift in radiological procedures, integrating AI into the workflow. However, the researchers did not provide reasons for not using AI, highlighting the necessity for further investigation into the potential impact of AI on the radiologist–patient relationship.[30]

Artificial Intelligence Versus Human Radiologists: Insights from Scholarly Discourse

The diagnostic performance of AI has been extensively studied, revealing its comparability to that of radiologists across various medical imaging tasks. Tong and colleagues[82] reported sensitivity ranging from 73% to 94% and specificity ranging from 81% to 91% in thyroid nodule detection via ultrasonography, indicating AI's effectiveness in this domain. Conversely, in the assessment of thyroid nodules, Xu and colleagues[83] found that 2 radiologists demonstrated higher sensitivity than an AI system, albeit at the expense of significantly lower specificity. These findings underscore the variability in AI's diagnostic performance across different imaging modalities and pathologies.

Furthermore, in the evaluation of suspected pulmonary embolism, Cheikh and colleagues[84] observed that AI exhibited higher sensitivity and negative predictive values, while radiologists demonstrated superior specificity and positive predictive value. This highlights the complementary strengths of AI and human radiologists in achieving comprehensive diagnostic accuracy, emphasizing the potential for collaborative utilization in clinical settings.

In the context of chest radiographs for COVID-19, Sun and colleagues[85] noted gender-based variations in AI performance, with higher sensitivity observed in men and higher specificity in women. This underscores the importance of considering demographic factors in assessing AI performance and optimizing its utility in diverse patient populations.

Despite these advancements, challenges remain in demonstrating the superiority of AI over human radiologists in diagnostic tasks. Shaari and colleagues[86] highlighted limitations in DL algorithms for pediatric brain tumor imaging, shedding light on the complexities AI faces in this specialized field. Similarly, skepticism among radiologists regarding AI's potential to replace human interpretation, particularly in the context of COVID-19 diagnosis and monitoring, has been noted.[87]

While ML holds promise for improving diagnostic accuracy, concerns persist regarding the scarcity of evidence demonstrating AI's superiority over human radiologists.[88] To address these challenges, advocates emphasize the importance of standardization and evaluation frameworks for AI software in radiology,[22] as well as the necessity of considering clinical requirements in AI studies within the field.[89] Furthermore, understanding the roles of radiologists in AI development is essential for comprehending the evolving dynamics between AI and human experts.[90]

Addressing Artificial Intelligence Inaccuracy: Strategies for Effective Implementation

When considering the reliability of AI systems, particularly in diagnostic imaging, it becomes evident that even the most advanced algorithms are not infallible. A comprehensive analysis of 503 studies reveals that while the receiver operating characteristic area under the curve for diagnostic imaging typically ranges from 0.864 to 0.937 for lung nodules or lung cancer on chest CT and chest radiographic examinations, specific metrics such as sensitivity and specificity demonstrate inherent limitations.[91] For instance, a specificity of 0.89 implies that AI may produce false-positive diagnoses in approximately 11 out of 100 true-negative cases, while a sensitivity of 0.87 suggests that false-negative diagnoses could occur in approximately 13 out of 100 true-positive cases.[92] Despite enhancing radiologist performance, the incorporation of AI does not guarantee flawless accuracy.

The implications of inaccurate AI outputs prompt important inquiries regarding their influence on radiologist decision-making processes. A study by Alberdi and colleagues[93] indicates that the presence of CAD can influence interpretations of mammograms, potentially leading to incorrect conclusions. When CAD feedback erroneously identifies cases as false negatives, a statistically significant proportion of readers under the CAD condition fail to recognize cancer, contrasting with a higher accuracy rate in the absence of CAD. This underscores the importance of assessing how AI feedback presentation can influence diagnostic outcomes. An essential consideration in mitigating the adverse effects of inaccurate AI feedback lies in refining the implementation of AI systems. This objective aligns with the aims of the ACR's Data Science Institute to enhance medical care through the development and integration of AI applications in radiology.[94] While substantial efforts have been directed toward AI algorithm refinement, insufficient attention has been given to investigating the potential negative impacts of AI on radiologist decision-making processes.

One notable approach under exploration involves deferring the display of AI-generated results until after a radiologist has reviewed the medical images. This method has demonstrated potential in reducing bias in AI interpretations.[95] The strategy aims to capitalize on the strengths of both AI technology and human expertise by allowing radiologists to independently analyze the images before being influenced by AI-generated findings. Through this sequential approach, where the radiologist's assessment precedes the AI analysis, there exists a potential to enhance the accuracy and reliability of diagnostic interpretations while mitigating inherent biases in AI algorithms. This innovative method not only highlights evolving strategies in AI utilization in medical imaging but also emphasizes the significance of maintaining a balance between technological advancements and human oversight to optimize patient care and outcomes.

To optimize patient outcomes, it is imperative to not only enhance the AI algorithms themselves but also to carefully consider how AI feedback is integrated into clinical workflows. Bernstein and colleagues[77] found that false positives decreased when radiologists were informed the inaccurate AI findings would be deleted from patient records, rather than retained. The theory is that radiologists may be reluctant to contradict AI when a permanent record of disagreement exists. Additionally, visually outlining suspicious regions found by AI reduced false-negative interpretations. This visual cue may lessen cognitive load and assist radiologists in catching incorrect AI results. Taken together, thoughtful integration of AI feedback presentation, such as deleting demonstrably inaccurate insights and clearly denoting areas of concern, can mitigate the potential negative impacts of imperfect AI on radiology performance. The findings underscore the need to carefully consider human factors when developing clinical AI tools, not just focus on the algorithm itself. Following these AI implementation strategies could safeguard against diagnostic errors when AI is flawed.

These obstacles and restrictions highlight the complexities and essential aspects related to integrating AI in radiology, stressing the necessity for thoughtful and ethical deliberation in the adoption of AI technologies within clinical practices.

CLINICAL EVIDENCE SUPPORTING ARTIFICIAL INTELLIGENCE IN RADIOLOGY
Overview of Studies and Trials

The clinical evidence for AI in radiology is grounded in a growing collection of studies and trials showcasing the potential of AI applications in enhancing diagnostic accuracy and patient care. Hosny and colleagues[17] offer a comprehensive review article outlining the challenges in clinical implementation and suggesting ways to advance the field. Gampala and colleagues[13] further illuminate the practical application of AI in radiology, especially in clinical settings, highlighting its transformative potential. Additionally, Strohm and colleagues[18] emphasize the importance of having evidence regarding the clinical benefits of AI in radiology for successful implementation, indicating ongoing endeavors to validate and integrate AI applications into clinical practices.

Comparative Analyses

Comparative analyses have been instrumental in assessing the clinical evidence endorsing AI in radiology, offering valuable insights into the effectiveness and influence of AI applications. Codari and colleagues[76] stress the importance of top-notch data for ensuring precise results and the effective transition of AI systems from research environments to clinical use. Additionally, Bahakeem and colleagues[96] present optimistic viewpoints regarding the integration of AI in radiology, underscoring the capability of AI to improve diagnostic proficiency and patient care.

Real-World Implementation Examples

Instances of real-world implementation have provided valuable insights into the clinical support for AI in radiology, showcasing practical demonstrations of AI applications in actual clinical settings. Chiwome and colleagues[2] underscore the transformative potential of AI in radiology, illustrating the significant progress AI has made in the field. Additionally, Tanguay and colleagues[22] present a framework for validating and evaluating AI software in radiology, emphasizing the endeavors to ensure the successful integration of AI applications into clinical practices. Furthermore, the study by Laborie and colleagues[14] highlights the establishment of a dedicated task force for AI in pediatric radiology, illustrating the real-world incorporation of AI in clinical settings.

One specific software is BoneXpert (Visiana, Denmark), renowned for its implementation in AI applications for radiology.[18] BoneXpert specializes in automated determination of skeletal maturity, aiding in bone age assessment from hand radiographs, particularly in pediatric patients. However, the landscape of AI applications in radiology extends far beyond BoneXpert to encompass a diverse array of software products catering to various radiological needs. Among these, Quibim Precision[97] stands out, offering advanced quantitative imaging solutions for analyzing and interpreting medical images across different modalities. Quibim Precision (Quibim, Valencia, Spain) is notable for its applications in cancer clinical trials, facilitating precise quantitative assessments of tumor characteristics and treatment responses. Another noteworthy software is the vessel occlusion detection software, which has garnered attention for its evaluation in acute stroke scenarios, showcasing the transformative potential of AI in radiology.[98] This software specializes in automated detection of intracranial vessel occlusions on computed tomography angiography (CTA), aiding in the rapid diagnosis and treatment of acute ischemic stroke. Its cost-effectiveness and accuracy make it a valuable tool in stroke management protocols, highlighting the diverse applications of AI in radiology beyond traditional imaging interpretation.

CASE STUDIES
Highlighting Successful Implementations

Instances of application through case studies have showcased successful incorporations of AI in radiology, illustrating the significant impact of AI applications in actual clinical scenarios. Wang and colleagues[99] evaluated the influence of AI on radiological education, emphasizing the necessity for comprehensive summaries detailing the perspectives, opportunities, and challenges presented by AI at various stages of radiologists' training. Additionally, Codari and colleagues[76] conducted a EuroAIM survey within the European Society of Radiology, revealing a generally positive attitude toward AI and indicating successful implementations with favorable outcomes. Moreover, Laborie and colleagues[14] established a task force dedicated to AI in pediatric radiology, offering a tangible example of the successful integration of AI tools in clinical settings and highlighting AI's potential to improve diagnostic capabilities and patient care.

Addressing Challenges Faced

Case studies have also delved into the difficulties faced in implementing AI in radiology, providing insights into the intricacies and factors linked to AI applications. Furthermore, Brandes and colleagues[100] investigated the influence of AI on the selection of radiology as a specialty by medical students, emphasizing worries about the possible challenges AI might pose to radiological practice and its effects on career decisions. These case studies highlight the importance of addressing challenges and apprehensions related to the incorporation of AI in radiology.

FUTURE PERSPECTIVES
Emerging Technologies

The future trajectory of AI in radiology is intricately connected to the advancement and incorporation of cutting-edge technologies. The utilization of AI in radiology is anticipated to progress, with emerging technologies such as DL and NLP playing a crucial role in augmenting diagnostic precision and efficiency. The examination conducted by Hosny and colleagues[17] underscores the notable advancements of AI algorithms, particularly DL, in tasks related to image recognition, highlighting the potential of emerging technologies to transform radiological procedures. Additionally, the Canadian Association of Radiologists White Paper on Artificial Intelligence in Radiology[10] accentuates the capacity of advancing technologies to propel measures promoting interoperability for AI-based applications in radiology, indicating the continuous evolution of technology and its implications for the future landscape of radiology.

Evolving Regulatory Landscape

The future of AI in radiology is also influenced by the changing regulatory environment, marked by ongoing endeavors to tackle regulatory and ethical concerns linked to AI applications. The analysis by Pesapane and colleagues[101] underscores the importance of standardizing AI software specifications, classifications, and evaluations to ensure the effective integration of AI applications in clinical practice, reflecting the dynamic nature of the regulatory landscape and its effects on the future of radiology. Additionally, the collaborative statement by European and North American multisociety on the ethics of artificial intelligence in radiology[102] highlights the necessity for ethical governance and transparency in AI applications, shedding light on the evolving regulatory environment and its implications for the future of radiology.

SUMMARY
Summary of Key Findings

The integration of AI in radiology has brought about substantial advancements and transformative potential in diagnostic imaging practices. Key findings from the literature highlight the impact of AI on improving diagnostic accuracy, streamlining workflow, and enhancing patient care. Studies have also emphasized the challenges and complexities associated with the adoption of AI in radiology, underscoring the need for careful navigation and ethical considerations in the implementation of AI technologies in clinical practice.

Recommendations for Future Research

Future research in the field of AI in radiology should focus on addressing the challenges and limitations associated with AI applications, particularly in the areas of data quality and quantity, regulatory and ethical concerns, and integration with existing systems. Additionally, there is a need for further exploration of the potential cost savings and the impact of AI on the radiologist–patient relationship. Research efforts should also aim to validate and implement AI applications in clinical practice, providing evidence on the clinical added value of AI in radiology.

Closing Thoughts on the Present and Future Role of Artificial Intelligence in Radiology

The present and future role of AI in radiology holds great promise for enhancing diagnostic capabilities, improving workflow efficiency, and ultimately, advancing patient care. As AI continues to evolve and integrate with emerging technologies, it is anticipated to drive significant advances and trends that will shape the future of radiology. However, it is essential to address the challenges and complexities associated with the adoption of AI in radiology, ensuring ethical governance, transparency, and the successful integration of AI applications in clinical practice.

CLINICS CARE POINTS

Pearls:

- Using AI for CAD and diagnosis in radiology has been shown to improve diagnostic accuracy for conditions including pulmonary nodules, breast abnormalities, and tuberculosis when used in combination with radiologist interpretation.

- Radiomics utilize quantitative image features to develop personalized prediction models of prognosis and treatment response across diverse organs and imaging modalities.

- Implementation of AI workflows in radiology requires extensive validation using standardized datasets and close integration with existing clinical systems.

Pitfalls:

- Relying solely on AI diagnoses without radiologist supervision could lead to critical imaging findings being overlooked or misinterpreted.
- Insufficient clinical validation and lack of transparency around AI algorithms hampers real-world adoption in patient care settings due to ethical and accuracy concerns.
- AI applications trained on small or biased datasets struggle to generalize well to diverse patient populations seen in clinical practice.

DISCLOSURE

The authors have nothing to disclose.

REFERENCES

1. Kwee TC, Kwee RM. Workload of diagnostic radiologists in the foreseeable future based on recent scientific advances: growth expectations and role of artificial intelligence. Insights Imaging 2021. https://doi.org/10.1186/s13244-021-01031-4.
2. Chiwome L, Okojie OM, Rahman A, et al. Artificial intelligence: is it armageddon for breast radiologists? Cureus 2020. https://doi.org/10.7759/cureus.8923.
3. Kim HE, Kim HH, Han B, et al. Changes in cancer detection and false-positive recall in mammography using artificial intelligence: a retrospective, multireader study. Lancet Digit Heal 2020. https://doi.org/10.1016/s2589-7500(20)30003-0.
4. Dembrower K, Wåhlin EK, Liu Y, et al. Effect of artificial intelligence-based triaging of breast cancer screening mammograms on cancer detection and radiologist workload: a retrospective simulation study. Lancet Digit Heal 2020. https://doi.org/10.1016/s2589-7500(20)30185-0.
5. Olthof A, van Ooijen PMA, Mehrizi MHR. Promises of artificial intelligence in neuroradiology: a systematic technographic review. Neuroradiology 2020. https://doi.org/10.1007/s00234-020-02424-w.
6. Huber FA, Guggenberger R. AI MSK clinical applications: spine imaging. Skeletal Radiol 2021. https://doi.org/10.1007/s00256-021-03862-0.
7. Nishida N, Yamakawa M, Shiina T, et al. Artificial Intelligence (AI) models for the ultrasonographic diagnosis of liver tumors and comparison of diagnostic accuracies between ai and human experts. J Gastroenterol 2022. https://doi.org/10.1007/s00535-022-01849-9.
8. van Leeuwen KG, Schalekamp S, Rutten MJCM, et al. Artificial intelligence in radiology: 100 commercially available products and their scientific evidence. Eur Radiol 2021. https://doi.org/10.1007/s00330-021-07892-z.
9. Alelyani M, Alamri S, Alqahtani MS, et al. Radiology community attitude in Saudi Arabia about the applications of artificial intelligence in radiology. Healthcare 2021. https://doi.org/10.3390/healthcare9070834.
10. Tang A, Tam R, Cadrin-Chênevert A, et al. Canadian Association of Radiologists White Paper on Artificial Intelligence in Radiology. Can Assoc Radiol J 2018. https://doi.org/10.1016/j.carj.2018.02.002.
11. Ho CW-L, Soon D, Caals K, et al. Governance of automated image analysis and artificial intelligence analytics in healthcare. Clin Radiol 2019. https://doi.org/10.1016/j.crad.2019.02.005.
12. Liu Y, Chen J, Feng H, et al. Early identification of COVID-19 progression to its severe form using artificial intelligence. Iran J Radiol 2022. https://doi.org/10.5812/iranjradiol.112562.
13. Gampala S, Vankeshwaram V, Gadula SSP. Is artificial intelligence the new friend for radiologists? a review article. Cureus 2020. https://doi.org/10.7759/cureus.11137.
14. Laborie LB, Naidoo J, Pace E, et al. European society of paediatric radiology artificial intelligence taskforce: a new taskforce for the digital age. Pediatr Radiol 2022. https://doi.org/10.1007/s00247-022-05426-3.
15. Syed A, Zoga AC. Artificial intelligence in radiology: current technology and future directions. Semin Musculoskelet Radiol 2018. https://doi.org/10.1055/s-0038-1673383.
16. Mei X, Lee H-C, Diao K, et al. Artificial intelligence–enabled rapid diagnosis of patients with COVID-19. Nat Med 2020. https://doi.org/10.1038/s41591-020-0931-3.
17. Hosny A, Parmar C, Quackenbush J, et al. Artificial intelligence in radiology. Nat Rev Cancer 2018. https://doi.org/10.1038/s41568-018-0016-5.
18. Strohm LGD, Hehakaya C, Ranschaert E, et al. Implementation of artificial intelligence (ai) applications in radiology: hindering and facilitating factors. Eur Radiol 2020. https://doi.org/10.1007/s00330-020-06946-y.
19. Tajaldeen A, Al-Ghamdi SG. Evaluation of radiologist's knowledge about the artificial intelligence in diagnostic radiology: a survey-based study. Acta Radiol Open 2020. https://doi.org/10.1177/2058460120945320.
20. Davendralingam N, Sebire NJ, Arthurs OJ, et al. Artificial intelligence in paediatric radiology: future opportunities. Br J Radiol 2021. https://doi.org/10.1259/bjr.20200975.
21. Mehrizi MHR, van Ooijen PMA, Homan M. Applications of artificial intelligence (ai) in diagnostic radiology: a technography study. Eur Radiol 2020. https://doi.org/10.1007/s00330-020-07230-9.
22. Tanguay W, Acar P, Fine B, et al. Assessment of radiology artificial intelligence software: a validation and

evaluation framework. Can Assoc Radiol J 2022. https://doi.org/10.1177/08465371221135760.

23. Chu LC, Ahmed T, Blanco A, et al. Radiologists' expectations of artificial intelligence in pancreatic cancer imaging: how good is good enough? J Comput Assist Tomogr 2023. https://doi.org/10.1097/rct.0000000000001503.

24. Abuzaid MM, Elshami W, McConnell J, et al. An extensive survey of radiographers from the middle east and india on artificial intelligence integration in radiology practice. Health Technol 2021. https://doi.org/10.1007/s12553-021-00583-1.

25. Matheny ME, Whicher D, Israni ST. Artificial intelligence in health care. JAMA 2020. https://doi.org/10.1001/jama.2019.21579.

26. Öztürk T, Talo M, Yildirim EA, et al. Automated detection of COVID-19 cases using deep neural networks with x-ray images. Comput Biol Med 2020. https://doi.org/10.1016/j.compbiomed.2020.103792.

27. Giansanti D, Rossi I, Monoscalco L. Lessons from the COVID-19 pandemic on the use of artificial intelligence in digital radiology: the submission of a survey to investigate the opinion of insiders. Healthcare 2021. https://doi.org/10.3390/healthcare9030331.

28. Aldhafeeri F. Perspectives of radiographers on the emergence of artificial intelligence in diagnostic imaging in Saudi Arabia. Insights Imaging 2022. https://doi.org/10.1186/s13244-022-01319-z.

29. Garwood ER, Tai R, Joshi G, et al. The use of artificial intelligence in the evaluation of knee pathology. Semin Musculoskelet Radiol 2020. https://doi.org/10.1055/s-0039-3400264.

30. Alsharif W, Qurashi AA, Toonsi F, et al. A qualitative study to explore opinions of saudi arabian radiologists concerning ai-based applications and their impact on the future of the radiology. Bjr|open 2022. https://doi.org/10.1259/bjro.20210029.

31. Dikici E, Bigelow MT, Prevedello LM, et al. Integrating AI into radiology workflow: levels of research, production, and feedback maturity. J Med Imaging 2020. https://doi.org/10.1117/1.jmi.7.1.016502.

32. Zhong Z, Yang W, Zhu C, et al. Role and progress of artificial intelligence in radiodiagnosing vascular calcification: a narrative review. Ann Transl Med 2023. https://doi.org/10.21037/atm-22-6333.

33. Choy G, Khalilzadeh O, Michalski M, et al. Current applications and future impact of machine learning in radiology. Radiology 2018. https://doi.org/10.1148/radiol.2018171820.

34. Barros DM da S, Moura JCC, Freire CR, et al. Machine learning applied to retinal image processing for glaucoma detection: review and perspective. Biomed Eng Online 2020. https://doi.org/10.1186/s12938-020-00767-2.

35. Montagnon E, Cerny M, Cadrin-Chênevert A, et al. Deep learning workflow in radiology: a primer. Insights Imaging 2020. https://doi.org/10.1186/s13244-019-0832-5.

36. Candemir S, Nguyen XV, Folio L, et al. Training strategies for radiology deep learning models in data-limited scenarios. Radiol Artif Intell 2021. https://doi.org/10.1148/ryai.2021210014.

37. Sung YS, Park B, Park HJ, et al. Radiomics and deep learning in liver diseases. J Gastroenterol Hepatol 2021. https://doi.org/10.1111/jgh.15414.

38. Turing AM. In: Epstein R, Roberts G, Beber G, editors. Computing machinery and intelligence BT - parsing the turing test: philosophical and methodological issues in the quest for the thinking computer. Dordrecht: Springer Netherlands; 2009. p. 23–65. https://doi.org/10.1007/978-1-4020-6710-5_3.

39. Wang Y, Mehrabi S, Sohn S, et al. Natural language processing of radiology reports for identification of skeletal site-specific fractures. BMC Med Inform Decis Mak 2019;19(3):73.

40. Pham A-D, Névéol A, Lavergne T, et al. Natural language processing of radiology reports for the detection of thromboembolic diseases and clinically relevant incidental findings. BMC Bioinf 2014;15(1):266.

41. Mitchell TM. Machine learning. New York, USA: McGraw-Hill; 1997.

42. LeCun Y, Bengio Y, Hinton G. Deep learning. Nature. England 2015;521(7553):436–44.

43. Ayer T, Ayvaci M, Liu ZX, et al. Computer-aided diagnostic models in breast cancer screening. Imaging Med 2010. https://doi.org/10.2217/iim.10.24.

44. Yoon H, Sohn I, Cho JH, et al. Decoding tumor phenotypes for ALK, ROS1, and RET fusions in lung adenocarcinoma using a radiomics approach. Medicine (Baltim) 2015. https://doi.org/10.1097/md.0000000000001753.

45. Pons E, Braun L, Hunink MGM, et al. Natural language processing in radiology: a systematic review. Radiology 2016. https://doi.org/10.1148/radiol.16142770.

46. Melendez J, Sánchez CI, Philipsen RHHM, et al. An automated tuberculosis screening strategy combining x-ray-based computer-aided detection and clinical information. Sci Rep 2016. https://doi.org/10.1038/srep25265.

47. Patel JS, Zhan S, Siddiqui ZA, et al. Automatic identification of self-reported covid-19 vaccine information from vaccine adverse events reporting system. Methods Inf Med 2023. https://doi.org/10.1055/s-0042-1760248.

48. Mashima Y, Tamura T, Kunikata J, et al. Using natural language processing techniques to detect adverse events from progress notes due to

chemotherapy. Cancer Inform 2022. https://doi.org/10.1177/11769351221085064.

49. Zirikly A, Desmet B, Newman-Griffis D, et al. Information extraction framework for disability determination using a mental functioning use-case. Jmir Med Informatics 2022. https://doi.org/10.2196/32245.

50. Kaufman DR, Sheehan B, Stetson PD, et al. Natural language processing–enabled and conventional data capture methods for input to electronic health records: a comparative usability study. Jmir Med Informatics 2016. https://doi.org/10.2196/medinform.5544.

51. Carrell D, Cronkite D, Shea M, et al. Clinical documentation of patient-reported medical cannabis use in primary care: toward scalable extraction using natural language processing methods. Subst Abus 2022. https://doi.org/10.1080/08897077.2021.1986767.

52. Chen R, Ho JC, Lin J-MS. Extracting medication information from unstructured public health data: a demonstration on data from population-based and tertiary-based samples. BMC Med Res Methodol 2020. https://doi.org/10.1186/s12874-020-01131-7.

53. Young M, Holmes NE, Kishore K, et al. Natural language processing diagnosed behavioral disturbance vs confusion assessment method for the intensive care unit: prevalence, patient characteristics, overlap, and association with treatment and outcome. Intensive Care Med 2022. https://doi.org/10.1007/s00134-022-06650-z.

54. Aramaki E, Wakamiya S, Yada S, et al. Natural language processing: from bedside to everywhere. Yearb Med Inform 2022. https://doi.org/10.1055/s-0042-1742510.

55. Çalışkan D, Zierk J, Kraska D, et al. First steps to evaluate an NLP tool's medication extraction accuracy from discharge letters. Stud Health Technol Inform 2021. https://doi.org/10.3233/shti210073.

56. Winder M, Owczarek A, Chudek J, et al. Are we overdoing it? changes in diagnostic imaging workload during the years 2010–2020 including the impact of the SARS-CoV-2 Pandemic. Healthcare 2021. https://doi.org/10.3390/healthcare9111557.

57. Ng KH, Tan CH. It is time to incorporate artificial intelligence in radiology residency programs. Korean J Radiol 2023. https://doi.org/10.3348/kjr.2022.1023.

58. Salemi S, Behzadi-Khormouji H, Rostami H, et al. Incremental deep learning training approach for lesion detection and classification in mammograms. Cybern Phys 2022. https://doi.org/10.35470/2226-4116-2022-11-4-234-245.

59. Novak RD, Novak NJ, Gilkeson RC, et al. A comparison of computer-aided detection (CAD) effectiveness in pulmonary nodule identification using different methods of bone suppression in chest radiographs. J Digit Imaging 2013. https://doi.org/10.1007/s10278-012-9565-4.

60. Wu N, Phang J, Park J, et al. Deep neural networks improve radiologists' performance in breast cancer screening. IEEE Trans Med Imaging 2020. https://doi.org/10.1109/tmi.2019.2945514.

61. Lehman CD, Wellman R, Buist DSM, et al. Diagnostic accuracy of digital screening mammography with and without computer-aided detection. JAMA Intern Med 2015. https://doi.org/10.1001/jamainternmed.2015.5231.

62. Gillies RJ, Schabath MB. Radiomics improves cancer screening and early detection. Cancer Epidemiol Biomarkers Prev 2020. https://doi.org/10.1158/1055-9965.epi-20-0075.

63. Rafferty EA, Park JM, Philpotts LE, et al. Assessing radiologist performance using combined digital mammography and breast tomosynthesis compared with digital mammography alone: results of a multicenter, multireader trial. Radiology 2013. https://doi.org/10.1148/radiol.12120674.

64. Fuchsjäger M. Is the future of breast imaging with AI? Eur Radiol 2019. https://doi.org/10.1007/s00330-019-06286-6.

65. Ah Y, Jang M, La Yun B, et al. Diagnostic performance of artificial intelligence-based computer-aided diagnosis for breast microcalcification on mammography. Diagnostics 2021. https://doi.org/10.3390/diagnostics11081409.

66. Xiao Y, Lin Y, Xia X, et al. A comparison of mammography and ultrasound in women with breast disease: a receiver operating characteristic analysis. Breast J 2012. https://doi.org/10.1111/j.1524-4741.2011.01219.x.

67. Lindsey R, Daluiski A, Chopra S, et al. Deep neural network improves fracture detection by clinicians. Proc Natl Acad Sci 2018. https://doi.org/10.1073/pnas.1806905115.

68. Skg O, Makmur A, Ayq S, et al. Attitudes toward artificial intelligence in radiology with learner needs assessment within radiology residency programmes: a national multi-programme survey. Singapore Med J 2021. https://doi.org/10.11622/smedj.2019141.

69. Seetharam K, Shrestha S, Sengupta PP. Cardiovascular imaging and intervention through the lens of artificial intelligence. Interv Cardiol Rev 2021. https://doi.org/10.15420/icr.2020.04.

70. Shao H, Chen X, Ma Q, et al. The feasibility and accuracy of machine learning in improving safety and efficiency of thrombolysis for patients with stroke: literature review and proposed improvements. Front Neurol 2022. https://doi.org/10.3389/fneur.2022.934929.

71. Mahoro E, Akhloufi MA. Applying deep learning for breast cancer detection in radiology. Curr Oncol 2022. https://doi.org/10.3390/curroncol29110690.

72. Tagliafico A, Piana M, Schenone D, et al. Overview of radiomics in breast cancer diagnosis and prognostication. Breast 2020. https://doi.org/10.1016/j.breast.2019.10.018.

73. Currie G, Rohren EM. The deep radiomic analytics pipeline. Vet Radiol Ultrasound 2022. https://doi.org/10.1111/vru.13147.

74. Sotoudeh H, Rezaei A, Godwin RC, et al. Radiomics outperforms clinical and radiologic signs in predicting spontaneous basal ganglia hematoma expansion: a pilot study. Cureus 2023. https://doi.org/10.7759/cureus.37162.

75. Li X, Lan M, Wang X, et al. Development and validation of a MRI-based combined radiomics nomogram for differentiation in chondrosarcoma. Front Oncol 2023. https://doi.org/10.3389/fonc.2023.1090229.

76. Codari M, Melazzini L, Morozov SP, et al. Impact of artificial intelligence on radiology: a euroaim survey among members of the european society of radiology. Insights Imaging 2019. https://doi.org/10.1186/s13244-019-0798-3.

77. Kaviani P, Kalra MK, Digumarthy SR, et al. Frequency of missed findings on chest radiographs (CXRs) in an International, Multicenter Study: Application of AI to Reduce Missed Findings. Diagnostics 2022. https://doi.org/10.3390/diagnostics12102382.

78. Recht MP, Dewey M, Dreyer K, et al. Integrating artificial intelligence into the clinical practice of radiology: challenges and recommendations. Eur Radiol 2020. https://doi.org/10.1007/s00330-020-06672-5.

79. Maaßen O, Fritsch S, Palm J, et al. Future medical artificial intelligence application requirements and expectations of physicians in German University Hospitals: web-based survey. J Med Internet Res 2021. https://doi.org/10.2196/26646.

80. Winfield JM, Blackledge M, Tunariu N, et al. Whole-Body MRI: a practical guide for imaging patients with malignant bone disease. Clin Radiol 2021. https://doi.org/10.1016/j.crad.2021.04.001.

81. Adams S, Henderson RDE, Xin Y, et al. Artificial intelligence solutions for analysis of x-ray images. Can Assoc Radiol J 2020. https://doi.org/10.1177/0846537120941671.

82. Tong W, Wu S, Cheng M, et al. Integration of artificial intelligence decision aids to reduce workload and enhance efficiency in thyroid nodule management. JAMA Netw Open 2023. https://doi.org/10.1001/jamanetworkopen.2023.13674.

83. Xu D, Wang Y, Wu H, et al. An artificial intelligence ultrasound system's ability to distinguish benign from malignant follicular-patterned lesions. Front Endocrinol 2022. https://doi.org/10.3389/fendo.2022.981403.

84. Cheikh A Ben, Gorincour G, Nivet H, et al. How artificial intelligence improves radiological interpretation in suspected pulmonary embolism. Eur Radiol 2022. https://doi.org/10.1007/s00330-022-08645-2.

85. Sun J, Peng L, Li T, et al. Performance of a chest radiograph AI diagnostic tool for COVID-19: A PROSPECTIVE OBSERVATIONAL STUdy. Radiol Artif Intell 2022. https://doi.org/10.1148/ryai.210217.

86. Shaari H, Kevrić J, Jukić S, et al. Deep learning-based studies on pediatric brain tumors imaging: narrative review of techniques and challenges. Brain Sci 2021. https://doi.org/10.3390/brainsci11060716.

87. Pankhania M. Artificial intelligence and radiology: Combating the COVID-19 conundrum. Indian J Radiol Imaging 2021;31(Suppl 1):S4–10. Germany.

88. DeJohn CR, Grant SR, Seshadri M. Application of machine learning methods to improve the performance of ultrasound in head and neck oncology: a literature review. Cancers 2022. https://doi.org/10.3390/cancers14030665.

89. Gong B, Salehi F, Hurrell C, et al. 2021 year in review. Can Assoc Radiol J 2022. https://doi.org/10.1177/08465371221083860.

90. Scheek D, Mehrizi MHR, Ranschaert E. Radiologists in the loop: the roles of radiologists in the development of AI applications. Eur Radiol 2021. https://doi.org/10.1007/s00330-021-07879-w.

91. Aggarwal R, Sounderajah V, Martin G, et al. Diagnostic accuracy of deep learning in medical imaging: a systematic review and meta-analysis. NPJ Digit Med 2021;4(1):65. England.

92. Bernstein MH, Atalay MK, Dibble EH, et al. Can incorrect artificial intelligence (AI) results impact radiologists, and if so, what can we do about it? A multi-reader pilot study of lung cancer detection with chest radiography. Eur Radiol 2023;33(11):8263–9. Germany.

93. Alberdi E, Povykalo A, Strigini L, et al. Effects of incorrect computer-aided detection (CAD) output on human decision-making in mammography. Acad Radiol 2004;11(8):909–18. United States.

94. American College of Radiology About ACR DSI. Available at: https://www.acrdsi.org/About-ACR-DSI. [Accessed 30 March 2022].

95. Liu L, Parker KJ, Jung S. Design and analysis methods for trials with AI-based diagnostic devices for breast cancer. J Pers Med 2021. https://doi.org/10.3390/jpm11111150.

96. Bahakeem BH, Alobaidi SF, Alzahrani AS, et al. The general population's perspectives on implementation of artificial intelligence in radiology in the Western Region of Saudi Arabia. Cureus 2023. https://doi.org/10.7759/cureus.37391.

97. Franco D, Granata V, Fusco R, et al. Artificial intelligence and radiation effects on brain tissue in glioblastoma patient: preliminary data using a quantitative tool. Radiol Med. Italy 2023;128(7): 813–27.

98. van Leeuwen KG, Meijer FJA, Schalekamp S, et al. Cost-effectiveness of artificial intelligence aided vessel occlusion detection in acute stroke: an early health technology assessment. Insights Imaging 2021. https://doi.org/10.1186/s13244-021-01077-4.

99. Wang C, Xie H, Wang S, et al. Radiological education in the era of artificial intelligence: a review. Medicine (Baltim) 2023. https://doi.org/10.1097/md.0000000000032518.

100. Brandes GIG, D'Ippólito G, Azzolini AG, et al. Impact of artificial intelligence on the choice of radiology as a specialty by medical students from the city of São Paulo. Radiol Bras 2020. https://doi.org/10.1590/0100-3984.2019.0101.

101. Pesapane F, Codari M, Sardanelli F. Artificial intelligence in medical imaging: threat or opportunity? radiologists again at the forefront of innovation in medicine. Eur Radiol Exp 2018. https://doi.org/10.1186/s41747-018-0061-6.

102. Geis JR, Brady AP, Wu CC, et al. Ethics of artificial intelligence in radiology: summary of the joint european and north american multisociety statement. Insights Imaging 2019. https://doi.org/10.1186/s13244-019-0785-8.

Iodine and Gadolinium Contrast Reactions
What Is the Risk and Role of Premedication, Abbreviated Protocols, Prior History of Reactions, and Cross-Reactivity?

Benjamin M. Mervak, MD[a,*], Jennifer S. McDonald, PhD[b]

KEYWORDS

- Iodinated contrast media • Gadolinium contrast media • Steroid premedication • Allergy
- Rapid premedication

KEY POINTS

- Data supporting the premedication of high-risk patients before intravenous (IV) low-osmolality contrast media are largely based on historical studies on high-osmolality contrast media. Information on premedication before IV gadolinium-based contrast media (GBCM) is limited and largely based on extrapolation.
- Direct risks of corticosteroid premedication are of limited clinical consequence. However, indirect risks can be substantial, particularly for inpatients. The number needed to treat to prevent one severe or lethal contrast reaction is very large.
- Recommendations on corticosteroid premedication from the American College of Radiology (ACR) and international organizations differ and are not always explicitly followed, so practices vary locally.
- The ACR recommends:
- a. Consideration of corticosteroid premedication only for high-risk patients with a prior history of reaction to the same category of contrast material.
- b. Not premedicating patients when a different class of contrast material is used (eg, GBCM in a patient with history of allergy to IV contrast media [iodinated contrast media]).
- c. Considering expedited IV corticosteroid premedication for some patient groups (eg, patients in the emergency department).
- Our knowledge about cross-reactivity within classes of contrast media and the potential for agent-switching to protect against reactions continues to evolve.

INTRODUCTION

Iodinated contrast media (ICM) and gadolinium-based contrast media (GBCM) are essential tools for the practice of radiology, allowing for improved visualization and characterization of anatomic structures and pathology. However, adverse reactions to ICM and GBCM occur in the form of both benign physiologic symptoms and immediate hypersensitivity reactions. While most reactions

[a] Department of Radiology, Michigan Medicine, 1500 East Medical Center Drive, B1D502, Ann Arbor, MI 48109, USA; [b] Department of Radiology, Mayo Clinic Rochester, 200 1st Street SW, Rochester, MN 55905, USA
* Corresponding author.
E-mail address: bmervak@med.umich.edu

Radiol Clin N Am 62 (2024) 949–957
https://doi.org/10.1016/j.rcl.2024.02.014
0033-8389/24/© 2024 Elsevier Inc. All rights reserved.

are mild and self-limited, life-threatening reactions do occur.

Several strategies including premedication and agent-switching have been studied and practiced as means to mitigate the risk of reactions. However, there are notable caveats: there are limitations to the historical studies on which premedication strategies are based, no strategy completely prevents breakthrough reactions, the efficacy of corticosteroid premedication has recently been brought into question, and the logistics of premedication or agent-switching may introduce supply difficulties for radiology departments or have other unintended consequences for patients. "Rapid" intravenous (IV) premedication protocols have become the norm in many emergency settings, although many of the same caveats apply to this expedited approach as well.

Although there is some common ground on patient populations considered higher risk for a contrast reaction, discrepancies in guidance still exist between major organizations, including recommendations from the American College of Radiology (ACR) versus international organizations, particularly the European Society of Urogenital Radiology (ESUR) and the UK's Royal College of Radiologists (RCR).

This article provides an in-depth look at the current knowledge and areas of controversy regarding corticosteroid premedication, abbreviated premedication protocols, factors that may influence the decision to premedicate a patient, and cross-reactivity within and between classes of contrast media.

DISCUSSION
Role of Premedication

Corticosteroid premedication strategies were initially described in the 1980s as an attempt to mitigate immediate hypersensitivity reactions to IV iodinated high-osmolality contrast media (HOCM).[1–3] At baseline, HOCM was found to result in an overall reaction rate as high as 12.7%, with a severe reaction rate of 0.22% in all patients.[4] Two teams were early in describing a protective effect of corticosteroids when given starting at least 12 hours in advance of an examination using IV HOCM, giving rise to 2 standardized premedication regimens (the "Greenberger" and "Lasser" preparations, named after the lead authors in those studies).[1,5]

1. *Greenberger*: prednisone 50 mg PO, given 13, 7, and 1 hour prior to the contrast-enhanced examination, plus diphenhydramine 50 mg PO, given 1 hour prior

2. *Lasser*: methylprednisolone 32 mg PO, given 12 and 2 hours prior to the contrast-enhanced examination

These studies resulted in a new paradigm for radiologists considering how to approach patients at risk for immediate hypersensitivity reactions to contrast media. Surveys conducted in 1995 and 2009 showed a substantial increase in the rates at which standardized premedication regimens (or substitution of a noncontrast examination) were used in high-risk patients, indicating incorporation into routine practice by radiologists across the United States.[6,7] However, several points of controversy have arisen due to the methodologies of the Greenberger and Lasser studies, changes in contrast agents over the last 30 years, and work to distinguish immediate hypersensitivity reactions from physiologic-type reactions, all of which have resulted in an ongoing discussion on whether these historical studies and their findings on the efficacy of premedication regimens are applicable to modern radiology practices and high-risk patient groups.

One major point of consideration is that since the 1980s, IV HOCM has been essentially completely replaced by IV low-osmolality contrast media (LOCM), which has a much lower baseline rate of immediate hypersensitivity reactions in all-comers ($\approx$ 0.6% in the general population for LOCM vs up to 12.7% for HOCM).[4,8] While Lasser and colleagues conducted a second study in 1994 on reactions to IV LOCM in average-risk patients with or without premedication, the study was underpowered. The investigators found a statistically significant decrease in total and mild reactions, although no difference was found in the rates of moderate or severe reactions,[9] which are the types of reactions likely to warrant urgent medical attention. This may have been due to a very small risk reduction, which would have required a very large number of additional patients to discern.

Another point of contention is that early studies often included both immune-mediated reactions (eg, hives, bronchospasm) and non-immune-mediated reactions or "intolerances" (eg, nausea, vomiting, and sneezing),[5,9] which may have artificially increased the measured reaction rates. While intolerances are known to occur, they are generally transient, are not life-threatening, and are not reduced by premedication regimens.[10] These are therefore now considered separate from immediate hypersensitivity reactions.

An additional weakness was the lack of assessment of specifically high-risk patients and the protective effect on this critical group, instead focusing on reducing the rate of reactions in all comers. As discussed in detail later, "high risk" remains incompletely defined,[10] and our understanding of which risk factors places patients in the "high-risk" group has evolved. However, at a minimum, patients who have had a previous reaction to the same class of contrast material are considered at a particular risk of immediate hypersensitivity reactions. The lack of direct consideration of high-risk patients by the Lasser studies and the lack of a nonpremedicated control group in the Greenberger study resulted in an unknown effect size of treatment for this group. Future studies would resort to surmising this treatment effect based on historical data.[11]

Recently, studies have added to the controversy on the role of corticosteroid premedication by refuting the idea that corticosteroid premedication reduces immediate hypersensitivity reactions and questioning routine practice. First, a group in Korea carried out a moderately sized multicenter study on patients with a prior moderate or severe reaction to IV LOCM ($n = 150$ patients with 328 re-exposures to ICM), some of whom were re-exposed without corticosteroid premedication.[12] No statistically significant difference in repeat reaction rate was found between the premedicated and nonpremedicated cohorts (reaction rate of 23.0% in premedicated and 16.5% in nonpremedicated patients). Limitations included a nonrandomized, retrospective design and lack of standardization with varying premedication regimens—some as short as 0.5 to 1 hour in length, which is not long enough to expect an effect. A second study conducted in the United States. more convincingly refuted the efficacy of corticosteroid premedication, retrospectively evaluating a larger number of patients ($n = 1973$) with a history of contrast reaction who later underwent IV contrast-enhanced computed tomography (CT) with either steroid premedication ordered, a different contrast agent than in the index reaction, or neither. Again, no statistically significant difference was found between the premedicated and nonpremedicated cohorts when they received the same contrast material as administered when the index reaction occurred (reaction rate of 26% in premedicated and 25% in nonpremedicated patients), within the limitations of a retrospective, nonrandomized study design and data obtained from a single medical center.

Regarding GBCM, an important point is that the protective effects of corticosteroid premedication on immediate hypersensitivity reactions to GBCM in high-risk patients have not been directly studied, and the widespread practice of premedication is essentially based on extrapolation from data on HOCM and LOCM, despite the study

limitations discussed earlier. The paucity of information may be in part because the baseline risk of immediate hypersensitivity reactions to GBCM is much lower than the corresponding risks to reactions to ICM, estimated to be 0.01% to 2.4%[13–17] with a severe reaction rate of 0.00008% to 0.0019%.[15,18] As a result, the number of patients that would be required to show a statistically significant difference after premedication would be extremely large, and the clinical impact would be lower.

Risks of Premedication

Even as the potential benefits of corticosteroid premedication were being explored, the potential risks of premedication were also considered, beginning with a focus on the direct risks such as transient leukocytosis, transient hyperglycemia, and the potential for an increased risk of infections.[19–21] As a result, we now know that direct risks of corticosteroid premedication are relatively small and of limited clinical importance.[10,19]

On the other hand, indirect risks of corticosteroid premedication were more difficult to measure but were eventually found to be substantial. Before these could be measured, information on the absolute risk reduction offered by steroid premedication and the resulting number needed to treat (NNT) was needed. A study in 2015 laid the groundwork by using historical data to estimate the rate of reactions in nonpremedicated high-risk patients (estimated at 3.5%) and comparing this to the rate of breakthrough reactions in premedicated high-risk patients.[11] Compatible with the Lasser 1994 study, a difference was found between premedicated patients and the expected reaction rate for nonpremedicated patients, although the protection was incomplete and the effect size was small (absolute risk reduction of $\approx 1.4\%$ for all reactions and 0.18% for severe reactions). This resulted in a large NNT to prevent a reaction of any type (NNT = 69) and a very large NNT to prevent a severe reaction (NNT = 569).[11]

A subsequent study in 2016 assessed the impact of premedication regimens on inpatients and the associated risks of prolonging hospitalization, specifically assessing for changes in the length of stay, time elapsed from an imaging order until the examination, additional hospital-acquired infections, and resulting monetary costs that could potentially stem from the administration of a 13 hour oral corticosteroid premedication regimen.[22] As mentioned earlier, the investigators found that indirect risks of such regimens were substantial for inpatients. When compared to matched controls, inpatients undergoing premedication before a CT experienced an increase in the median length of stay and time from order to CT (+25 hours vs controls for both) and rate of hospital-acquired infections (5.1% vs 3.1% in controls). Extrapolating from this using the daily cost of hospitalization and mortality risk from hospital-acquired infections, the investigators suggested that preventing one reaction of any severity would cost over $150,000 and result in 0.7 hospital-acquired infections and 0.04 infection-related deaths. Furthermore, preventing one severe reaction would cost over $131 million and result in 551 hospital-acquired infections and 32 infection-related deaths.

Notably, these indirect risks of corticosteroid premedication focus on inpatient populations who likely face higher risk in a hospital than would outpatients undergoing oral corticosteroid premedication at home. Indirect risks for an outpatient population have not been specifically studied, to our knowledge. Detailed information on indirect risks of corticosteroid premedication prior to GBCM-enhanced MR imaging has also not been directly assessed. However, given that the rate of reactions to GBCM is much lower than the rate of reactions to ICM at baseline, an even greater amount of indirect risk can be inferred from the inpatient population due to the smaller absolute risk reduction and larger NNT. Minor direct risks for corticosteroid premedication prior to GBCM would likely remain similar due to the identical premedication regimens administered.

The limitations of early studies supporting corticosteroid premedication, recent questions raised on efficacy, and the considerable disadvantages—at least in an inpatient population—have resulted in discrepancies in recommendations from the ACR versus European organizations including the ESUR and RCR, and between the ACR versus national organizations in other medical specialties, particularly Allergy and Immunology. The ACRs recommendations are somewhat vague, noting in the ACR Manual on Contrast Media v2023 that despite the drawbacks and gaps in knowledge on premedication of high-risk patients, corticosteroid premedication "may be considered," particularly in outpatients with a prior immediate hypersensitivity reaction to the same class of contrast medium, and "should be considered if feasible" in patients with a history of severe reaction to the same class of contrast medium when IV contrast material is necessary and there are no reasonable alternative tests.[10] Conversely, the ESUR has published Guidelines on Contrast Agents v10.0, which is much more decisive in recommending against routine corticosteroid premedication, including in patients at an increased risk of reaction, stating simply that "premedication is not recommended because there is not good evidence of its effectiveness."[23] In the UK's RCR document on Standards for Intravascular Contrast Agent Administration to Adult Patients similarly states that "there is no conclusive evidence of benefit for the prophylactic use of steroids in the prevention of severe reactions to contrast agents".[24] Finally, a 2020 update to practice parameters by the Joint Task Force on Practice Parameters for Allergy and Immunology in the United States recommended against routine corticosteroid premedication, even for high-risk patients, although a grading of the evidence behind this recommendation showed that the certainty was very low and the strength of recommendation was conditional.[25]

Despite a long period during which a consensus could have been reached and recent articles questioning the utility of premedication and suggesting a desire for standardization, the international community remains at odds with the US regarding recommendations on corticosteroid premedication.[26,27]

Abbreviated Protocols

The pharmacologic action of corticosteroids in the prevention of immediate hypersensitivity reactions is incompletely understood, although corticosteroids generally act by activating cellular receptors and triggering the intracellular assembly of enzymes, a process which takes at least several hours.[28] However, a pressing need for an IV contrast-enhanced CT or MR imaging may outweigh the benefits of a steroid premedication regimen lasting 12 hours or more, for example, inpatients in the emergency department. As a result, physicians have sought to find a "rapid" premedication regimen that balances the risk of immediate hypersensitivity reactions with the risk of waiting for a radiologic examination.

We know that very short premedication regimens have no statistically significant effect based on the landmark Lasser and colleagues' study in which they examined a standardized oral regimen 2 hours in length and found no significant decrease in reactions to HOCM.[5] The only direct evidence supporting premedication regimens shorter than 12 hours was also explored in the era of HOCM, when Greenberger and colleagues assembled a small case series of high-risk patients (n = 9) who were premedicated with IV hydrocortisone beginning "as soon as the procedure was judged essential" and every 4 hours thereafter until the procedure was completed. No patients experienced a breakthrough reaction. Notably, this study may not be fully translatable to modern radiology practice due to the use of HOCM, the very small number of patients pretreated, and the nonstandardized protocol with premedication durations ranging from 1 to 9 hours. Although no direct test of a standardized rapid premedication regimen prior to LOCM has been subsequently performed, a study in 2015 compared the breakthrough reaction rate following a 5 hour IV premedication regimen to a traditional 13 hour oral regimen and found no significant difference.[29] Despite the limited evidence, the ACR Manual on Contrast Media describes rapid IV regimens as a strategy to consider for some patient groups (eg, patients in the emergency department). In practice, rapid premedication regimens are widely used in the United States; a survey of US radiologists in 2020 showed that 70% of radiologists would recommend an IV regimen 4 to 6 hours in duration for patients in the ED and that the use of rapid premedication regimens has increased since a similar survey in 2009.[7,30] Again, there is no direct evidence to support rapid premedication for IV gadolinium, with current practices in rapid premedication extrapolated from the limited evidence on HOCM.

Establishing Patient Risk Stratification for Contrast Reaction

Deciding which patients to premedicate is also controversial as the occurrence of reactions can be unpredictable, even in high-risk patients. In general, the decision to premedicate is based on patient history rather than any laboratory or skin testing. It is recognized that the most substantial risk factor for a reaction to IV contrast media is a prior history of reaction to the same category of contrast media, resulting in approximately 5 times increased risk versus the general population.[4,10,31–33] However, several other potential risk factors have historically been explored. Atopic risk factors including asthma, allergic rhinitis, or allergies to other substances, particularly if severe, are also thought to increase a patient's risk of a contrast reaction by 2 to 3 times.[4,10] Despite this increased risk, a history of atopy is generally downplayed as the risk increase is less substantial; the ACR unambiguously recommends against premedication or restricting use of contrast material based solely on a patient history of unrelated allergies or asthma.[10] Middle-aged patients, women, and patients taking beta-blockers are also thought to have a modestly increased risk.[8,34,35] However, some studies exploring these risk factors were conducted more than 25 years ago, so data may not accurately reflect the risk when these patients receive LOCM. Shellfish allergy, other food/medication allergies, and iodine allergy have been studied but have not definitively found to be associated with an increased risk of contrast reactions.[36]

Despite clear statements on conditions that do not warrant premedication, the ACR Manual on Contrast media provides only some examples of settings in which corticosteroid premedication "may be considered." Specific inclusion criteria or a definition of "high-risk" are not given, which may contribute to heterogeneity in clinical practice. While some medical centers in the United States only premedicate patients for a history of contrast reactions, recent surveys of US radiologists have shown that substantial local variability remains and that utilization of steroid premedication has increased despite the improved risk profile of LOCM versus HOCM.[7,30]

Cross-Reactivity

Cross-reactivity between iodinated contrast media and gadolinium-based contrast media classes

When providers encounter a patient with a prior reaction to a class of contrast media, they may opt for an imaging examination using a different contrast class to avoid the risk of a repeat reaction. For example, a patient with a prior reaction to ICM may instead undergo an IV contrast-enhanced MR examination using GBCM. As there are major differences in the chemical structures of ICM and GBCM, cross-reactivity is unlikely, particularly when mediated by immunoglobulin E (IgE). The ACR Manual on Contrast Media does not recommend corticosteroid premedication when a different class of contrast media is used,[10] and there are several reports documenting the safe administration of GBCM in patients with prior severe reactions to ICM and vice versa.[37–39] Despite these facts, a recent survey found that many radiologists are hesitant to order an IV contrast-enhanced CT for a patient with a prior severe reaction to a GBCM.[30]

Conversely, one recent large study reported an increased risk of an allergic reaction to GBCM in patients with a prior reaction to ICM.[40] Potential contributing factors may include the hyperosmolarity of agents directly activating mast cells, inducing a reaction by both contrast classes. Patients with mastocytosis may also be more likely to have reactions to both ICM and GBCM. Another possibility is sensitivities to additives or contaminants that may be present in either ICM or GBCM, such as trometamol.[41] Finally, patients who have experienced a prior allergic-like reaction may be more cognizant of the symptoms and more likely to report symptoms regardless of the contrast class administered. Additional studies are needed to further explore these possibilities.

Cross-reactivity within iodinated contrast media or gadolinium-based contrast media class

Cross-reactivity within a particular contrast class is expected due to similar chemical structures. Cross-reactivity is observed more frequently between certain pairs of ICM including iodixanol, iohexol, iopentol, ioversol, and iomeprol, and particularly between iohexol and iodixanol.[8] Ioxaglate, iopamidol, iobitridol, and iopromide have been found to have limited cross-reactivity.

To further explore cross-reactivity, numerous skin testing studies have been conducted. Skin test sensitivity for ICM has been reported to range from 4% to 73%, with a similar range observed with GBCM.[42] This large range has been attributed to variability in skin testing protocols, including whether a skin prick test or intradermal test is performed, variable dilution of the contrast agent, inciting contrast agent, reaction severity (with prior moderate or severe reactions having increased sensitivity), and the time between reaction and testing (with longer delays decreasing the chance of a positive result[43]). Specificity for skin testing is approximately 95%.[44] Although the negative predictive value for ICM skin testing may be as high as 97%,[45] it decreases to 60% when drug provocation tests are performed.[46] The clinical utility of skin testing to assess allergy to ICM and GBCM is still uncertain, to our knowledge.

Some debate exists about the existence of true ICM cross-reactivity based on chemical structures. One systemic review of 25 studies classified 340 patients into those who had "polyvalent reactivity" or multiple positive skin test results across all ICM and those who had cross-reactivity or multiple positive skin test results within ICM with similar chemical structures.[47] The incidence of polyvalent reactivity was higher than the incidence of cross-reactivity, suggesting that individual reaction patterns to ICM may outweigh cross-reactivity patterns defined by chemical structure. Larger and more thorough studies are needed to better assess the mechanisms of cross-reactivity.

Cumulatively, cross-reactivity within the same class appears to occur in approximately a third of patients with a history of contrast reaction.[48,49] A recent study of 245 patients for prospective skin testing (209 ICM, 36 GBCM) reported cross-reactivity in 27% of ICM reaction and 50% of GBCM reaction patients.[50] Cross-reactivity rates were higher when undiluted contrast was used for skin testing (31% when diluted and 63% when undiluted).

Evidence regarding GBCM cross-reactivity and skin testing performance is more limited than evidence regarding ICM, as reactions to GBCM are far less frequent. Aside from the discussed earlier, much evidence comes from case reports and small case series; for example, a case series of 11 patients and 17 published cases reported that GBCM cross-reactivity was observed in one-third of cases.[51] Cross-reactivity has been reported within macrocyclic agents, within linear agents, and between macrocyclic and linear agents.

There are several limitations to the skin testing studies described earlier. Most notably, there is substantial variability in the specific testing protocol.[52] Skin testing results may also vary depending on whether the reaction was acute or delayed. As medical centers are often limited by the number of ICM or GBCM options stocked by that institution, a complete assessment of all relevant contrast agents is not always performed. Skin testing patients infrequently undergo drug provocation testing or undergo repeat imaging with an agent that caused a negative skin test result, making it challenging to assess the clinical relevance of skin testing. Repeat imaging using an agent that caused a positive skin test result is especially uncommon, as most providers believe such re-exposure has too high of a risk. Finally, most studies are limited by small sample sizes as immediate hypersensitivity reactions to contrast are uncommon and skin testing is not routinely performed following a reaction.

Cross-reactivity and repeat immediate hypersensitivity reactions

Cross-reactivity within a contrast class can be indirectly assessed by examining repeat reaction rates in patients exposed to different ICM or GBCM than the one that caused their prior reaction. Retrospective studies have found that using a different ICM or GBCM than the one that caused the prior reaction was associated with a reduced risk of repeat reaction than using the same agent, even with steroid premedication.[53–55] Substitution does not eliminate the risk of repeat reaction due to presumed cross-reactivity in a subset of patients.

A large study of over 9000 IV contrast-enhanced CT examinations performed in patients with a prior reaction to ICM reported that the rate of repeat reactions varied with certain ICM combinations. The investigators did not find evidence of ICM cross-reactivity, suggesting that the side chain structure of ICM is not an important risk factor for repeat reactions.[56] Sohn and colleagues reported that patients with a severe prior reaction showed cross-reactivity between ICM with common side chains and repeat reaction rates were reduced in these patients by avoiding ICM without common side chains and selecting ICM with negative skin test results. However, these findings were not observed in patients with nonsevere prior reactions.[48] A meta-analysis of 8 GBCM studies reported that repeat reaction rates were similar between patients who underwent skin testing workup and patients who received the same GBCM and corticosteroid prep.[57] A case series of 11 patients and 17 published cases found that no repeat reactions were observed in the few cases of re-exposure to a GBCM with a negative skin test result.[51] Additional studies are needed to assess the correlation between skin testing results and ICM or GBCM re-exposure and repeat reaction rates.

SUMMARY

Immediate hypersensitivity reactions to ICM and GBCM can be life-threatening, and no mitigation strategy completely prevents breakthrough reactions. While some historical studies indicate that corticosteroid premedication reduces risk, there are limitations to these older studies and the efficacy of corticosteroid premedication with modern contrast agents has recently been questioned. "Rapid" IV premedication protocols have become the norm in many emergency settings, although many of the same caveats also apply to this expedited approach. While the direct risks of premedication are limited, to our knowledge, indirect risks are substantial, particularly for inpatient populations, and the risk–benefit ratio continues to be questioned and investigated.

Although there is some common ground on patient populations considered at-risk for contrast reactions, discrepancies in recommendations still exist between major radiological organizations in the United States versus those in Europe, and between recommendations from the ACR versus organizations focused on the disciplines of allergy and immunology.

Chemical differences between ICM and GBCM result in limited cross-reactivity; some evidence suggests that cross-reactions may be due to osmolality or additives common to both classes of contrast media. Several gaps in knowledge exist regarding the utility of skin testing for ICM or GBCM sensitivities, potential mechanisms of cross-reactivity, and how this information can help reduce repeat reactions.

CLINICS CARE POINTS

- Data supporting corticosteroid premedication before IV LOCM are largely based on historical studies on HOCM from the 1980s and 1990s; premedication before IV GBCM is largely based on extrapolation from data on ICM, with little direct evidence.

- Recommendations on corticosteroid premedication from the ACR and international organizations differ and are not always explicitly followed, so practices vary locally.

- The ACR recommends:
  a. Considering corticosteroid premedication only for high-risk patients with a prior history of reaction to the same category of contrast material.
  b. Not premedicating patients when a different class of contrast material is used (eg, GBCM in a patient with history of allergy to ICM).
  c. Considering expedited IV corticosteroid premedication for some patient groups (eg, patients in the emergency department).

- Our knowledge about cross-reactivity within classes of contrast media continues to evolve; agent-switching may be an effective strategy when feasible.

DISCLOSURE

J.S. McDonald reports investigator-initiated research grants and consulting work with GE Healthcare independent of the current review.

REFERENCES

1. Greenberger PA, Patterson R, Radin RC. Two pretreatment regimens for high-risk patients receiving radiographic contrast media. J Allergy Clin Immunol 1984;74:540–3, 4, Part 1.
2. Greenberger PA, Michael Halwig J, Patterson R, et al. Emergency administration of radiocontrast media in high-risk patients. J Allergy Clin Immunol 1986;77(4):630–4.
3. Greenberger PA, Patterson R. The prevention of immediate generalized reactions to radiocontrast media in high-risk patients. J Allergy Clin Immunol 1991;87(4):867–72.
4. Katayama H, Yamaguchi K, Kozuka T, et al. Adverse reactions to ionic and nonionic contrast media. A report from the Japanese Committee on the Safety of Contrast Media. Radiology 1990;175(3):621–8.

5. Lasser EC, Berry CC, Talner LB, et al. Pretreatment with corticosteroids to alleviate reactions to intravenous contrast material. N Engl J Med 1987; 317(14):845–9.

6. Cohan RH, Ellis JH, Dunnick NR. Use of low-osmolar agents and premedication to reduce the frequency of adverse reactions to radiographic contrast media: a survey of the Society of Uroradiology. Radiology 1995;194(2):357–64.

7. O'Malley RB, Cohan RH, Ellis JH, et al. A Survey on the use of premedication prior to iodinated and gadolinium-based contrast material administration. J Am Coll Radiol 2011;8(5):345–54.

8. Wang CL, Cohan RH, Ellis JH, et al. Frequency, outcome, and appropriateness of treatment of nonionic iodinated contrast media reactions. Am J Roentgenol 2008;191(2):409–15.

9. Lasser EC, Berry CC, Mishkin MM, et al. Pretreatment with corticosteroids to prevent adverse reactions to nonionic contrast media. AJR Am J Roentgenol 1994;162(3):523–6.

10. American College of Radiology - Committee on Drugs and Contrast Media. ACR manual on contrast media. American College of Radiology. 2023. Available at: https://www.acr.org/-/media/ACR/Files/Clinical-Resources/Contrast_Media.pdf. [Accessed 1 November 2023].

11. Mervak BM, Davenport MS, Ellis JH, et al. Rates of breakthrough reactions in inpatients at high risk receiving premedication before contrast-enhanced CT. Am J Roentgenol 2015;205(1):77–84.

12. Park HJ, Park JW, Yang MS, et al. Re-exposure to low osmolar iodinated contrast media in patients with prior moderate-to-severe hypersensitivity reactions: A multicentre retrospective cohort study. Eur Radiol 2017;27(7):2886–93.

13. Hao D, Ai T, Goerner F, et al. MRI contrast agents: Basic chemistry and safety. J Magn Reson Imag 2012;36(5):1060–71.

14. Li A, Wong CS, Wong MK, et al. Acute adverse reactions to magnetic resonance contrast media – gadolinium chelates. BJR 2006;79(941):368–71.

15. Jung JW, Kang HR, Kim MH, et al. Immediate hypersensitivity reaction to gadolinium-based MR Contrast Media. Radiology 2012;264(2):414–22.

16. Dillman JR, Ellis JH, Cohan RH, et al. Frequency and severity of acute allergic-like reactions to gadolinium-containing IV contrast media in children and adults. Am J Roentgenol 2007;189(6):1533–8.

17. Forsting M, Palkowitsch P. Prevalence of acute adverse reactions to gadobutrol—A highly concentrated macrocyclic gadolinium chelate: Review of 14,299 patients from observational trials. Eur J Radiol 2010;74(3):e186–92.

18. Prince MR, Zhang H, Zou Z, et al. Incidence of immediate gadolinium contrast media reactions. Am J Roentgenol 2011;196(2):W138–43.

19. Lasser E. Pretreatment with corticosteroids to prevent reactions to i.v. contrast material: overview and implications. Am J Roentgenol 1988;150(2):257–9.

20. Davenport MS, Cohan RH, Caoili EM, et al. Hyperglycemic consequences of corticosteroid premedication in an outpatient population. AJR Am J Roentgenol 2010;194(6):W483–8.

21. Davenport MS, Cohan RH, Khalatbari S, et al. Hyperglycemia in hospitalized patients receiving corticosteroid premedication before the administration of radiologic contrast medium. Acad Radiol 2011; 18(3):384–90.

22. Davenport MS, Mervak BM, Ellis JH, et al. Indirect Cost and Harm Attributable to Oral 13-Hour Inpatient Corticosteroid Prophylaxis before Contrast-enhanced CT. Radiology 2016;279(2):492–501.

23. European Society of Urogenital Radiology (ESUR). Guidelines on Contrast Agents v10.0. 2018. Available at: https://www.esur.org/esur-guidelines-on-contrast-agents/. [Accessed 17 November 2023].

24. The Royal College of Radiologists. Standards for intravascular contrast agent administration to adult patients, Second edition. 2010.

25. Shaker MS, Wallace DV, Golden DBK, et al. Anaphylaxis—a 2020 practice parameter update, systematic review, and Grading of Recommendations, Assessment, Development and Evaluation (GRADE) analysis. J Allergy Clin Immunol 2020;145(4):1082–123.

26. Davenport MS, Cohan RH. The Evidence for and Against Corticosteroid Prophylaxis in At-Risk Patients. Radiol Clin North Am 2017;55(2):413–21.

27. Davenport MS, Weinstein S. (Still) Wondering If We Should Stop Giving Steroid Preps. Radiology 2021; 301(1):141–3.

28. Morcos SK. Acute serious and fatal reactions to contrast media: our current understanding. BJR 2005;78(932):686–93.

29. Mervak BM, Cohan RH, Ellis JH, et al. Intravenous Corticosteroid Premedication Administered 5 Hours before CT Compared with a Traditional 13-Hour Oral Regimen. Radiology 2017;285(2):425–33.

30. Sodagari F, Davenport MS, Asch D, et al. A survey of practicing radiologists on the use of premedication before intravenous iodinated contrast medium administration. J Am Coll Radiol 2023. https://doi.org/10.1016/j.jacr.2023.04.024.

31. Bettmann MA, Heeren T, Greenfield A, et al. Adverse events with radiographic contrast agents: results of the SCVIR Contrast Agent Registry. Radiology 1997;203(3):611–20.

32. Brockow K, Christiansen C, Kanny G, et al. Management of hypersensitivity reactions to iodinated contrast media. Allergy 2005;60(2):150–8.

33. Mortelé KJ, Oliva MR, Ondategui S, et al. Universal use of nonionic iodinated contrast medium for CT: Evaluation of safety in a large urban teaching hospital. Am J Roentgenol 2005;184(1):31–4.

34. Callahan MJ, Poznauskis L, Zurakowski D, et al. Nonionic iodinated intravenous contrast material-related reactions: incidence in large urban children's hospital–retrospective analysis of data in 12,494 patients. Radiology 2009;250(3):674–81.

35. Lang DM, Alpern MB, Visintainer PF, et al. Elevated risk of anaphylactoid reaction from radiographic contrast media is associated with both beta-blocker exposure and cardiovascular disorders. Arch Intern Med 1993;153(17):2033–40.

36. Boehm I. Seafood allergy and radiocontrast media: are physicians propagating a myth? Am J Med 2008;121(8):e19.

37. Benzon HT, Schechtman J, Zheng SC, et al. Patients with a history of hypersensitivity reaction to iodinated contrast medium and given iodinated contrast during an interventional pain procedure. Reg Anesth Pain Med 2019;44(1):118–21.

38. Guragai N, Roman S, Vasudev R, et al. Gadolinium-based coronary angiography in a patient with prior known anaphylaxis to iodine-based dye. J Community Hosp Intern Med Perspect 2021;11(2):286–8.

39. Juneman E, Saleh L, Thai H, et al. Successful coronary angiography with adequate image acquisition using a combination of gadolinium and a power injector in a patient with severe iodine contrast allergy. Exp Clin Cardiol 2012;17(1):17–9.

40. Ahn YH, Kang DY, Park SB, et al. Allergic-like hypersensitivity reactions to gadolinium-based contrast agents: An 8-year Cohort Study of 154 539 Patients. Radiology 2022;303(2):329–36.

41. Lukawska J, Mandaliya D, Chan AWE, et al. Anaphylaxis to trometamol excipient in gadolinium-based contrast agents for clinical imaging. J Allergy Clin Immunol Pract 2019;7(3):1086–7.

42. Rosado Ingelmo A, Dona Diaz I, Cabanas Moreno R, et al. Clinical Practice Guidelines for Diagnosis and Management of Hypersensitivity Reactions to Contrast Media. J Investig Allergol Clin Immunol 2016;26(3):144–55. quiz 2 p following 155.

43. Fernandez TD, Torres MJ, Blanca-Lopez N, et al. Negativization rates of IgE radioimmunoassay and basophil activation test in immediate reactions to penicillins. Allergy 2009;64(2):242–8.

44. Brockow K, Garvey LH, Aberer W, et al. Skin test concentrations for systemically administered drugs – an ENDA/EAACI Drug Allergy Interest Group position paper. Allergy 2013;68(6):702–12.

45. Caimmi S, Benyahia B, Suau D, et al. Clinical value of negative skin tests to iodinated contrast media. Clin Exp Allergy 2010;40(5):805–10.

46. Salas M, Gomez F, Fernandez TD, et al. Diagnosis of immediate hypersensitivity reactions to radiocontrast media. Allergy 2013;68(9):1203–6.

47. Schmid AA, Morelli JN, Hungerbuhler MN, et al. Cross-reactivity among iodinated contrast agents: should we be concerned? Quant Imag Med Surg 2021;11(9):4028–41.

48. Sohn KH, Seo JH, Kang DY, et al. Finding the Optimal Alternative for Immediate Hypersensitivity to Low-Osmolar Iodinated Contrast. Invest Radiol 2021;56(8):480–5.

49. Yoon SH, Lee SY, Kang HR, et al. Skin tests in patients with hypersensitivity reaction to iodinated contrast media: a meta-analysis. Allergy 2015;70(6):625–37.

50. Clement O, Dewachter P, Mouton-Faivre C, et al. Immediate Hypersensitivity to Contrast Agents: The French 5-year CIRTACI Study. EClinicalMedicine 2018;1:51–61.

51. Grueber HP, Helbling A, Joerg L. Skin test results and cross-reactivity patterns in IgE- and T-Cell-mediated allergy to gadolinium-based contrast agents. Allergy Asthma Immunol Res 2021;13(6):933–8.

52. Saenz de Santa Maria R, Labella M, Bogas G, et al. Hypersensitivity to gadolinium-based contrast. Curr Opin Allergy Clin Immunol 2023;23(4):300–6.

53. McDonald JS, Larson NB, Kolbe AB, et al. Prevention of allergic-like reactions at repeat CT: steroid pretreatment versus contrast material substitution. Radiology 2021;301(1):133–40.

54. Umakoshi H, Nihashi T, Takada A, et al. Iodinated contrast media substitution to prevent recurrent hypersensitivity reactions: a systematic review and meta-analysis. Radiology 2022;305(2):341–9.

55. Walker D, McGrath TA, Glikstein R, et al. Empiric switching of gadolinium-based contrast agents in patients with history of previous immediate hypersensitivity reaction to GBCA: A prospective single-center, single-arm efficacy trial. Invest Radiol 2021;56(6):369–73.

56. Kim SR, Son NH, Park HJ, et al. Differences in the recurrence rate of immediate adverse drug reactions according to the components of alternative contrast media: analysis of repetitive computed tomography cases in a single tertiary hospital. Drug Saf 2022;45(9):995–1002.

57. Walker DT, Davenport MS, McGrath TA, et al. Breakthrough hypersensitivity reactions to gadolinium-based contrast agents and strategies to decrease subsequent reaction rates: a systematic review and meta-analysis. Radiology 2020;296(2):312–21.

Iodinated Contrast and Nephropathy
Does It Exist and What Is the Actual Evidence?

Robert J. McDonald, MD, PhD, Jennifer S. McDonald, PhD*

KEYWORDS

- Iodinated contrast material • Contrast-induced acute kidney injury • Contrast safety
- Contrast-induced nephropathy • CT contrast • Acute kidney injury

KEY POINTS

- Controlled studies are critical for distinguishing between true cases of contrast-induced acute kidney injury (CI-AKI) and contrast-associated AKI (CA-AKI), or AKI concurrent with, but causally unrelated to, iodinated contrast material (ICM) exposure.
- The incidence and severity of CI-AKI has been greatly overstated by prior uncontrolled studies; recent controlled studies find no risk of CI-AKI for patients with an estimated glomerular filtration rate (eGFR) of 45 mL/min or greater. The risk of CI-AKI in patients with an eGFR less than 30 mL/min is still debated.
- Controlled studies have not found an increased risk of longer term morbidity, including chronic kidney disease, emergent dialysis, or mortality, from CI-AKI, even among patients with an eGFR less than 30 mL/min.
- No patient group has a complete contraindication for ICM use; instead, an individualized approach should be taken to determine if the important clinical benefits of ICM administration outweigh the potential risk of CI-AKI.

INTRODUCTION

Iodinated contrast material (ICM) has revolutionized radiologic examinations and the fields of radiology and medicine, via improved conspicuity of soft tissues, and differentiation between normal and diseased tissues. The clinical utility of these agents is underscored by their extensive utilization in medical practice, with an estimated over 1 billion doses administered worldwide since the initial development in the 1920s.[1] Since the initial discovery, the chemical structure and properties of ICMs have evolved from earlier generation high-osmolar, ionic agents, to modern-day low-osmolar and iso-osmolar nonionic agents with fewer side effects and increased patient tolerance. The reported nephrotoxic effects of ICMs, or contrast-induced acute kidney injury (CI-AKI), were once considered a universally accepted risk of ICM exposure; however, the reported incidence, severity, and even existence of this complication has become increasingly controversial over the past 2 decades. The genesis of this controversy came about after closer examination of prior studies of CI-AKI, and the fact that the causal relationship between ICM exposure and nephrotoxicity has not been proven with sufficient scientific rigor. Further, as CI-AKI was originally reported following the administration of older, high-osmolar ICM with far greater nephrotoxic potential, the reported incidence and risk of

Department of Radiology, Mayo Clinic, Rochester, MN, USA
* Corresponding author. Department of Radiology, Mayo Clinic, 200 1st Street SouthWest, Rochester, MN 55905.
E-mail address: mcdonald.jennifer@mayo.edu

Radiol Clin N Am 62 (2024) 959–969
https://doi.org/10.1016/j.rcl.2024.03.001
0033-8389/24/© 2024 Elsevier Inc. All rights reserved.

CI-AKI has likely been greatly overstated in modern practice, as more "kidney-friendly" low-osmolar and iso-osmolar agents have replaced these older agents.

Recent studies have challenged the existence of CI-AKI, even among patients considered at highest risk for this feared complication. These findings have led to an unexpected consensus across medical disciplines that the incidence and severity of CI-AKI have been overstated in most patients. Controversy remains over whether CI-AKI is either an uncommon causal complication from ICM exposure among patients with pre-existing renal dysfunction or a causal fallacy; a phenomenon of temporal concurrence whereby ICM is administered at the inflection point in a patient's health and underlying disease(s) at the same time other causative factors are adversely affecting renal function. This review will summarize recent changes in CI-AKI nomenclature, provide an overview of the evidence for and against the existence of CI-AKI, and discuss the most recent findings regarding long-term outcomes of CI-AKI, prophylaxis efficacy, CI-AKI biomarkers and screening, and risk stratification.

INTRAVASCULAR CONTRAST-ASSOCIATED AKI AND INTRAVASCULAR CONTRAST-INDUCED AKI

The term "contrast-induced nephropathy" has previously been extensively used to describe nephrotoxicity due to contrast administration. However, this term has been used to define both contrast-dependent AKI and contrast-independent AKI that occurs following intravascular contrast exposure. Newer terminology was, therefore, needed to clearly distinguish these 2 phenomena. In 2020, the American College of Radiology and the National Kidney Foundation endorsed using the terms "contrast-associated AKI" (CA-AKI) and "contrast-induced AKI" (CI-AKI) to avoid this confusion.[2]

CA-AKI encompasses all AKI that occurs 48 to 72 hours following intravascular ICM administration, including both contrast-dependent and contrast-independent AKI (ie, AKI caused by hypovolemia, compromised cardiac function, or nephrotoxic medications). CA-AKI is a correlative diagnosis instead of a causal relationship between ICM exposure and AKI, which can, in improperly designed studies, be mistaken for CI-AKI. In contradistinction, CI-AKI is a contrast-dependent AKI that occurs within 48 to 72 hours of intravascular ICM administration in the absence of other causes. CI-AKI is, therefore, a causative diagnosis. The terms CA-AKI and CI-AKI cannot be used interchangeably.

Uncontrolled studies should use the term CA-AKI, as they are incapable of discriminating between CA-AKI and CI-AKI. Only properly designed controlled studies are capable of distinguishing between these 2 phenomena.

Most studies of the potential nephrotoxicity of ICM have focused on intra-arterial (IA) administration of ICM over intravenous (IV) administration. IA studies of nephrotoxicity are limited as they are universally uncontrolled; they lack a control group of patients who underwent similar invasive procedures without ICM exposure, as doing so would be unethical or unfeasible. Accordingly, these IA studies are unable to discriminate between CI-AKI and CA-AKI.[3] Further, the reported incidence and risk of CA-AKI from IA procedures and interventions cannot be extrapolated to IV ICM procedures and examinations due to procedural differences (eg, higher total and effective renal artery ICM dose), differences in patient characteristics, higher AKI risk (eg, higher risk of hemodynamic instability), and increased risk of iatrogenesis from catheter-associated atheroembolic renal ischemia.[3,4] This review will, therefore, focus on CA-AKI and CI-AKI following IV administration of ICM.

HISTORICAL CONTEXT OF CONTRAST-INDUCED ACUTE KIDNEY INJURY

The first reported case of CA-AKI in 1954 described acute anuria in a patient with multiple myeloma after the administration of iodopyracet, an early ionic ICM agent.[5] Subsequent uncontrolled studies of older high-osmolar agents reported a CA-AKI rate as high as 20% in the general population, and even higher with certain comorbidities.[6,7] Most of these uncontrolled studies were affected by the post hoc fallacy; they attributed all cases of AKI to ICM exposure instead of other, and often more likely, contrast-independent causes of AKI. The inability of these studies to disentangle CI-AKI from CA-AKI cases precludes their assessment of the causal relationship between ICM exposure and deteriorating renal function.[3] Further, other uncontrolled studies did not find evidence of CA-AKI after exposure to IV or IA ICM.[8,9] These conflicting findings suggested that ICM exposure was not universally nephrotoxic to renally impaired patients.

EVIDENCE AGAINST THE EXISTENCE OF CONTRAST-INDUCED ACUTE KIDNEY INJURY
Retrospective Controlled Studies

Controlled studies of IV ICM that directly compared contrast-exposed patients to unexposed control patients were first published 35 years ago.[10] These studies refuted prior uncontrolled studies and reported no elevated risk of AKI following ICM exposure.[11] Paradoxically, these studies often reported a higher rate of AKI in control patients (not exposed to ICM) compared to ICM-exposed patients. This finding was a substantial source of criticism, and suggested either a nephroprotective effect of ICM exposure, an unlikely possibility, or that these studies were affected by substantial selection bias; a bias where patients with more severe baseline renal disease were steered away from receiving ICM, creating demographic differences and heterogeneity between unexposed control and contrast-exposed groups. This phenomenon, known as "renalism,"[12] ultimately results in ICM unexposed patient groups with more severe renal dysfunction compared to ICM-exposed groups.

Renalism alone does not account for why unexposed patients have higher AKI rates than ICM-exposed patients. Patients with severe renal dysfunction are more likely to have other confounders that adversely affect renal function (ie, more likely to be on nephrotoxic medications, suboptimal fluid balance or oral intake, and higher prevalence of other comorbidities including congestive heart failure, coronary artery disease, or renal artery stenosis). Despite improvements in demographic heterogeneity, retrospective studies that accounted for these variables still observed higher rates of AKI in unexposed patient groups.[13,14] Another explanation for this observation is the positive correlation between physiologic variability in serum creatinine (SCr) and severity of baseline renal dysfunction; patients with more severe renal dysfunction have higher variability in SCr that can confound laboratory diagnosis of CI-AKI. Two studies of the temporal course of renal function among hospitalized patients not exposed to contrast reported a positive correlation between worsening renal function and renal function variability over a 48 hour period.[15,16] In many cases, this variability would have met the technical criteria for CI-AKI had contrast been administered. The term "hospital-induced nephropathy" was coined to demonstrate that much, if not all, of what had previously been termed CI-AKI in the hospitalized setting were actually misattributed cases of CA-AKI confounded by variability in SCr.[17]

Retrospective Controlled Studies Using Propensity Score Adjustment

An increasing number of controlled retrospective studies have been published in the past decade that utilized the statistical approach of propensity score adjustment to address selection bias and

renalism limitations of earlier retrospective studies. Propensity score adjustment simulates the randomization enrollment event of a prospective randomized controlled trial, creating more homogenous and comparable populations of unexposed and exposed patients with regard to the clinical decision factors associated with ICM administration, minimizing selection bias.[18] Most of these propensity score controlled studies found no increased risk of AKI among ICM-exposed patients compared to unexposed, clinically similar control patients, even in subgroups of patients with estimated glomerular filtration rate (eGFR) less than 30 mL/min and other comorbidities believed to increase the risk of CI-AKI.[13,19–21] The current authors of this article also performed an additional counterfactual analysis that failed to suggest a casual relationship between ICM exposure and nephrotoxicity after comparing AKI rates among patients that underwent both nonenhanced and IV contrast-enhanced computed tomographic (CT) examinations over the study timeframe.[22] Cumulatively, these controlled studies suggest that there is no causal association between ICM exposure and AKI.

EVIDENCE SUPPORTING THE EXISTENCE OF CONTRAST-INDUCED ACUTE KIDNEY INJURY

Over the decades, animal model studies have suggested several potential mechanisms of ICM-mediated nephrotoxicity including (1) direct free-radical mediated tubular toxicity, (2) renal ischemia from reduced afferent arteriolar blood flow, and (3) renal ischemia from excessive ICM-mediated osmolar load in the renal tubule.[23] Such findings validate theoretic concerns over ICM-mediated nephrotoxicity, although the clinical translation of these findings to patients receiving standard doses of ICM remains a topic of debate, as the severity of renal injury necessary in these animal models to express a CI-AKI phenotype exceeds that which is observed in nonanuric patients with severe renal impairment.

To date, 7 controlled propensity score-matched retrospective studies have reported an increased risk of CI-AKI in specific patient subgroups.[24–30] Increased risk was observed in patients with baseline eGFR less than 30 mL/min in some studies, with an absolute increase in risk of 4%.[24–27] In other studies, there was either a marginally statistically significant and/or comorbidity-dependent risk of CI-AKI among patients with baseline eGFR 30 to 44 mL/min.[25,27] A meta-analysis of 21 propensity score-adjusted controlled studies agreed that patients with an eGFR less than 30 mL/min were at increased risk of CI-AKI.[14] However, studies of patients with an eGFR less than 30 mL/min are limited by small sample sizes and difficulties matching exposed and control patients. Larger studies specifically focused on this patient subset are needed to better assess the true risk of CI-AKI.

INCIDENCE OF CONTRAST-INDUCED ACUTE KIDNEY INJURY AND CONTRAST-ASSOCIATED ACUTE KIDNEY INJURY

Historical studies, predominantly of IA ICM, reported AKI incidences of 0% to 5% in the general population, and up to 30% among patients with pre-existing renal dysfunction and other comorbidities.[31–33] As these studies were uncontrolled, these incidences largely reflected CA-AKI instead of CI-AKI cases. More recent controlled studies are now able to disambiguate CI-AKI from CA-AKI and define CI-AKI as the absolute increase in AKI incidence between ICM-exposed and unexposed patients. These studies have reported CI-AKI rates of 0% to 2% in the general population and up to 17% among patients with severe renal dysfunction.[13,14]

POTENTIAL LONG-TERM RISKS OF IODINATED CONTRAST MATERIAL EXPOSURE

Historical studies have suggested a high risk of permanent renal injury from CI-AKI manifesting as chronic kidney disease, emergent dialysis, and inhospital and longer-term mortality.[34–36] However, as these studies were uncontrolled, they were unable to assess causality. Most recent controlled studies refute these claims and found no association between ICM administration and more severe outcomes,[37–42] but a few controlled studies reported an increased risk of certain adverse outcomes. A retrospective controlled study of patients with chronic kidney disease (CKD) by Takura and colleagues reported marginally greater decreases in renal function over a 4 to 5 year observation window among ICM-exposed patients versus unexposed patients (eGFR change 7.9 vs 4.7 mL/min/1.73 m²/y).[43] Huang and colleagues performed a propensity score-adjusted analysis of dialysis-dependent patients with CKD and reported an increased risk of adverse cardiovascular events from ICM exposure over a 10 year period when compared to clinically similar unexposed patients.[44]

Assessing the potential causal relationship between ICM exposure and longer term outcomes is more challenging than examining acute, short-term outcomes. Studies of longer term outcomes are subject to additional confounders of outcomes that are introduced over longer study timeframes, most notably the clinical indication and underlying diseases that prompted an IV contrast-enhanced CT examination. For example, if a patient receives such an examination to diagnose malignancy, subsequent renal dysfunction may be a result of chemotherapeutic use, declining clinical condition, poor self-care, or the malignancy itself. While propensity score adjustment can minimize bias over a short-term period, this approach is less effective when examining longer time periods and cannot guarantee that exposed and control groups remain similar. Accordingly, results from long-term outcome studies need to be interpreted with caution.

POTENTIAL CONTRAST-ASSOCIATED ACUTE KIDNEY INJURY AND CONTRAST-INDUCED ACUTE KIDNEY INJURY RISK FACTORS

Risk factors for CA-AKI include renal and cardiovascular comorbidities and other conditions that are associated with a general increased risk of AKI, including chronic kidney disease, diabetes mellitus, hypovolemia, exposure to other nephrotoxic agents, hypotension, albuminuria, and heart failure.[45–48] However, the only consistent risk factor for CI-AKI reported in controlled studies is pre-existing CKD.[24–26] Other renal and cardiovascular conditions have not been consistently found to be independent CI-AKI risk factors in these studies.[13,20,42,49–51] No controlled study published to date to our knowledge has found an increased risk of CI-AKI in patients with normal renal function to mild renal dysfunction (eGFR ≥45 mL/min).

Accordingly, the medical community now widely accepts that patients with normal renal function or mild renal dysfunction (CKD stages 1–2) are not at risk of CI-AKI. The risk in patients with more severe renal dysfunction remains uncertain due to limited and conflicting evidence. Patient groups that are potentially considered at higher risk of CI-AKI include patients with severe renal dysfunction (CKD stages 4–5, eGFR <30 mL/min), patients with concurrent AKI, and dialysis patients with residual renal function.

Recent studies examining patients with stages 4 to 5 CKD not undergoing maintenance hemodialysis have had conflicting results, with some meta-analyses and controlled studies not finding evidence of CI-AKI even in this patient population,[13,19–21] while other controlled studies and meta-analyses reporting an increased risk of CI-AKI.[14,24–26] Studies of this subgroup are particularly challenging due to the small number of stages 4 to 5 patients with CKD that receive ICM and the higher likelihood of confounding.

Limited and conflicting evidence also exists for patients who have pre-existing AKI at the time of

ICM administration. Ehmann and colleagues reported that patients with pre-existing AKI were not at an increased risk of prolonged AKI or dialysis following IV ICM exposure, even in a subset of critical care patients.[52] Another controlled study of inpatients with AKI exposed to ICM found no increased risk of worsened renal function, dialysis, or mortality.[53] Conversely, a controlled study of contrast CT recipients who developed AKI in the 72 hour window before and after ICM exposure reported that cumulative ICM doses greater than 100 mL were independently associated with major adverse kidney events.[29]

Nonanuric patients on maintenance dialysis are also considered at higher risk for CI-AKI and subsequent further loss of renal function. No IV ICM studies have yet been performed in this population, to our knowledge. However, 3 controlled studies of IA ICM or a combination of IA and IV ICM have previously demonstrated no long-term effects of ICM on residual renal function.[54–56] One additional study suggests that dialysis patients with hypoalbuminemia may be at an increased risk of CA-AKI following IA ICM.[57]

Some providers also view pediatric patients as a potentially vulnerable population for CI-AKI. Four retrospective controlled studies of pediatric and neonatal cohorts did not find evidence of CI-AKI following IV ICM exposure.[58–61] However, as most of these patients had normal renal function, it is unknown whether renal insufficiency increases the risk of CI-AKI in pediatric patients. Additional controlled studies focused on pediatric patients with renal insufficiency are needed to better assess the risk in this patient population.

Finally, administering multiple ICM doses within a short timeframe is widely considered to increase the risk of CI-AKI; however, scant evidence exists supporting this assumption, to our knowledge. Larger studies comparing patients who receive 1 ICM dose to clinically similar patients who receive multiple doses are needed. However, such a study will be challenged by confounding bias from the varied indications and associated differences clinical status of patients requiring 1 versus multiple IV contrast-enhanced CT examinations over a short period.

SCREENING FOR CONTRAST-INDUCED ACUTE KIDNEY INJURY

Current clinical practice guidelines recommend performing renal function screening in all patients prior to ICM administration to identify potential at-risk individuals.[62] Most screening recommendations are derived from studies examining other causes of AKI instead of studies specifically focused on CI-AKI.[63] For screenings that utilize renal biomarker testing, eGFR measurements are recommended instead of SCr as the former provides a more accurate assessment of renal function. The race-independent chronic kidney disease epidemiology collaboration (CKD-EPI) creatinine equation is currently recommended by the American Society of Nephrologists and the National Kidney Foundation for calculating eGFR.[64] The American College of Radiology (ACR) notes that no specific cutoffs exist where ICM use is absolutely contraindicated; however, a cutoff of eGFR less than 30 mL/min is commonly viewed as the point at which ICM use may cause an excess risk of CI-AKI.[62] The potential risk of CI-AKI in high-risk patients is a relative, rather than absolute, contraindication to ICM exposure. ICM administration for a life-threatening diagnosis should not be withheld based solely on compromised renal function.

Utilizing patient surveys or medical chart reviews to screen for the presence of specific clinical conditions that may increase the risk of CI-AKI is controversial and of uncertain benefit. Studies examining the utility of screening surveys have found that a history of kidney disease (ie, CKD, history of AKI or renal surgery, albuminuria) is the strongest predictor of renal dysfunction.[65,66] Screening for other factors including diabetes mellitus, age, or hypertension has not been predictive of elevated AKI risk.

PREVENTION OF CONTRAST-INDUCED ACUTE KIDNEY INJURY

While numerous studies have been published that have examined the effectiveness of various prophylactic measures in preventing CI-AKI, the vast majority arise from uncontrolled IA ICM studies. These studies cannot disambiguate the ability of these measures to prevent true CI-AKI versus CA-AKI. It is impossible to determine if a favorable result indicates that the prophylactic measure mitigated CI-AKI alone, CA-AKI in general, or globally affected/altered biomarker results, thereby masking any true effect on AKI rates. Any observed benefits of prophylactic measures may instead be for general CA-AKI instead of specifically CI-AKI. While there is an obvious benefit in reducing overall AKI rates, the effectiveness of preventative measures reported in these uncontrolled studies should not be attributed to reducing CI-AKI alone.

Fewer studies have specifically examined the effects of preventative measures on IV ICM administration. Several recent randomized studies of patients with renal dysfunction exposed to IV ICM have failed to show a benefit of hydration in the reduction of CA-AKI. The AMACING trial (n = 660, 341 received IV ICM) randomized patients with eGFR 30 to 59 mL/min to a 4 to 12 hour 0.9% NaCl infusion protocol or no fluids and reported no difference in CA-AKI between groups.[67] The KOMPAS trial (n = 523), randomized patients with eGFR 30 to 59 mL/min and diabetes mellitus or at least 2 other risk factors to a 1 hour sodium bicarbonate infusion protocol or no fluids and also reported no difference in CA-AKI between groups.[68] Finally, a retrospective study compared matched patients with eGFR less than 30 mL/min who did or did not receive IV hydration prior to CECT and also reported no differences in CA-AKI, dialysis, or mortality between groups.[69] Further, as endpoints in many of these studies are simply reductions in SCr, prophylactic measures that involve post-ICM fluid administration may simply reflect nothing more than an expected physiologic response to increased intravascular volumes with an improved urine output and decreased or diluted SCr.

These findings indicate that IV hydration is not effective at preventing CA-AKI after IV ICM administration in patients with moderate renal dysfunction. However, evidence supporting this hypothesis is currently limited to observational studies in patients with severe renal dysfunction (eGFR <30 mL/min). Randomized studies are needed in this patient subset to better assess the effectiveness of hydration in preventing CA-AKI following IV administration of ICMs.

Numerous prior studies have also purported the effectiveness of other prophylactic agents, most notably N-acetylcysteine, sodium bicarbonate, and statins, in preventing CA-AKI.[70] However, newer and larger studies of these agents have questioned their effectiveness following IV administration of ICMs. A recent large meta-analysis of 101 studies found that substantial study heterogeneity and publication bias led to the misleading conclusion that N-acetylcysteine was effective.[71] When the analysis was restricted to large (n > 500) randomized controlled trials, no benefit was observed. Other studies have not found a benefit in administering sodium bicarbonate or statins prior to IV ICM administration.

Newer CA-AKI preventative measures, including the RenalGuard System (RenalGuard Solutions Inc., Milford, MA), a device that modulates IV fluid delivery based on urine output, and remote ischemic preconditioning, which involves applying brief episode(s) of nonlethal ischemia and reperfusion to remote tissue, show early promise in reducing AKI.[72–74] However, most of these studies focused on IA ICM administration, raising questions about their effectiveness on preventing CA-AKI after IV administration of ICMs and overall ability to mitigate CI-AKI versus CA-AKI.

CREATININE AND NEWER CONTRAST-INDUCED ACUTE KIDNEY INJURY BIOMARKERS

Across all fields, SCr remains the most common diagnostic AKI biomarker as it is extremely cost-effective and readily available. However, there are many limitations with SCr as a marker of renal function and injury, including limited sensitivity, inability to distinguish between CI-AKI and CA-AKI, delayed response to renal injury, and nonlinear variance with gender, age, and muscle mass. Improved AKI biomarkers have been identified over the past decades, including neutrophil gelatinase-associated lipocalin (NGAL), kidney injury molecule-1 (KIM-1), tissue inhibitor of metalloproteinases 2 (TIMP-2), insulin-like growth factor-binding protein 7 (IGFBP-7), interleukin 18 (IL-18), and liver fatty acid-binding protein (L-FABP).[75] Recent studies have also suggested that certain microRNAs biomarkers may also be useful in the diagnosis of CI-AKI.[76] However, research focused on these newer biomarkers is limited as these studies typically use SCr as the reference standard, amplifying the issues with SCr described earlier. Renal biopsy results may need to be utilized in comparison with newer biomarkers to better assess their sensitivity and specificity for CA-AKI and CI-AKI.

Numerous studies have assessed the effectiveness of these newer markers for diagnosing general AKI; however, evidence is more limited regarding their effectiveness at specifically detecting CI-AKI. In addition, some studies reported differences in biomarkers between AKI patients and non-AKI patients[77,78] while others reported no differences.[79,80] No controlled studies reported to date have to our knowledge compared ICM-exposed patients to unexposed patients to properly discriminate between CA-AKI and CI-AKI. Further, no AKI biomarkers specific to ICM exposure have been identified that could be assessed in an unexposed patient group or a group that developed AKI independently of ICM. Such controlled studies are necessary to identify specific CI-AKI biomarkers; such biomarkers would enable the assessment of the true incidence of CI-AKI.

Some researchers have suggested that future studies should transition away from traditional biomarker-defined CI-AKI outcomes to more clinically relevant outcomes, including acute dialysis, development or progression of CKD, and renal-related mortality.[71] Biomarkers are ultimately a surrogate outcome of AKI, and substantial heterogeneity exists in biomarker studies due to the lack of a standardized definition of AKI.[81] In addition, it has been demonstrated that interventions that either cause or prevent biomarker-defined AKI ultimately did not affect the risk of chronic kidney disease or mortality.[82,83]

FUTURE CONSIDERATIONS

The reference standard to determine causality is a prospective randomized controlled trial. Such randomization has, to date, been impossible for IA administration of ICM, as contrast administration is typically required for such procedures, and there is no clinically equivalent nonenhanced procedure. However, an increased interest in and utilization of intravenously administered carbon dioxide as an alternative to ICM for endovascular angiography and interventional procedures could revolutionize our understanding of the incidence and severity of IA CI-AKI. Studies that randomize patients to traditional IA ICM versus zero-contrast carbon dioxide would be able to better assess the true renal effects of IA ICM. Smaller, observational studies report decreased AKI with carbon dioxide imaging versus ICM[84,85]; however, larger, matched observational studies and prospective randomized controlled trials are needed to better assess the effects of IA-ICM.

No properly controlled randomized prospective studies of CI-AKI from IV ICM use have been published to date, to our knowledge. Additional challenges have impeded performing randomized studies of IV CI-AKI. Most notably, there are potential ethical issues regarding the decision to intentionally administer or withhold ICM from patients during routine care. Such studies would also require large numbers of patients if the study design is noninferiority and the hypothesis is that ICM does not affect renal function. Finally, many providers and patients are resistant to randomization due to concerns that ICM causes AKI and still believe that administering ICM would cause unnecessary risk, or because they are convinced ICM does not cause AKI and withholding ICM would cause unnecessary risk. One possible alternative to CI-AKI randomized-controlled trials may be to identify randomized controlled trials that are focused on comparing the diagnostic accuracy of IV contrast-enhanced examinations to an alternative examination that does not utilize ICM. Renal function testing could be included in such studies as a secondary outcome to collect more data about CI-AKI.

CURRENT RECOMMENDATIONS FOR IODINATED CONTRAST MATERIAL USE

Evidence published in the past decade has caused professional societies including the ACR and National Kidney Foundation (NKF) to conclude that the risk of CI-AKI is much lower than what had previously been suggested. Such a conclusion represents a monumental paradigm shift in clinical practice; instead of viewing ICMs as potentially pan-nephrotoxic to all patients, now over 95% of hospitalized and ambulatory patients can safely receive ICM without concern for AKI. The risk of AKI-related long-term outcomes also appears to be substantially overstated in all patients. However, debate continues regarding the risk of CI-AKI in a small subset of patient groups (ie, eGFR <30 mL/min and other potential risk factors discussed earlier). Due to this ongoing uncertainty, it is advised to use caution when considering ICM administration in these patient groups. It is important to note that no patient group has a complete contraindication for ICM use; instead, an individualized approach should be taken to determine if the important clinical benefits of ICM administration outweigh the potential risk of CI-AKI.

SUMMARY

Numerous studies published over the past decade have markedly changed our understanding of the potential nephrotoxic risks associated with intravenously administered ICM. Prior clinical guidelines that viewed all ICM administration as potentially nephrotoxic with an increased risk of negative long-term outcomes has been replaced by a more nuanced understanding and risk-stratified approach to ICM administration. Radiologists and nephrologists today collectively view modern ICM use in patients with normal-to-moderately compromised renal function (eGFR ≥30 mL/min) as safe, with no increased risk of AKI or AKI-related adverse outcomes. CI-AKI risk may still exist for patients with severe renal dysfunction (eGFR <30 mL/min); however, the incidence and severity of these risks have been overstated by prior uncontrolled studies. The risk of CI-AKI should not be viewed as an absolute contraindication to ICM administration, even in patients with severe renal dysfunction and particularly in emergent clinical situations or circumstances where the benefits of ICM use outweigh the risks of this clinical phenomenon.

CLINICS CARE POINTS

- Recent evidence has caused a paradigm shift in clinical practice where over 95% of hospitalized and ambulatory patients can now safely receive ICM without concern for CI-AKI.

- The risk of CI-AKI-related long-term outcomes appears to be substantially overstated in all patients.

- Debate continues regarding the risk of CI-AKI in a small subset of patient groups (i.e. eGFR < 30 ml/min and other potential risk factors). Due to this ongoing uncertainty, judicious use of ICM is warranted in these patient groups.

- No risk factor alone poses an absolute contraindication for ICM use; instead, an individualized approach should be taken to determine if the important clinical benefits of ICM administration outweigh the small risk of CI-AKI.

DISCLOSURE

J.S. McDonald and R.J. McDonald report investigator-initiated research grants with GE Healthcare, United Kingdom. J.S. McDonald and R.J. McDonald serve as consultants and scientific advisors for GE Healthcare regarding preclinical and clinical studies.

REFERENCES

1. Koeppel DR, Boehm IB. Shortage of iodinated contrast media: status and possible chances - a systematic review. Eur J Radiol 2023;164:110853.

2. Davenport MS, Perazella MA, Yee J, et al. Use of intravenous iodinated contrast media in patients with kidney disease: consensus statements from the american college of radiology and the national kidney foundation. Radiology 2020;294:660–8.

3. Katzberg RW, Newhouse JH. Intravenous contrast medium-induced nephrotoxicity: is the medical risk really as great as we have come to believe? Radiology 2010;256:21–8.

4. Stratta P, Bozzola C, Quaglia M. Pitfall in nephrology: contrast nephropathy has to be differentiated from renal damage due to atheroembolic disease. J Nephrol 2012;25:282–9.

5. Bartels ED, Brun GC, Gammeltoft A, et al. Acute anuria following intravenous pyelography in a patient with myelomatosis. Acta Med Scand 1954; 150:297–302.

6. Taliercio CP, Vlietstra RE, Fisher LD, et al. Risks for renal dysfunction with cardiac angiography. Ann Intern Med 1986;104:501–4.

7. McCullough PA, Wolyn R, Rocher LL, et al. Acute renal failure after coronary intervention: incidence, risk factors, and relationship to mortality. Am J Med 1997;103:368–75.

8. Quader MA, Sawmiller C, Sumpio BA. Contrast-induced nephropathy: review of incidence and pathophysiology. Ann Vasc Surg 1998;12:612–20.

9. Katzberg RW, Lamba R. Contrast-induced nephropathy after intravenous administration: fact or fiction? Radiol Clin North Am 2009;47:789–800.

10. McDonald JS, McDonald RJ, Comin J, et al. Frequency of acute kidney injury following intravenous contrast medium administration: a systematic review and meta-analysis. Radiology 2013;267:119–28.

11. Katzberg RW, Barrett BJ. Risk of iodinated contrast material–induced nephropathy with intravenous administration. Radiology 2007;243:622–8.

12. Chertow GM, Normand SL, McNeil BJ. "Renalism": inappropriately low rates of coronary angiography in elderly individuals with renal insufficiency. J Am Soc Nephrol 2004;15:2462–8.

13. Lee YC, Hsieh CC, Chang TT, et al. Contrast-induced acute kidney injury among patients with chronic kidney disease undergoing imaging studies: a meta-analysis. AJR Am J Roentgenol 2019;213: 728–35.

14. Obed M, Gabriel MM, Dumann E, et al. Risk of acute kidney injury after contrast-enhanced computerized tomography: a systematic review and meta-analysis of 21 propensity score-matched cohort studies. Eur Radiol 2022;32:8432–42.

15. Bruce RJ, Djamali A, Shinki K, et al. Background fluctuation of kidney function versus contrast-induced nephrotoxicity. AJR Am J Roentgenol 2009;192:711–8.

16. Newhouse JH, Kho D, Rao QA, et al. Frequency of serum creatinine changes in the absence of iodinated contrast material: implications for studies of contrast nephrotoxicity. AJR Am J Roentgenol 2008;191:376–82.

17. Baumgarten DA, Ellis JH. Contrast-induced nephropathy: contrast material not required? AJR Am J Roentgenol 2008;191:383–6.

18. McDonald RJ, McDonald JS, Kallmes DF, et al. Behind the numbers: propensity score analysis-a primer for the diagnostic radiologist. Radiology 2013;269:640–5.

19. Ehrmann S, Quartin A, Hobbs BP, et al. Contrast-associated acute kidney injury in the critically ill: systematic review and Bayesian meta-analysis. Intensive Care Med 2017;43:785–94.

20. McDonald JS, McDonald RJ, Carter RE, et al. Risk of intravenous contrast material-mediated acute kidney injury: a propensity score-matched study stratified by baseline-estimated glomerular filtration rate. Radiology 2014;271:65–73.

21. Tao SM, Kong X, Schoepf UJ, et al. Acute kidney injury in patients with nephrotic syndrome undergoing contrast-enhanced CT for suspected venous thromboembolism: a propensity score-matched retrospective cohort study. Eur Radiol 2018;28: 1585–93.

22. McDonald RJ, McDonald JS, Bida JP, et al. Intravenous contrast material-induced nephropathy: causal

or coincident phenomenon? Radiology 2013;267: 106–18.

23. Kiss N, Hamar P. Histopathological evaluation of contrast-induced acute kidney injury rodent models. BioMed Res Int 2016;2016:3763250.

24. Davenport MS, Khalatbari S, Cohan RH, et al. Contrast material-induced nephrotoxicity and intravenous low-osmolality iodinated contrast material: risk stratification by using estimated glomerular filtration rate. Radiology 2013;268:719–28.

25. Ellis JH, Khalatbari S, Yosef M, et al. Influence of clinical factors on risk of contrast-induced nephrotoxicity from iv iodinated low-osmolality contrast material in patients with a low estimated glomerular filtration rate. AJR Am J Roentgenol 2019;213: W188–93.

26. Gorelik Y, Bloch-Isenberg N, Yaseen H, et al. Acute kidney injury after radiocontrast-enhanced computerized tomography in hospitalized patients with advanced renal failure: a propensity-score-matching analysis. Invest Radiol 2020;55: 677–87.

27. Lee CC, Chan YL, Wong YC, et al. Contrast-enhanced CT and acute kidney injury: risk stratification by diabetic status and kidney function. Radiology 2023;307:e222321.

28. Su TH, Hsieh CH, Chan YL, et al. Intravenous CT contrast media and acute kidney injury: a multicenter emergency department-based study. Radiology 2021;301:571–81.

29. Chua HR, Low S, Murali TM, et al. Cumulative iodinated contrast exposure for computed tomography during acute kidney injury and major adverse kidney events. Eur Radiol 2021;31:3258–66.

30. Kene M, Arasu VA, Mahapatra AK, et al. Acute kidney injury after CT in emergency patients with chronic kidney disease: a propensity score-matched analysis. West J Emerg Med 2021;22:614–22.

31. Bartholomew BA, Harjai KJ, Dukkipati S, et al. Impact of nephropathy after percutaneous coronary intervention and a method for risk stratification. Am J Cardiol 2004;93:1515–9.

32. McCullough PA, Adam A, Becker CR, et al. Risk prediction of contrast-induced nephropathy. Am J Cardiol 2006;98:27K–36K.

33. Rihal CS, Textor SC, Grill DE, et al. Incidence and prognostic importance of acute renal failure after percutaneous coronary intervention. Circulation 2002;105:2259–64.

34. Diprose WK, Sutherland LJ, Wang MTM, et al. Contrast-associated acute kidney injury in endovascular thrombectomy patients with and without baseline renal impairment. Stroke 2019;50:3527–31.

35. Fukushima Y, Miyazawa H, Nakamura J, et al. Contrast-induced nephropathy (CIN) of patients with renal dysfunction in CT examination. Jpn J Radiol 2017;35:427–31.

36. Lakhal K, Ehrmann S, Chaari A, et al. Acute kidney injury network definition of contrast-induced nephropathy in the critically ill: incidence and outcome. J Crit Care 2011;26:593–9.

37. Aycock RD, Westafer LM, Boxen JL, et al. Acute kidney injury after computed tomography: a meta-analysis. Ann Emerg Med 2018;71:44–53 e44.

38. Ehrmann S, Badin J, Savath L, et al. Acute kidney injury in the critically ill: is iodinated contrast medium really harmful? Crit Care Med 2013;41:1017–26.

39. Miyamoto Y, Iwagami M, Aso S, et al. Association between intravenous contrast media exposure and non-recovery from dialysis-requiring septic acute kidney injury: a nationwide observational study. Intensive Care Med 2019;45:1570–9.

40. McDonald JS, McDonald RJ, Williamson EE, et al. Post-contrast acute kidney injury in intensive care unit patients: a propensity score-adjusted study. Intensive Care Med 2017;43:774–84.

41. McDonald JS, McDonald RJ, Williamson EE, et al. Is intravenous administration of iodixanol associated with increased risk of acute kidney injury, dialysis, or mortality? a propensity score-adjusted study. Radiology 2017;285:414–24.

42. McDonald RJ, McDonald JS, Carter RE, et al. Intravenous contrast material exposure is not an independent risk factor for dialysis or mortality. Radiology 2014;273:714–25.

43. Takura T, Nitta K, Tsuchiya K, et al. Long-term effects of contrast media exposure on renal failure progression: a retrospective cohort study. BMC Nephrol 2023;24:135.

44. Huang ST, Yu TM, Chen CH, et al. Risk of major cardiovascular disease after exposure to contrast media: a nationwide population-based cohort study on dialysis patients. Metabolites 2023;13(2):266.

45. Ho YF, Hsieh KL, Kung FL, et al. Nephrotoxic polypharmacy and risk of contrast medium-induced nephropathy in hospitalized patients undergoing contrast-enhanced CT. AJR Am J Roentgenol 2015;205:703–8.

46. Huang MK, Hsu TF, Chiu YH, et al. Risk factors for acute kidney injury in the elderly undergoing contrast-enhanced computed tomography in the emergency department. J Chin Med Assoc 2013;76:271–6.

47. Arayan A, Nigogosyan MA, Van Every MJ. A retrospective review of contrast nephropathy in a general population. Wis Med J 2015;114:95–9.

48. Moore A, Dickerson E, Dillman JR, et al. Incidence of nonconfounded post-computed tomography acute kidney injury in hospitalized patients with stable renal function receiving intravenous iodinated contrast material. Curr Probl Diagn Radiol 2014;43: 237–41.

49. Parfrey PS, Griffiths SM, Barrett BJ, et al. Contrast material-induced renal failure in patients with diabetes mellitus, renal insufficiency, or both. A

prospective controlled study. N Engl J Med 1989; 320:143–9.

50. Tong GE, Kumar S, Chong KC, et al. Risk of contrast-induced nephropathy for patients receiving intravenous vs. intra-arterial iodixanol administration. Abdom Radiol (NY) 2016;41:91–9.

51. Safi W, Rauscher I, Umgelter A. Contrast-induced acute kidney injury in cirrhotic patients. A retrospective analysis. Ann Hepatol 2015;14:895–901.

52. Ehmann MR, Mitchell J, Levin S, et al. Renal outcomes following intravenous contrast administration in patients with acute kidney injury: a multi-site retrospective propensity-adjusted analysis. Intensive Care Med 2023;49:205–15.

53. Yan P, Zhang NY, Luo XQ, et al. Is intravenous iodinated contrast medium administration really harmful in hospitalized acute kidney injury patients: a propensity score-matched study. Eur Radiol 2022;32:1163–72.

54. Moranne O, Willoteaux S, Pagniez D, et al. Effect of iodinated contrast agents on residual renal function in PD patients. Nephrol Dial Transplant 2006;21:1040–5.

55. Dittrich E, Puttinger H, Schillinger M, et al. Effect of radio contrast media on residual renal function in peritoneal dialysis patients–a prospective study. Nephrol Dial Transplant 2006;21:1334–9.

56. Janousek R, Krajina A, Peregrin JH, et al. Effect of intravascular iodinated contrast media on natural course of end-stage renal disease progression in hemodialysis patients: a prospective study. Cardiovasc Intervent Radiol 2010;33:61–6.

57. Hassan K, Fadi H. Is hypoalbuminemia a prognostic risk factor for contrast-induced nephropathy in peritoneal dialysis patients? Ther Clin Risk Manag 2014; 10:787–95.

58. Bedoya MA, White AM, Edgar JC, et al. Effect of intravenous administration of contrast media on serum creatinine levels in neonates. Radiology 2017;284:530–40.

59. Gilligan LA, Davenport MS, Trout AT, et al. Risk of acute kidney injury following contrast-enhanced CT in hospitalized pediatric patients: a propensity score analysis. Radiology 2020;294:548–56.

60. McDonald JS, McDonald RJ, Tran CL, et al. Postcontrast acute kidney injury in pediatric patients: a cohort study. Am J Kidney Dis 2018;72:811–8.

61. Calle-Toro J, Viteri B, Ballester L, et al. Risk of acute kidney injury following contrast-enhanced CT in a cohort of 10 407 children and adolescents. Radiology 2023;307:e210816.

62. ACR Committee on Drugs and Contrast Media. ACR Manual on Contrast Media. 2022. Available at: https://www.acr.org/-/media/ACR/Files/Clinical-Resources/Contrast_Media.pdf.

63. Davenport MS, Khalatbari S, Cohan RH, et al. Contrast medium-induced nephrotoxicity risk assessment in adult inpatients: a comparison of serum creatinine level- and estimated glomerular filtration rate-based screening methods. Radiology 2013;269:92–100.

64. Delgado C, Baweja M, Crews DC, et al. A unifying approach for GFR estimation: recommendations of the NKF-ASN task force on reassessing the inclusion of race in diagnosing kidney disease. J Am Soc Nephrol 2021;32:2994–3015.

65. Choyke PL, Cady J, DePollar SL, et al. Determination of serum creatinine prior to iodinated contrast media: is it necessary in all patients? Tech Urol 1998; 4:65–9.

66. Too CW, Ng WY, Tan CC, et al. Screening for impaired renal function in outpatients before iodinated contrast injection: Comparing the Choyke questionnaire with a rapid point-of-care-test. Eur J Radiol 2015;84:1227–31.

67. Nijssen EC, Rennenberg RJ, Nelemans PJ, et al. Prophylactic hydration to protect renal function from intravascular iodinated contrast material in patients at high risk of contrast-induced nephropathy (AMACING): a prospective, randomised, phase 3, controlled, open-label, non-inferiority trial. Lancet 2017;389:1312–22.

68. Timal RJ, Kooiman J, Sijpkens YWJ, et al. Effect of No prehydration vs sodium bicarbonate prehydration prior to contrast-enhanced computed tomography in the prevention of postcontrast acute kidney injury in adults with chronic kidney disease: the kompas randomized clinical trial. JAMA Intern Med 2020;180:533–41.

69. Yan P, Duan SB, Luo XQ, et al. Effects of intravenous hydration in preventing post-contrast acute kidney injury in patients with eGFR < 30 mL/min/1.73 m(2). Eur Radiol 2023;33(12):9434–43.

70. Subramaniam RM, Wilson RF, Turban S, et al. Contrast-Induced Nephropathy: Comparative Effectiveness of Preventive Measures. Rockford MD: Agency for Healthcare Research and Quality; 2016.

71. Magner K, Ilin JV, Clark EG, et al. Meta-analytic techniques to assess the association between n-acetyl-cysteine and acute kidney injury after contrast administration: a systematic review and meta-analysis. JAMA Netw Open 2022;5:e2220671.

72. Deng J, Lu Y, Ou J, et al. Remote ischemic preconditioning reduces the risk of contrast-induced nephropathy in patients with moderate renal impairment undergoing percutaneous coronary angiography: a meta-analysis. Kidney Blood Press Res 2020;45:549–64.

73. Mattathil S, Ghumman S, Weinerman J, et al. Use of the RenalGuard system to prevent contrast-induced AKI: A meta-analysis. J Interv Cardiol 2017;30:480–7.

74. Wang Y, Guo Y. RenalGuard system and conventional hydration for preventing contrast-associated

acute kidney injury in patients undergoing cardiac interventional procedures: A systematic review and meta-analysis. Int J Cardiol 2021;333:83–9.

75. Zou C, Wang C, Lu L. Advances in the study of subclinical AKI biomarkers. Front Physiol 2022;13: 960059.

76. Liu X, Li Y, Zhu X, et al. MicroRNA as an early diagnostic biomarker for contrast-induced acute kidney injury. Drug Chem Toxicol 2022;45:1552–7.

77. Breglia A, Godi I, Virzi GM, et al. Subclinical contrast-induced acute kidney injury in patients undergoing cerebral computed tomography. Cardiorenal Med 2020;10:125–36.

78. Filiopoulos V, Biblaki D, Lazarou D, et al. Plasma neutrophil gelatinase-associated lipocalin (NGAL) as an early predictive marker of contrast-induced nephropathy in hospitalized patients undergoing computed tomography. Clin Kidney J 2013;6:578–83.

79. Kooiman J, van de Peppel WR, Sijpkens YW, et al. No increase in kidney injury molecule-1 and neutrophil gelatinase-associated lipocalin excretion following intravenous contrast enhanced-CT. Eur Radiol 2015;25:1926–34.

80. Rouve E, Lakhal K, Salmon Gandonniere C, et al. Lack of impact of iodinated contrast media on kidney cell-cycle arrest biomarkers in critically ill patients. BMC Nephrol 2018;19:308.

81. Thomas ME, Blaine C, Dawnay A, et al. The definition of acute kidney injury and its use in practice. Kidney Int 2015;87:62–73.

82. Coca SG, Zabetian A, Ferket BS, et al. Evaluation of short-term changes in serum creatinine level as a meaningful end point in randomized clinical trials. J Am Soc Nephrol 2016;27:2529–42.

83. Legrand M, Bagshaw SM, Koyner JL, et al. Optimizing the design and analysis of future AKI trials. J Am Soc Nephrol 2022;33:1459–70.

84. Ghumman SS, Weinerman J, Khan A, et al. Contrast induced-acute kidney injury following peripheral angiography with carbon dioxide versus iodinated contrast media: A meta-analysis and systematic review of current literature. Catheter Cardiovasc Interv 2017;90:437–48.

85. Wagner G, Glechner A, Persad E, et al. Risk of contrast-associated acute kidney injury in patients undergoing peripheral angiography with carbon dioxide compared to iodine-containing contrast agents: a systematic review and meta-analysis. J Clin Med 2022;11(23):7203.

Potpourri of Contrast Controversies and Myths
Where Is the Actual Evidence?

Miltiadis Tembelis, MD[a,*], Gregg Blumberg, DO[a], Luis Colon-Flores, MD[a],
Julie Hong, MD[b,1], Jason C. Hoffmann, MD, FSIR[a],
Douglas S. Katz, MD, FACR, FASER, FSAR[a]

KEYWORDS

- Contrast material • Iodinated contrast • Barium contrast • Gadolinium contrast • Patient safety
- Evidence-based radiology

KEY POINTS

- Much of what we do in our radiologic practice, particularly regarding contrast usage, is based on routines learned in training, often without much thought about the evidence supporting our decisions.
- Knowledge of the current contrast-related misconceptions, the origin of such misconceptions, and which engrained practices can be challenged, can help radiologists provide higher quality care to their patients.
- Nephrogenic systemic fibrosis is an extremely rare complication, associated with intravenous (IV) gadolinium agents no longer commonly utilized in medical practice.
- A history of a shellfish allergy is not a contraindication for IV iodinated contrast administration.

INTRODUCTION

Much of what we do in our daily practice as physicians, including in radiologic practice, is based on routines learned in training, often without much thought about the evidence supporting our decisions. Often, these practices are based on out-of-date or limited data without much actual evidence. In the realm of radiology, the administration of contrast agents is essential to diagnosing disease, but unfortunately contrast cannot be freely administered to all patients for a multitude of reasons. Some of these reasons either may not be backed by valid data we assume exist or may, in fact, have already been proven to be false. The goal of this review article, therefore, is to address several commonly encountered controversies behind the administration of contrast material and to bring attention to the actual data behind these controversies and where misunderstandings may stem from. Knowledge of the current misconceptions, the origin of such misconceptions, and which ingrained practices can be challenged, can help radiologists provide patients with the most appropriate scan protocols, ease referring physicians' hesitance to use specific contrast material and contrast protocols, and help guide discussions with concerned patients. Among these controversies we will discuss is the use of iodinated intravenous (IV) contrast in patients with shellfish allergies, barium peritonitis, the use of iodinated IV contrast in patients with a solitary

[a] Department of Radiology, NYU Grossman Long Island School of Medicine, NYU Langone Hospital - Long Island, 259 First Street, Mineola, NY 11501, USA; [b] Department of Surgery, New York-Presbyterian Queens Hospital, Flushing, NY, USA
[1] Present address: 222 Station Plaza North, Suite 501, Mineola, NY 11501.
* Corresponding author. 132 Island Parkway North, Island Park, NY 11558.
E-mail address: tembelismd@gmail.com

Radiol Clin N Am 62 (2024) 971–978
https://doi.org/10.1016/j.rcl.2024.04.007
0033-8389/24/© 2024 Elsevier Inc. All rights reserved.

kidney, the role of hemodialysis in patients receiving IV contrast, the effects of iodine contrast on pediatric thyroid function, and the use of low-osmolality contrast in patients with a history of contrast reactions. We will also briefly discuss the risk of nephrogenic systemic fibrosis (NSF) in patients receiving gadolinium and contrast-induced kidney injury.

THE EVIDENCE BEHIND BARIUM PERITONITIS

Controversies behind the administration of contrast exist beyond IV agents. Perhaps, one of the oldest and ingrained rules of radiology is "do not administer barium to patients who may have a bowel perforation." Many trainees hear this from a more seasoned radiologist, and it will become assimilated into their practice without an understanding of the literature actually supporting this statement. Additionally, much concern can arise either when a patient undergoing a barium examination is unexpectedly found to have a perforation or when a patient inadvertently has a perforation during such an examination.

Barium peritonitis was first described by Zheutlin and colleagues in 1952, who described 53 cases of intraperitoneal spread of barium.[1] Although this case series showed a 51% mortality, most of these cases occurred in the 1940s, nearly 80 years ago, before modern surgical interventions and antibiotic treatments existed. Since then, to our knowledge, only case reports and small case series of barium peritonitis have been published. It should be noted that uneventful introduction of barium into the abdominal cavity is unlikely to be reported.

A much more recent case series by Ghahremani and colleagues, which included 18 patients aged 6 months to 80 years and followed these patients for up to 17 years after moderate-to-large volume intraperitoneal barium leakage, brought barium peritonitis into serious question.[2] None of the patients in this study developed clinically significant symptoms due to barium leakage into the peritoneum, although 2 of the patients were noted to have adhesions during abdominal surgery performed for unrelated reasons. All patients had urgent surgery for perforation, with peritoneal lavage, and were treated with appropriate antibiotics.

The ability of barium to cause peritonitis in isolation was also brought into question by Kleinsasser and Warshaw, who injected either barium and/or sterile fecal matter into the peritoneum of dogs years ago. None of the dogs suffered a barium-related death, while the 2 dogs whose peritoneal cavity was injected with feces and barium both died.[3] On the contrary, a similar study, but also similarly very old, by Almond and colleagues revealed that there was 70% mortality among 10 dogs that received barium alone and 100% among the 3 dogs that received feces and barium.[4]

Although the causation of peritonitis by barium introduction into the abdomen can be substantially questioned, there is at least a theoretic long-term risk for intra-abdominal adhesions, and since there are other, water-soluble agents which can be used for diagnosis, it is best to exercise caution when assessing a patient with a potential bowel leak.

IODINATED CONTRAST USE IN PATIENTS WITH A SHELLFISH ALLERGY

The common misconception of the link between a history of shellfish allergies and increased risk of iodinated contrast allergy likely originated from studies in the early 1970s. For example, in 1973, Witten and colleagues reported that IV contrast allergic reactions were seen in 6% of patients with a prior history of seafood allergy.[5] However, medical literature in the last 2 decades has debunked this myth, and demonstrated that no such relationship actually exits.[6] Hypersensitivity reactions can be classified as immunoglobulin E (IgE)-mediated or non-IgE-mediated. IgE-mediated allergic reactions require an antigen, and iodine is a chemical element; therefore, it does not play such a role and cannot elicit an immune response. Allergic reactions to seafood are due to specific proteins, such as parvalbumins or tropomyosins.[7] Reactions to IV contrast are most likely related to some other component of the contrast media and not the iodine itself. Ultimately, the strongest predictor of future contrast reactions is a history of prior contrast reaction, which confers a 5 fold higher risk.[7]

Despite all the evidence, to this date many physicians and other health care providers, including radiologists, still inquire about shellfish allergies prior to ordering or administering IV contrast. For example, in a 2008 study, 65% of radiologists and 88% of interventional cardiologists reported inquiring about history of seafood and/or shellfish allergy, and 37% of radiologists and 50% of interventional cardiologists would not administer contrast, or recommend pretreatment in patients who reported seafood allergies.[8] Similar results were seen in a 2014 study by Baig and colleagues, which surveyed 100 cardiologists and discovered that 66% asked about a shellfish allergy.[9] Among these cardiologists, 56% reported that they pretreated the patients with steroids and antihistamines prior to the angiogram.[9] Another study in 2014, by Callahan and colleagues, which surveyed

88 members of the Society for Pediatric Radiology, noted that 24% of respondents believed that asking for shellfish allergies is mandatory before IV contrast administration.[10]

As a consequence of this very commonly encountered misconception, many patients are affected by either undergoing suboptimal nonenhanced imaging examinations or receiving unnecessary premedication treatment protocols. This problem becomes more relevant in the context of the estimated 2.3% prevalence of seafood allergy in the United States, which translates to approximately 6.6 million Americans.[8] With the goal of better serving this population and eradicating this myth, a more robust and continuous education is required for both health care providers and radiology staff.

IODINATED CONTRAST USE IN PATIENTS WITH A SOLITARY KIDNEY

For many years, the American College of Radiology (ACR) Manual on Contrast Media listed the presence of solitary kidney as an indicator that a patient should get screened with a serum creatinine level before the administration of IV contrast. However, this risk was always theoretical, as to the best of our knowledge, no clinical study existed that supported the validity of this claim.

Further, a 2016 study by McDonald and colleagues investigated the incidence of acute kidney injury (AKI) following contrast administration in 264 patients with a solitary kidney. When compared to patients with 2 kidneys, the authors found that these patients are not at any greater risk for developing AKI.[11] Additionally, the rate of emergent dialysis was very low (0.8%) and was similar to the control group (0.4%).

The most recent ACR guidelines no longer catalog solitary kidney as a risk factor.[12] Thus, patients with a single kidney should be managed similarly to patients with 2 functional kidneys. The decision to administer or withhold IV contrast should be always made solely on the basis of the renal function, that is, based on the estimated glomerular filtration rate (eGFR), and the presence of a solitary kidney should not be used to alter this decision.

THE ROLE OF PROPHYLACTIC HEMODIALYSIS IN PATIENTS WITH CHRONIC RENAL DISEASE IN THE PREVENTION OF CONTRAST-INDUCED NEPHROPATHY

For many years, there has been a misconception regarding the capacity of hemodialysis in reducing adverse effects related to the administration of IV contrast. It was thought that prophylactic hemodialysis (HD) could be used as a means to reduce the incidence of contrast-induced nephropathy in high-risk patients. Although it has been demonstrated that hemodialysis can effectively remove contrast media from the blood, there is no evidence that it decreases the incidence of contrast-induced nephropathy (CIN). Several studies during the last 2 decades have demonstrated that hemodialysis has failed to provide any benefit as a prophylactic alternative.[13]

There are 2 hypothetical concerns that are potential indications for receiving emergent HD following IV contrast administration. The first is the possibility of turning an oliguric dialysis patient into an anuric state. The second concern is inducing pulmonary edema and anasarca due to the osmotic load from IV contrast. However, these remain speculative, since there are no clinical studies confirming their veracity, to the best of our knowledge. The latter could have represented a problem a few decades ago, when high osmolality contrast media (HOCM) was more frequently used. However, HOCM are no longer used intravenously and have been replaced with low osmolality contrast media (LOCM). The safety of LOCM was evaluated in a study of Takebayashi and colleagues, which followed 1287 patients on chronic HD after receiving IV contrast, and none of the patients had serious adverse reactions that warranted dialysis before the next routine scheduled session.[14] Additionally, a meta-analysis in 2020 by Okolo and colleagues concluded that IV contrast does not statistically significantly reduce the residual renal function in dialysis patients.[15]

Therefore, given the lack of benefits, potential risks, and cost, the 2023 ACR Manual on Contrast Media recommends that patients' routine hemodialysis schedule should not be altered solely on recent IV contrast administration.[12]

INTRAVENOUS CONTRAST ADMINISTRATION DURING PREGNANCY AND LACTATION

Both CT and MR imaging can be used in pregnant patients and may require the use of IV contrast agents in order to achieve superior diagnostic accuracy. Despite the advantages of IV contrast agents for diagnosis, there is still uncertainty surrounding their use during pregnancy due to potential teratogenic effects and the lack of well-controlled trials in humans.

Concerns about iodine-based contrast agents, in particular, revolve around IV contrast-induced neonatal hypothyroidism. This concern is heightened in pregnant patients during the second and third trimesters, when the fetal thyroid is fully formed and functioning. Although hypothyroidism can cause intellectual disabilities, there is a substantial lack of literature to our knowledge supporting this potential theoretical complication.

A 1976 study reported 6 of 7 neonates exposed to iodine in utero had hypothyroidism, but this was after the use of a combination of water-soluble and fat-soluble agents for aminofetography.[16] These results were not reproducible, as a similar study failed to show any effect of aminofetography on neonatal thyroid function when using only water-soluble agents. A 2012 study, with 64 neonates who were exposed to IV iodinated contrast agents while in utero, found only one neonate to have hypothyroidism and that neonate was born at 25 weeks gestation.[17] A larger, 2010 study by Bourkeily and colleagues with 343 fetuses exposed to a single high-dose water-soluble iodine load, demonstrated only 1 case of transient hypothyroidism, which was confounded by maternal drug exposure.[18] Because of the lack of evidence, the ACR does not recommend withholding iodinated contrast in pregnant women.[12]

On the other hand, the ACR advises IV gadolinium for MR imaging to be used with caution in pregnant patients or potentially pregnant patients, and only be used if its addition is potentially critical to aid in diagnosis.[12] At most institutions, and practices, to our knowledge, gadolinium is almost always avoided in pregnant patients. The concern behind the use of gadolinium during pregnancy is due to the fact that gadolinium crosses the placenta and accumulates in the amniotic fluid. As it stays in the amniotic fluid, it begins to dechelate, exposing the fetus for prolonged periods, and theoretically raising the risk for NSF.[19] This concern is further heightened when linear ionic agents are used. Despite this, a very large 2022 study with 4,692,744 pregnant patients showed that approximately 0.12% of pregnant patients are inadvertently given gadolinium without any issue.[20]

A groundbreaking 2016 Canadian study, with 1.4 million deliveries, in which 397 neonates were exposed to gadolinium in utero, found a higher rate of stillbirth and neonatal death in those exposed to gadolinium in comparison to those who were not exposed to MR imaging at all, with a relative risk of 3.7 (1.55–8.85).[21] Additionally, there was an increase in rheumatological, inflammatory, and infiltrative skin conditions within 4 years of birth in those who were exposed to gadolinium as opposed to those who did not undergo an MR imaging, with a hazards ratio of 1.36 (1.09–1.69).[21] It should be noted that the prevalence of rheumatological, inflammatory, and infiltrative skin conditions in those who were not exposed to MR imaging in utero was 27%, which is considerably high, bringing into question the clinical relevance of the skin conditions as well as their associations with MR imaging/IV gadolinium exposure in utero. A more recent 2022 study with 782 neonates exposed to gadolinium in utero found no increased risk of fetal or neonatal death, or neonatal intensive care unit admissions, in the group exposed to gadolinium contrast agents, in comparison to those who underwent MR imaging examination but did not receive gadolinium.[22]

It used to be recommended that lactating women who receive an IV dose of gadolinium express their breast milk for 24 hours before resuming breastfeeding, but more recent data have shown only 0.04% of gadolinium contrast is excreted into breast milk, and only a small percentage of that is absorbed by the gastrointestinal tract, and so this is no longer recommended.[23]

CONTRAST OSMOLALITY AND THE RISK OF INTRAVENOUS CONTRAST ALLERGY

Iodinated contrast utilized in medical imaging can be classified into high, low, or iso-osmolality in relationship to human plasma. While both high-osmolality contrast media (LOCM) and low-osmolality contrast media (LOCM) are tri-iodinated benzoic acid derivatives, LOCMs have fewer ionizing moieties (eg, contain an amide or amine group, rather than a carboxyl group), requiring less salt for dissolution.[24] Examples of HOCMs include diatrizoate and iothalamate, while examples of LOCMs include ioxaglate, iohexol, and iopromide. Compared to HOCMs, LOCMs can attain similar concentrations of iodine for radiographic visualization with less salt. Dimers of LOCMs can be used to form iso-osmolality contrast media (IOCM) where 6 iodine moieties are present per molecule. Due to lower concentrations required for IOCM to meet adequate iodine concentrations, lower levels of salt are required to hold IOCM in solution.

Although anaphylactic reactions have been reported more frequently following HOCM over LOCM administration, these reactions are often not true allergies. Surveys of patients with reactions to contrast media reveal that many of these reactions are not IgE-mediated and rarely appear in diagnostic skin testing.[25] Instead, histamine release from mast cells and basophils can be initiated by osmolality, the complement system, or by direct bradykinin formation.[26,27]

While LOCMs are less concentrated in comparison to HOCMs and may be associated with fewer nonallergic anaphylactoid reactions, the prevalence of LOCM use as well as reports of true LOCM allergies have been increasing.[28]

Additionally, large population-based studies investigating rates of adverse reactions between patients receiving HOCMs and LOCMs reveal that the incidence of mild-to-moderate adverse reactions were higher in the HOCM group (2.2% vs 0.6%; HOCM vs LOCM), but there was no statistically significant difference in severe adverse reactions (0.08% vs 0.05%; HOCM vs LOCM), and the overall rate of reaction was low in both groups.[29]

IODINATED CONTRAST ADMINISTRATION AND THYROID FUNCTION OF PEDIATRIC PATIENTS

In 2015, the Food and Drug Administration (FDA) announced that all newborns and children aged under 3 years may be more susceptible to temporary or permanent thyroid suppression after IV administration of iodinated contrast.[30] This was based on the Wolff–Chaikoff effect, where excess free iodine can lead to decreased thyroid hormone production, due to feedback mechanisms.[31] Independent review of this statement by the ACR found that such incidents were rarely reported in literature, and that the studies cited by the FDA were concerning for selection bias and limited generalizability due to focus on unique subgroups, such as congenital heart disease and very low birthweight premature infants.[32] Articles not included in the FDA report but included in the 2022 ACR review included retrospective studies using a large general population, and methods such as propensity matching to ensure that the control cohort was comparable with the very rare disease cohort, as well as a small randomized control trial.[33–35] Updated guidelines by the FDA in 2022 and 2023 now communicate that most cases of hypothyroidism following iodinated contrast media have been subclinical and transient, with thyroid hormone derangements lasting from 8.5 to 138 days, and recommend that thyroid monitoring following the administration of IV iodine contrast be performed on a case-by-case basis.[36]

GADOLINIUM-BASED CONTRAST AGENTS AND NEPHROGENIC SYSTEMIC FIBROSIS

NSF is a disorder associated with gadolinium-based contrast agents (GBCAs), which, while rare, is of high concern due to the poor prognosis. A total of 1603 cases of NSF have been reported as of 2013, peaking at 500 cases in 2010, and markedly decreasing since then.[37] Although the pathophysiology of NSF still remains unclear to our knowledge, there is a clear association between NSF and 3 factors: the class of GBCAs, the administered dose,

and both acute and chronic kidney disease (CKD). Initial cases associating GBCAs with NSF were published in 2006; however, cases have gone down markedly, as noted, since 2008, presumably due to mitigation strategies of the aforementioned factors, and the introduction of newer contrast agents.[38] Despite of this, referring physicians are often hesitant to order MR examinations with IV gadolinium in patients with renal disease due to the concern of NSF.

Over 99% of the reported cases of NSF are primarily associated with the linear group I class agents listed in **Table 1**. The use of group I agents has decreased since the introduction of the now more widely used Group II macrocyclic agents, for which only 5 unconfounded cases have been reported thus far, to our knowledge.[40] Group I agents are associated with a 190 fold increase in risk of NSF, in comparison to group II agents.[38] A meta-analysis performed in 2020 containing 4931 patients with stage 4 or 5 CKD showed *0 cases* of NSF in patients receiving group II agents.[41] On the other hand, one review of 519 patients exposed to group I agents showed higher rates of NSF, especially in patients with CKD. In that study, patients with stage 4 or 5 advanced kidney disease (CKD) (eGFR 15–30 or <15, respectively) had a 1% to 7% chance of developing NSF after one or more exposures to group 1 GBCAs, and among those who developed NSF, 80.9% of patients were already dialysis dependent. There were few reports of patients with stage 3 CKD, and none with stage 2 or stage 1.[42]

Group III agents have no known association with NSF, presumably due to hepatobiliary excretion, though the data are limited, and caution should still be utilized.[12]

Many cases of presumed gadolinium-induced NSF were found in patients who received single doses of gadolinium above the standard diagnostic dose of 0.1 mmol per kilogram of body weight. One study showed that of 74,124 patients who received a standard dose, none developed

Table 1
Gadolinium-based contrast agent and the percentage of nephrogenic systemic fibrosis they account for[39]

Group I GBCA	Reported NSF Cases (%)
Gadodiamide	70
Gadopentetate dimeglumine	25
Gadoversetamide	4.8

Gadolinium-Based Contrast Agents (GBCAs) and the NSF Risk: Regulatory Update. Food and Drug Administration - 2019.

NSF, while of 8997 patients who received 2 to 4× the standard dose, 15 cases were reported (~0.17%).[43] Additionally, this study by Prince and colleagues found that of 5725 patients who received multiple standard doses over the course of the 10 year study, none developed NSF, although cumulative doses reached in excess of 100 mL.[43] It should be noted that this study was conducted from 1997 to 2007, while group I agents were still in common use.

Although much of the risk of gadolinium-induced NSF is mitigated by the use of group II contrast agents, the ACR considers patients receiving group I agents who are on dialysis, have an eGFR of less than 30 (stage 4 or 5), or AKI, "at risk," making it best practice to screen for kidney disease when using group I agents or high-dose GBCA examinations, such as MR angiography.

THE ROLE OF HEMODIALYSIS AFTER THE ADMINISTRATION OF GADOLINIUM-BASED CONTRAST AGENTS

Referring providers will commonly attempt to coordinate contrast-enhanced MR scans with dialysis in order to prevent NSF in patients with CKD. The efficacy of dialysis in the removal of GBCAs from the body is questionable and not completely elucidated, to the best of our knowledge. Although hemodialysis can reduce serum gadolinium levels by 75% to 98%, studies have only assessed the serum levels of gadolinium and not total gadolinium removal.[44] Even though hemodialysis is effective at removing GBCA from the serum, dialysis is not considered prophylaxis for NSF and provides only a theoretical reduction in the risk of NSF.[45,46] A 2023 study of 1129 patients with end-stage renal disease (ESRD) on dialysis demonstrated no cases of NSF, regardless if they received dialysis urgently after gadolinium administration, or one to 2 days after the administration of gadolinium.[47] Additionally, performing dialysis on 2 or more consecutive days after the administration of gadolinium was deemed unnecessary.[47] With this in mind, a joint statement by the ACR and National Kidney Foundation recommends timing the GBCA administration before a hemodialysis session as it is regularly scheduled if medically feasible.[12] If for some reason this is not possible, patients should undergo the examination if necessary and continue their regular dialysis schedule, particularly if they are receiving a group II agent.[12]

SUMMARY

The ingrained habits we have in our medical and radiologic practices are often passed down from generation to generation, with little thought about the actual evidence supporting these practices. It is important to understand the research and confirmed evidence in order to optimize our clinical practice and to provide better input when consulted by patients or referring physicians, including best practices for the use of contrast agents for imaging examinations. Additionally, one may be surprised to learn that the dogma and long held beliefs in the subspecialty of radiology are not always necessarily true, and may have been debunked by newer and stronger medical evidence, and the severity or true incidence of potential complications may be very different than how they are actually perceived.

CLINICS CARE POINTS

- The severity of complications from the spillage of barium into the peritoneum may be overstated in medical training.
- Shellfish allergies do not put patients at an increased risk for iodinated contrast allergy.
- There is no additional risk to administering iodine contrast agents in patients with a solitary kidney as opposed to two kidneys.
- Prophylactic hemodialysis does not prevent contrast-induced nephropathy in patients with chronic kidney disease.
- The administration of gadolinium-based and iodinated contrast is safe in breast feeding patients.
- Hypothyroidism after iodine contrast administration to pediatric patients is rare and is often only seen in patients with congenital heart disease or very low birth weight.
- The now widely used Group II gadolinium-based contrast agents have largely mitigated the risk of nephrogenic systemic fibrosis.

DISCLOSURE

The authors do not have any relevant financial or nonfinancial interest to disclose. The authors did not receive funding for this article.

REFERENCES

1. Zheutlin N, Lasser EC, Rigler LG. Clinical studies on effect of barium in the peritoneal cavity following rupture of the colon. Surgery 1952;32(6):967–79.
2. Ghahremani GG, Gore RM. Intraperitoneal barium from gastrointestinal perforations: reassessment of the prognosis and long-term effects. Am J Roentgenol 2021;217(1):117–23.

3. Kleinsasser LJ, Warshaw H. Perforation of the sigmoid colon during barium enema: report of a case with review of the literature, and experimental study of the effect of barium sulfate injected intraperitoneally. Ann Surg 1952;135(4):560–5.

4. Almond CH, Cochran DQ, Shucart WA. Effects of various radiographic contrast media. Ann Surg 1961;154(Suppl 6):219–24.

5. Witten DM, Hirsch FD, Hartman GW. Acute reactions to urographic contrast medium: incidence, clinical characteristics and relationship to history of hypersensitivity states. Am J Roentgenol Radium Ther Nucl Med 1973;119(4):832–40.

6. Schabelman E, Witting M. The relationship of radiocontrast, iodine, and seafood allergies: a medical myth exposed. J Emerg Med 2010;39(5):701–7.

7. Bruen R, Stirling A, Ryan M, et al. Shelling the myth: allergies to Iodine containing substances and risk of reaction to Iodinated contrast media. Emerg Radiol 2022;29(1):67–73.

8. Beaty AD, Lieberman PL, Slavin RG. Seafood allergy and radiocontrast media: are physicians propagating a myth? Am J Med 2008;121(2):158.e1–4.

9. Baig M, Farag A, Sajid J, et al. Shellfish allergy and relation to iodinated contrast media: United Kingdom survey. World J Cardiol 2014;6(3):107–11.

10. Callahan MJ, Servaes S, Lee EY, et al. Practice patterns for the use of iodinated i.v. contrast media for pediatric CT studies: a survey of the Society for Pediatric Radiology. AJR Am J Roentgenol 2014;202(4):872–9.

11. McDonald JS, Katzberg RW, McDonald RJ, et al. Is the presence of a solitary kidney an independent risk factor for acute kidney injury after contrast-enhanced CT? Radiology 2016;278(1):74–81.

12. American College of Radiology, Committee on Drugs and Contrast Media. ACR Manual On Contrast Media. 2023. Available at: https://www.acr.org/-/media/ACR/Files/Clinical-Resources/Contrast_Media.pdf. [Accessed 13 February 2024].

13. Weisbord SD, Palevsky PM. Iodinated contrast media and the role of renal replacement therapy. Adv Chronic Kidney Dis 2011;18(3):199–206.

14. Takebayashi S, Hidai H, Chiba T. No need for immediate dialysis after administration of low-osmolarity contrast medium in patients undergoing hemodialysis. Am J Kidney Dis 2000;36(1):226.

15. Oloko A, Talreja H, Davis A, et al. Does iodinated contrast affect residual renal function in dialysis patients? a systematic review and meta-analysis. Nephron 2020;144(4):176–84.

16. Rodesch F, Camus M, Ermans AM, et al. Adverse effect of amniofetography on fetal thyroid function. Am J Obstet Gynecol 1976;126(6):723–6.

17. Kochi MH, Kaloudis EV, Ahmed W, et al. Effect of in utero exposure of iodinated intravenous contrast on neonatal thyroid function. J Comput Assist Tomogr 2012;36(2):165–9.

18. Bourjeily G, Chalhoub M, Phornphutkul C, et al. Neonatal thyroid function: effect of a single exposure to iodinated contrast medium in utero. Radiology 2010;256(3):744–50.

19. Oh KY, Roberts VHJ, Schabel MC, et al. Gadolinium chelate contrast material in pregnancy: fetal biodistribution in the nonhuman primate. Radiology 2015;276(1):110–8.

20. Bird ST, Gelperin K, Sahin L, et al. First-trimester exposure to gadolinium-based contrast agents: a utilization study of 4.6 million U.S. pregnancies. Radiology 2019;293(1):193–200.

21. Ray JG, Vermeulen MJ, Bharatha A, et al. Association between MRI exposure during pregnancy and fetal and childhood outcomes. JAMA 2016;316(9):952–61.

22. Winterstein AG, Thai TN, Nduaguba S, et al. Risk of fetal or neonatal death or neonatal intensive care unit admission associated with gadolinium magnetic resonance imaging exposure during pregnancy. Am J Obstet Gynecol 2023;228(4):465.e1–11.

23. Guidelines for diagnostic imaging during pregnancy and lactation. Available at: https://www.acog.org/en/clinical/clinical-guidance/committee-opinion/articles/2017/10/guidelines-for-diagnostic-imaging-during-pregnancy-and-lactation. [Accessed 24 September 2022].

24. Jean-Marc I, Emmanuelle P, Philippe P, et al. Allergy-like reactions to iodinated contrast agents. A critical analysis. Fund Clin Pharmacol 2005;19(3):263–81.

25. Trcka J, Schmidt C, Seitz CS, et al. Anaphylaxis to iodinated contrast material: nonallergic hypersensitivity or IgE-mediated allergy? Am J Roentgenol 2008;190(3):666–70.

26. Laroche D, Vergnaud MC, Lefrançois C, et al. Anaphylactoid reactions to iodinated contrast media. Acad Radiol 2002;9(2, Supplement):S431–2.

27. Gueant-Rodriguez RM, Romano A, Barbaud A, et al. Hypersensitivity reactions to iodinated contrast media. Curr Pharmaceut Des 2006;12(26):3359–72.

28. Kang DY, Lee SY, Ahn YH, et al. Incidence and risk factors of late adverse reactions to low-osmolar contrast media: A prospective observational study of 10,540 exposures. Eur J Radiol 2022;146:110101.

29. Valls C, Andía E, Sánchez A, et al. Selective use of low-osmolality contrast media in computed tomography. Eur Radiol 2003;13(8):2000–5.

30. Research C for DE and. FDA Drug Safety Communication: FDA advises of rare cases of underactive thyroid in infants given iodine-containing contrast agents for medical imaging. FDA. 2022. Available at: https://cacmap.fda.gov/drugs/drug-safety-and-availability/fda-drug-safety-communication-fda-advises-rare-cases-underactive-thyroid-infants-given-iodine. [Accessed 22 July 2022].

31. Lee SY, Rhee CM, Leung AM, et al. A review: radiographic iodinated contrast media-induced thyroid

dysfunction. J Clin Endocrinol Metabol 2015;100(2): 376–83.

32. Dillman JR, Forbes-Amrhein MM, Wang CL, et al. ACR statement on use of iodinated contrast material for medical imaging in young children and need for thyroid monitoring. J Am Coll Radiol 2022;19(7): 849–53.

33. Jick SS, Hedderson M, Xu F, et al. Iodinated contrast agents and risk of hypothyroidism in young children in the United States. Invest Radiol 2019;54(5):296.

34. Gilligan LA, Dillman JR, Su W, et al. Primary thyroid dysfunction after single intravenous iodinated contrast exposure in young children: a propensity score matched analysis. Pediatr Radiol 2021;51(4):640–8.

35. Rath CP, Thomas M, Sullivan D, et al. Does the use of an iodine-containing contrast agent to visualise the PICC tip in preterm babies cause hypothyroidism? A randomised controlled trial. Arch Dis Child Fetal Neonatal Ed 2019;104(2):F212–4.

36. Research C for DE and. FDA recommends thyroid monitoring in babies and young children who receive injections of iodine-containing contrast media for medical imaging. FDA. 2023. Available at: https:// www.fda.gov/drugs/drug-safety-and-availability/fda-recommends-thyroid-monitoring-babies-and-young-children-who-receive-injections-iodine-containing. [Accessed 14 April 2024].

37. Mathur M, Jones JR, Weinreb JC. Gadolinium deposition and nephrogenic systemic fibrosis: a radiologist's primer. Radiographics 2020;40(1):153–62.

38. Davenport MS. Virtual elimination of nephrogenic systemic fibrosis: a medical success story with a small asterisk. Radiology 2019;292(2):387–9.

39. Krefting I. Gadolinium-Based Contrast Agents (GBCAs) and the NSF Risk: Regulatory Update.

40. Research C for DE and. FDA Drug Safety Communication: FDA warns that gadolinium-based contrast agents (GBCAs) are retained in the body; requires new class warnings. FDA. 2023. Available at: https:// www.fda.gov/drugs/drug-safety-and-availability/fda-drug-safety-communication-fda-warns-gadolinium-based-contrast-agents-gbcas-are-retained-body. [Accessed 1 February 2024].

41. Shankar PR, Davenport MS. Risk of nephrogenic systemic fibrosis in stage 4 and 5 chronic kidney disease following group ii gadolinium-based contrast agent administration: subanalysis by chronic kidney disease stage. Radiology 2020; 297(2):447–8.

42. Elmholdt TR, Pedersen M, Jørgensen B, et al. Nephrogenic systemic fibrosis is found only among gadolinium-exposed patients with renal insufficiency: a case-control study from Denmark. Br J Dermatol 2011;165(4):828–36.

43. Prince MR, Zhang H, Morris M, et al. Incidence of nephrogenic systemic fibrosis at two large medical centers. Radiology 2008;248(3):807–16.

44. Rudnick MR, Wahba IM, Leonberg-Yoo AK, et al. Risks and options with gadolinium-based contrast agents in patients with CKD: a review. Am J Kidney Dis 2021;77(4):517–28.

45. Yee J. Prophylactic hemodialysis for protection against gadolinium-induced nephrogenic systemic fibrosis: A Doll's House. Adv Chron Kidney Dis 2017;24(3):133–5.

46. Joffe P, Thomsen HS, Meusel M. Pharmacokinetics of gadodiamide injection in patients with severe renal insufficiency and patients undergoing hemodialysis or continuous ambulatory peritoneal dialysis. Acad Radiol 1998;5(7):491–502.

47. Lee Y, Kim J, Kwon S, et al. The need for prophylactic hemodialysis to protect against nephrogenic systemic fibrosis in patients with end-stage renal disease receiving gadolinium-based contrast agents. Acta Radiol 2023;64(8):2492–6.

Vertebral Augmentation for Osteoporotic Vertebral Compression Fractures
What is the Current Evidence Pro and Con?

Tarik Gozel, MD*, A. Orlando Ortiz, MD, MBA

KEYWORDS

- Percutaneous vertebral augmentation • Osteoporotic vertebral compression fracture
- Vertebroplasty • Kyphoplasty

KEY POINTS

- In addition to nonoperative management or spine surgery, image-guided percutaneous vertebral augmentation procedures are an alternative treatment option for painful osteoporotic vertebral compression fractures.
- Though their efficacy has been questioned, a substantial body of evidence now supports the benefits of vertebral augmentation compared to nonoperative management.
- New devices and injectable agents that are used in vertebral augmentation procedures show great potential with respect to biomechanical advantages that translate into patient clinical improvement.

INTRODUCTION

Percutaneous vertebral augmentation (PVA) refers to a growing number of image-guided percutaneous procedures that have been developed to treat painful osteoporotic or pathologic vertebral compression fractures by accessing the damaged vertebral body with some type of bone needle or cannula system, and by placing 1 or more implants within this vertebral body to stabilize it, and, where possible, to restore the vertebral body height and morphology. These procedures can be performed on an inpatient or outpatient basis with varying levels of anesthesia (local, moderate sedation, or general anesthesia) based on operator and patient preferences. In the vertebroplasty procedure (VP), which was first clinically introduced in the United States in 1993, radio-opaque bone cement is injected into the vertebral body (**Fig. 1**).[1] Kyphoplasty (KP), or balloon-assisted VP, was clinically introduced a few years later, and entails the temporary inflation of a balloon tamp within the damaged vertebral body, to create a working cavity for subsequent bone cement injection (**Fig. 2**).[2] The bone cement that has been used for these procedures is an acrylic agent, polymethylmethacrylate, which is combined with barium sulfate to permit its visualization during injection under imaging guidance. The main modification to commercially available cement preparations over the past 2 decades consists of increasing the cement's viscosity to reduce the likelihood of cement extravasation beyond the vertebral body. The latter can be associated with potentially adverse complications. These are rare, but include pulmonary cement embolism and spinal cord or nerve root compression. Some of these acrylic cement formulations have such high viscosity that a hydraulic system is used to inject the very thick cement into the vertebral body. Another development consists of inserting a calibrated leak mesh implant that is subsequently injected with acrylic bone cement

Department of Radiology, Albert Einstein College of Medicine, Jacobi Medical Center, 1400 Pelham Pkwy South, Bronx, NY 10461, USA
* Corresponding author.
E-mail address: gozelt@nychhc.org

Radiol Clin N Am 62 (2024) 979–991
https://doi.org/10.1016/j.rcl.2024.03.004

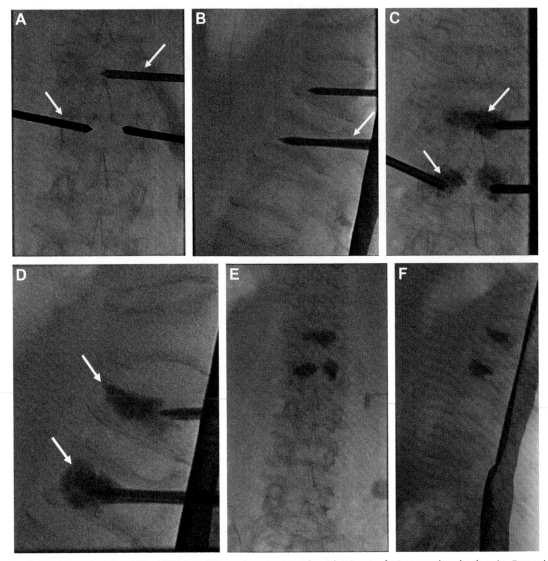

Fig. 1. VP for acute L1 and L2 oVCFs in a 46F on chronic steroids with 10 out of 10 severe low back pain. Frontal (*A*) and lateral (*B*) fluoroscopic images show the transpedicular insertion of bone needles (*arrows*) into each vertebral body. Radio-opaque acrylic bone cement was then carefully injected into each vertebral body using meticulous fluoroscopy. Note the cement location within each vertebral body on the frontal (*C*) and lateral (*D*) fluoroscopic images. Patient's symptoms were relieved and she remained stable clinically and radiographically up to and beyond her 1 year follow-up as shown on these frontal (*E*) and lateral (*F*) fluoroscopic images.

with a small amount of cement being allowed to extrude slowly into the anterior aspect of the vertebral body (**Fig. 3**).[3] Other injectable agents were developed, especially for the VP procedure, which consist of more biocompatible cements including calcium derivatives and a bioceramic agent,[4] Cortoss (Stryker), which simulates the biomechanical characteristics of the vertebral body trabecular structure and better integrates with the osseous matrix, serving as scaffolding for osteogenesis.[5]

The development of new devices for vertebral augmentation (VA) paralleled a fundamental change

in treatment approach due to an increased understanding of the biomechanical effects of an osteoporotic vertebral compression fracture (oVCF) upon the adjacent osteoporotic vertebra, the facet joints and on sagittal spinal alignment.[6] That a majority of oVCFs occur within the mid-thoracic spine (T5–T8) and at the thoraco-lumbar junction (T10–L2), spinal segments associated with increased load stress due to anterior column loading in the mid-thoracic spine and flexion at the thoracolumbar junction, is consistent with these biomechanical concepts (**Fig. 4**). Additionally, the

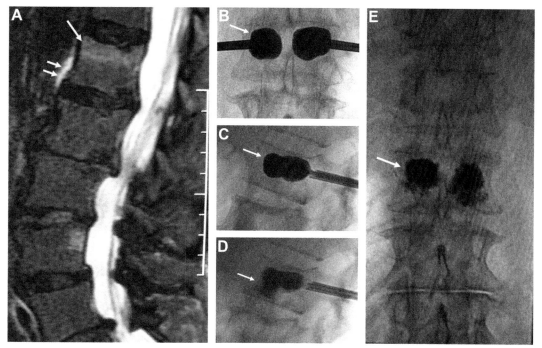

Fig. 2. L1 KP in 91F with acute oVCF and 8 out of 10 low back pain × 2 weeks. Short tau inversion recovery (STIR) sagittal image (*A*) shows superior endplate edema (*arrow*) and prevertebral soft tissue swelling (*double arrow*). Frontal (*B*) and lateral (*C*) fluoroscopic images show bilateral inflation of the balloon tamps (*arrows*) within the vertebral body. Lateral (*D*) and frontal (*E*) fluoroscopic images following the injection of bone cement (*arrows*). The patient experienced complete pain relief in 1 day and was pain free at all follow-up visits to 1 year.

importance of the disc/vertebral–endplate complex, which is usually compromised in osteoporotic fractures, as a component of the functional spine unit, and the alteration of intradiscal pressures following osteoporotic fractures, placed new emphasis on restoring the integrity of the vertebral endplate.[7,8] This heralded innovative percutaneous approaches,

so called vertebral body reconstruction, with the use of curettes, modified balloon inflation techniques, and ultimately, polyether ether ketone (PEEK) and metallic stent implants.[9–11]

When these implants are utilized, a working channel is first created with a twist drill and, in some cases, a bone curette. The implant is then

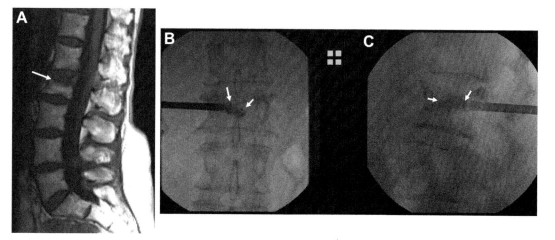

Fig. 3. 61F acute L2 oVCF with superior endplate involvement; 10 out of 10 low back pain (LBP). T1 sagittal image (*A*) shows superior endplate fracture with edema (*arrow*). Frontal (*B*) and lateral (*C*) fluoroscopic images during cement injection into a mesh implant show cement within the implant just beneath the fractured endplate (*arrows*).

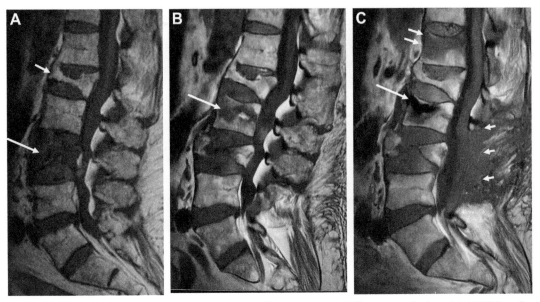

Fig. 4. T1-weighted sagittal images show, serial oVCFs: (*A*) Acute L3 oVCF (*large arrow*), chronic L1 VCF (*small arrow*), (*B*) One year later, acute L2 oVCF (*arrow*) located between 2 oVCFs, a high fracture risk situation. The L2 oVCF was subsequently treated with VA. (*C*) Six months later: laminectomy (*small arrows*), L2 VA (*arrow*), acute T12 oVCF (*double arrows*) located above the chronic L1 oVCF and the augmented L2 oVCF.

inserted coaxially over a guide device into the vertebral body. Subsequently, radio-opaque acrylic bone cement is injected, using a coaxially placed bone cannula, around the implant. In one system, cement is injected into the center of a spiral PEEK implant that contains calibrated leak holes in its center to facilitate central cement extrusion within the implant with some cement extending around it.[10] In another system, a metallic implant is inserted through each pedicle and then each implant is gradually expanded by a mechanical twisting process, like that of a car jack.[11] The plates of this implant effectively elevate and realign the depressed, fractured endplate. Cement is then injected into the vertebral body to enhance the stabilizing effect of the implant. The objectives of implant use are to restore the vertebral body height in the anterior column of the spine as much as possible, to realign the vertebral endplates of the collapsed vertebral body, and to reduce the injected cement volume. Vertebral body height restoration, in turn, reduces kyphotic angulation. This decreases biomechanical stress on the adjacent vertebra (anteriorly and posteriorly) and improves sagittal balance. All these treatment objectives ideally translate into a more favorable patient outcome with respect to pain relief, better balance, and endurance when standing or walking, and decreased adjacent level fracture risk. The use of less bone cement also reduces the likelihood of symptomatic cement extravasation. The technical aspects for performing image-guided percutaneous VP have been made available to all operators to increase the efficacy and safety of the procedure.[1] The procedure was even extended to the sacrum for the treatment of painful sacral insufficiency fractures.[12] Multiple medical societies have developed guidelines for the performance of image-guided PVA procedures.[13,14]

It must be emphasized that prior to the development of these percutaneous interventions for treating painful oVCFs, the standard treatment entailed nonoperative management (**Table 1**). Nonoperative management for painful oVCF consists of one or more of a combination of bedrest, analgesics, back brace or orthosis, and varying amounts of physical therapy. This treatment option, however, has historically had variable success, even with respect to pain relief.[15] Indeed, the morbidity and mortality associated with what is a common condition in the older adult population is substantial.[16–18] These patients may become even more frail and prone to falls because of prolonged bedrest, which also tends to decrease muscle and bone mass. The use of narcotic analgesics in elderly patients is a challenging clinical scenario. Moreover, oVCFs alter the patient's sagittal balance, making their ambulation much more difficult. A negative feedback loop ensues, as the alteration of the vertebral body morphology and the destabilizing impact of

Table 1
Advantages and disadvantages of currently available treatments for painful osteoporotic vertebral compression fractures

	Advantages	Disadvantages
Nonsurgical Management Bedrest Analgesics Bracing Physical therapy	No surgical risk Improved pain with bedrest No anesthesia requirement	Narcotic use Prolonged pain Prolonged hospitalization Imbalance Accelerated demineralization Muscular atrophy Fracture progression Adjacent level fracture Pulmonary embolism Infections (pneumonia, urinary tract infection) New fractures Death
VA Vertebroplasty KP Implant-assisted augmentation	Pain relief Decreased narcotic use Resumption of daily activities Restore sagittal balance Prevent fracture collapse Facilitate hospital discharge	Anesthesia/surgical risk Symptomatic cement leakage Pulmonary embolism Spinal canal compression Adjacent level fracture
Surgery Spine instrumentation	Stabilization Decompression	Anesthesia risk Prolonged recovery Implant failure New fractures

Boldface text used to distinguish 3 major types of currently available treatments for painful osteoporotic vertebral compression fractures

the fracture, in turn, lead to further height loss of the affected vertebra, especially in the anterior column of the spine, which predispose to further kyphosis and more vertebral fractures, either adjacent or remote to the initially fractured vertebra. The deteriorating oVCF may progressively collapse with osseous retropulsion into the spinal canal resulting in spinal cord compression (Fig. 5A, B). This structural insult to the vertebral column, with or without analgesics on board, also compromises the thoracic and/or abdominal cavities with an adverse impact on pulmonary function and/or gastrointestinal function, respectively. With such an immediate impact due to the fracture and such a prolonged recuperation with nonoperative treatments, it is common for these patients to suffer from depression, as they are unable to properly engage in their activities of daily living.

The other treatment alternative for these patients is open surgical repair and stabilization of their fractures.[19] Many elderly patients with painful oVCF are neither surgical or anesthesia candidates due to the presence of major comorbidities. Additionally, many surgeons are reluctant to instrument osteoporotic bone given a high likelihood

of construct failure. For those few patients who are surgical and anesthesia candidates and who elect to undergo open surgical repair, a prolonged recuperation is likely. Nevertheless, open surgical repair may be a required treatment option in those patients who suffer from osteoporotic fractures that acutely compromise the spinal canal and cause spinal cord compression.

DISCUSSION
Controversies

In the setting of this background with 2 treatment options, conservative medical (nonsurgical) management (NSM), or open surgical intervention, it appeared as if there was finally a viable treatment alternative for patients with debilitating, painful osteoporotic fractures of the spine and sacrum. In 2009, 2 studies that compared VP to a sham intervention and 1 study that compared VP to NSM with respect to pain and quality of life outcome measures showed equivalency of these treatment options over a short follow-up period.[20-22] The VP procedure subsequently came under intense scrutiny by both the medical community and insurance carriers. A decrease in

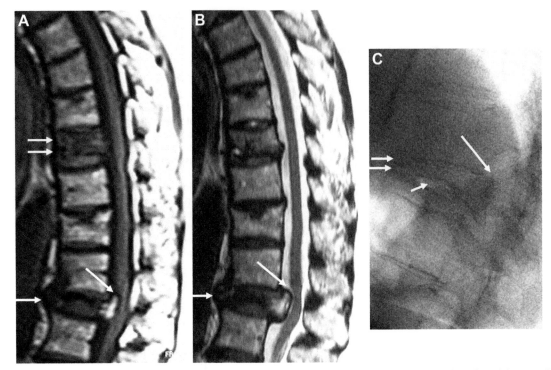

Fig. 5. 70F T8 and T12 oVCF presents with back pain and lower extremity weakness. T1 (*A*) and T2 (*B*) sagittal images show acute T8 oVCF with marrow edema (*double arrow*) and T12 vertebra plana deformity (*small arrow*) with osseous retropulsion and spinal cord compression (*large arrow*). Lateral fluoroscopic image (*C*) shows the severe impacted T12 oVCF (*double arrow*) with a gas containing cleft (*small arrow*) and retropulsed bone fragment (*large arrow*).

requests and approvals for this procedure, to the dismay of patients suffering from painful oVCFs and the operators who perform the procedure, promptly ensued. The KP procedure eluded some of these repercussions, as in the same year, a randomized-controlled trial showed superiority of KP over NSM with respect to both pain relief and quality of life measures at 12 months follow-up.[23] Nonetheless, the efficacy of all these percutaneous interventions was being questioned and the operators who performed them, along with their respective medical societies, commenced with their response. This controversy would continue for approximately the following decade, as the scenario shifted from vertebroplasty trials, to "vertebroplasty on trial" (**Table 2**).

It is reasonable that the initial outcome measures for VA procedures were defined by pain reduction parameters and disability measures. Indeed, the indication and objective of these procedures was to relieve the pain that originated from the fractured vertebra, and to allow the patient to resume their usual activities of daily living. In 1 of the previously mentioned trials, VP accelerated patient discharge from the hospital by 4 days.[22] Comparing the VA procedure to NSM

or medical management was also a reasonable approach, as the latter was the prevalent treatment option available to this patient group (see **Table 2**). An earlier study that used this approach compared VP to NSM in patients with early subacute osteoporotic fractures (>6 weeks) at several time points including the immediate postoperative period and up to 1 year after their intervention.[25] This study found a statistically significant improvement in pain scores and in quality of life (measured

Table 2			
Vertebral augmentation trials, favorable and unfavorable			
		Favorable	*Unfavorable*
VP	vs:		
	NOM	VERTOS II[24]	Alvarez[25]
			Rousing[22]
	SHAM	VAPOUR[26]	Buchbinder[20]
		VERTOS V[27]	INVEST[21]
		VOPE[28]	VERTOS IV[29]
KP	vs:		
	NOM	FREE[23]	—
	STENT	SAKOS[11]	—

by a validated tool: 36 item short-form survey of basic quality-of-life measures [SF-36]) favoring VP, but only in the first 3 months after the patient's intervention. After that, at 6 and 12 months, there was no statistically significant difference in these outcomes. A smaller study using a similar outcomes approach except in patients with acute osteoporotic fractures, found no statistically significant difference in between VP and NSM up to 12 months after the intervention.[22]

In the INVEST trial, a randomized control study, the authors compared VP (68 patients) to a sham (63 patients) procedure that consisted of a paraspinous lidocaine injection in patients with acute, subacute, or chronic fractures.[21] The outcome measures in this study included pain relief, disability (measured by the Roland Morris questionnaire), and quality of life (SF-36 and Euro-QOL is a simple questionnaire formeasuring quality of life in 5 dimensions [EQ-5D] questionnaires, 2 validated tools that address basic quality of life measures), with follow-up performed via telephone communication. Patient crossover from one intervention to the other was allowed in this study. The authors found no statistically significant differences between the 2 interventions at 1 month postprocedure but noted a trend favoring VP with respect to pain relief (64% in the VP group compared to 48% in the sham group, P = .06). The authors also noted that the crossover rate from the sham group (43%) was significantly higher (P < .001) than from the VP group (12%). A second similar randomized control trial comparing VP (38 patients) to a sham (40 patients) intervention in patients with acute or subacute fractures showed no significant difference between the 2 interventions with respect to pain relief, disability, and quality of life outcomes up to 6 months after the initial intervention.[20]

The favorable trend that was reported in the Invest trial led another group of investigators to repeat a similar type of randomized-control trial, VERTOS IV.[29] Using a larger sample size (180 patients), the authors randomized patients with acute vertebral fractures into either a VP procedure (91 patients) or a sham procedure (89 patients), with the objective of achieving statistical significance with respect to pain relief. As with the other sham studies, there was no statistically significant difference between the 2 treatment groups up to 12 months after the initial intervention.

All studies have limitations, and these trials were no exception. Critics, especially those individuals who perform these procedures and could not reconcile their anecdotal favorable patient experiences with the results of these studies, cited several concerns about the validity of these results. With respect to the sham procedure, many operators believe that a paraspinal lidocaine injection is a treatment of back pain. For instance, 1 study showed that facet joint injections could not only provide pain relief for patients suffering from painful oVCF but can also be used for patient selection for VA procedures.[30] Approximately one-third of facet joint injection patients experienced pain relief of at least 8 weeks duration in this study. Clearly these are not sham procedures, but therapeutic injections with albeit temporary relief as well as a confounding intervention from the perspective of all these sham trials. Those patients who did not respond to facet joint injections went on to undergo successful VP.[30] The significant crossover rate by sham patients who wanted to have the procedure was also a point of concern. Patient selection was called into question based upon the lack of a consistent imaging algorithm; not all patients had an MR imaging result showing marrow edema at the fracture level. Furthermore, patient follow-up via telephone also raised concerns, as it is difficult to localize and characterize pain without a direct patient facing clinical visit. This, however, was not a deviation from the standard of practice at the time of the study. Many VP practitioners are from the interventional radiology community, and this is how many interventional patients received their postprocedure follow-up. Only if there was a concern for a procedure complication or if there was a complaint of new severe back pain would a patient be scheduled for an in-person visit.

There are challenges with using pain relief as an outcome in this patient population. Not all back pain is the same, not all vertebral compression fractures are the same. First back pain is quite common in the elderly, even in patients without oVCF. It is one of the most frequent complaints that lead patients to seek medical attention and/or alternative therapies. Patients often have more than one, if not multiple pain generators responsible for their unique back pain profiles. Sorting this out on the diagnostic side requires detailed clinical evaluation, including pain diagrams, lists of medications, and prior therapeutic interventions and physical examination, combined with the appropriate imaging examinations. The treatment aspect requires judicious use of medications in this patient group as well as other treatment modalities, including physical therapy, and clinically appropriate spine interventions. It is common for the post-VA patient to experience back pain. Post-VA back pain was seen in 23% of patients in 1 series.[31] VA treats only the fracture that is causing vertebrogenic pain. In most cases, the back pain will be related neither to their treated fracture nor to a new fracture, but to another pain generator such as an irritated facet or sacroiliac joint.[31] The pain could also originate from innervated joints, ligaments, and muscles that may also be injured at the time of an acute vertebral compression fracture. The various origins of back pain emphasize the importance of performing in-person post-VA procedure patient follow-up. Given the increased frequency of back pain episodes in the elderly and the number of potential back pain generators, some of which are triggered by the vertebral fracture event, it is quite possible for a patient to attribute their back pain to a failed procedure. This could certainly confound the outcome in any study that does not discriminate between the sources of back pain and merely groups the response as only 1 type of pain. The question with respect to treatment efficacy, therefore, should be specific to pain relief from the fracture repair, not just back pain relief.

With the observation that many patients with oVCF improve over time with conservative management, the decision of when to intervene with VA has also been a source of controversy as oVCFs are not all the same. They differ not only with respect to location and morphology but also with respect to height loss, matrix (including avascular necrosis with vertebral cleft development), endplate involvement, and associated disc injury. They may occur in isolation, in association with prior or chronic fractures, or with 1 or more fractures in patients with varying amounts of bone density compromise in the context of their osteoporosis, especially those patients requiring chronic steroid use. In these latter conditions, the fracture may progress quickly over time (measured in days to a week or two), with respect to height loss, kyphosis, and even osseous retropulsion into the spinal canal. They also differ with respect to "age" or time of clinical presentation relative to when the fracture occurred. Given that patients with acute fractures may improve without a VA procedure, it is understandable that NSM may be equivalent to VA with respect to pain relief in some patients and in certain types of fractures. After all, that is what some of the previously discussed equivalency trials are showing—no statistically significant difference. In the double blind placebo-controlled trial of percutaneous vertebroplasty (VOPE) double-blind randomized-control trial, 22 patients had VP and 24 patients had a "sham" procedure, essentially a percutaneous spine biopsy with paraspinous anesthetic infiltration, for a fracture age of 8 weeks or less and MR imaging evidence of bone marrow edema.[28] At 1 year follow-up, there was a statistically higher pain score in the sham group.[28] Perhaps, the more

favorable outcome for VP in this study compared to the other sham procedure studies is based on the requirement for more detailed patient selection using MR imaging criteria. The VERTOS V trial, a single-center randomized control trial similar to the VERTOS IV trial except for the fracture age, compared VP (40 patients) to a spine injection (40 patients) in patients with chronic (>3 months) oVCFs.[27] Not surprisingly, the outcome for the 2 interventions was similar with respect to pain relief at 1 month, again demonstrating the temporary benefit of a paraspinal injection procedure. At 1 year, however, VP showed a statistically significant improvement with respect to both pain relief and quality of life measures as compared to the spine injection procedure. This study indicated the importance of procedure timing with respect to chronic painful oVCF.[27] The VAPOUR trial looked at early acute oVCF of less than 6 weeks of duration.[26] In this multicenter randomized control trial, 61 patients underwent VP, and 59 patients underwent a placebo or mock VP short of any paraspinous needle placement or anesthetic infiltration. VP showed statistically significant pain relief compared to the placebo intervention up to 6 months after the intervention. In this study, both the fracture age and the lack of a paraspinous intervention were controlled variables. In VERTOS II, a randomized control trial, 101 patients underwent VP, and 101 patients underwent NSM for their acute oVCFs.[24] The VP group showed statistically significant improvement at 1 year with respect to pain relief and quality of life measures. The ability to intervene on an oVCF acutely is appealing to both operators and patients, as this strategy observes the standard operating principle for orthopedic interventions in extremity fractures whereby early intervention and stabilization produce better biomechanical, morphologic, and functional outcomes in addition to pain relief.

At the core of this controversy is the use of outcome measures (pain relief, analgesic reduction, disability scores, and quality of life measures), inclusion criteria for patient selection (fracture age–procedure timing, vertebral marrow edema on MR imaging, clinical confirmation of vertebrogenic pain, and diagnosis of osteoporosis using bone density testing) and patient follow-up (including clinical evaluation/examination, osteoporosis management, and physical therapy gait/balance training). Study sample size may also be an important factor, as some of these trials involve small numbers of patients. Several meta-analyses have shown a benefit for VA over NSM with the caveat of inclusion of heterogeneous patient samples. A meta-analysis that included a comparison of VP, KP, and NSM found 27 articles with level 1 or 2 evidence up to the beginning of 2011, which met stringent inclusion criteria for the analysis.[32] These authors concluded that VA procedures provided greater pain relief than NSM. A second meta-analysis was performed for studies performed over a 5 year period after the prior meta-analysis.[33] This second meta-analysis included 25 prospective comparative level 1 or level 2 studies in patients who underwent either KP, VP, VA with implant, or NSM. This analysis showed that KP provided statistically significantly better pain relief than NSM, while VP tended to show better pain relief than NSM. KP also showed significant pain reduction and improvement in disability scores compared to VA with implant.[33] A third meta-analysis assessed level 1 randomized control trials, 16 total, with pain reduction and quality of life improvement as the outcome variables: 8 studies compared VP to nonoperative management (NOM), 3 studies compared VP to a sham procedure, 4 studies compared VP to KP, and 1 study compared KP to NOM.[34] Of the 8 studies comparing VP to NOM, 7 favored VP and 1 showed no statistical difference between the VP and NOM groups. As previously discussed, all 3 studies that compared VP to a sham paraspinal injection showed no statistical difference in outcome between the 2 interventions. Three of the 4 studies comparing KP and VP showed no significant difference between these procedures with respect to pain relief. KP showed statistically significant improvements with respect to pain relief and quality of life measures as compared to NOM. An additional level 1 randomized control trial comparing VP to a sham paraspinal injection that was not included in this meta-analysis, because it was not yet published, the VERTOS V study favored the VP procedure.[27]

When subjective outcome measures such as pain relief and quality of life are replaced by objective outcome measures, the case for performing VA in appropriately selected patients becomes much stronger.[35] One objective measure that has been studied in this patient population is mortality. It is known that vertebral compression fractures, as with hip fractures, can have an adverse impact on life expectancy in patients with osteoporosis. NOM is a treatment decision and as such is not without its associated risks. Multiple studies assessing Medicare databases for either 1 or more years and comparing either VP or KP to NOM have shown a statistically significant increase in mortality in patients who have not undergone the VA procedure.[36,37] Moreover, a meta-analysis of 7 studies that includes over 2 million patients with oVCF who either underwent VA or NSM, showed that patients who underwent

VA were 22% less likely to die at up to 10 years after their treatment.[38] To better assess the treatment impact of VA relative to life preservation, a calculation of the number of patients needed to treat to save 1 life at 1 year, in patients with oVCF, is 15.[39] These authors compared this epidemiologic measurement result to those of other treatments such as intravenous tissue plasminogen activatior (tPA) for acute ischemic stroke (number needed to treat [NNT] = 15), statins for cardiovascular event (NNT = 250), and aspirin for heart attack (NNT = 1667) or stroke (NNT = 3000), all clinically accepted standard of care interventions.

Another objective outcome measure for VA is whether there is a favorable biomechanical impact as a result of the procedure. The performance of vertebral body reconstruction, which includes balloon-assisted KP and vertebral implants, is an area that remains under active investigation. For instance, KP has been shown to provide height restoration in acute vertebral compression fractures. This in turn leads to kyphosis correction and restoration of sagittal alignment. As previously stated, one level 1 randomized controlled trial showed a statistically significant improvement in outcomes with respect to pain relief, disability scores, and quality of life measures.[23] Vertebral body reconstruction facilitates vertebral endplate stabilization, and this, in turn, contributes to pain relief reflected by improved load transfer. A review of the meta-analyses on these procedures clarifies the potential of these procedures for height correction and maintenance. An initial meta-analysis concluded that KP provides statistically significantly greater height restoration and kyphosis angle correction when compared to VP.[32] A follow-up meta-analysis found that KP tended to show better, but not statistically significant, anterior height restoration and kyphosis angle correction when compared to VP.[33] Of 14 studies (8 KP, 6 VP) that reported on kyphosis angle correction, the majority(10 studies) showed definite improvement, and 4 showed little or no improvement.[32] More importantly, none showed deterioration with respect to kyphosis angle, which is what is observed in patients with untreated oVCFs. Furthermore, the restored height is maintained over the long term in both VA procedures.[40] Maintaining the height of the vertebral body is certainly more desirable than the progressive vertebral body collapse that often occurs in nonaugmented oVCF. In those studies that compared VA procedures to either NSM or sham interventions, noticeable height loss was reported in the control or nonaugmented group.[33]

Vertebral body height restoration and maintenance are critical because an existing oVCF is associated with a greater risk for subsequent fracture within 3 vertebral levels of the initially fractured vertebra.[41] A recent study showed that this fracture risk is related to factors beyond what could be explained by low bone mineral density alone.[42] Early on in the VA literature, it was initially reported that VP was associated with a substantial increased incidence of adjacent level vertebral compression fractures in patients with osteoporosis.[43] The authors noted a subsequent fracture rate of 12.4% in 177 patients treated with VP, with 24 of the 36 new fractures (67%) located adjacent to the previously treated vertebra. These new fractures occurred within 1 month following VP in 67% of the patients.[43] It was believed that the acrylic bone cement increased the stiffness of the vertebral body and subjected the adjacent vertebra, which was already weakened by osteoporosis, to increased biomechanical stress. This evolved into a controversial topic and was used as an argument against performing VA. The concern over adjacent level fracture risk also led to the development of alternative, more biocompatible cement preparations and implants.[9,44] In one prospective randomized control trial, Cortoss, a bioceramic cement, was shown to be associated with a 43.4% lower adjacent level fracture rate (10.3%) as compared to acrylic bone cement (18.2%).[44]

It has been previously reported that the incidence of a new oVCF within 1 year in women who just experienced a fracture was 19.2%.[45] In addition, the incidence of new fractures increased to 24% when more than 2 or more pre-existing vertebral compression fractures were present.[45] These data not only illustrate the natural history of a patient with an oVCF but also shed light on an oVCF's adverse biomechanical impact on the axial skeleton. In other words, more vertebral compression fractures lead to greater spinal deformity and increased stress on an already weakened skeleton.[45] Low bone mineral density and pre-existing vertebral compression fractures are associated with an increased fracture risk (Fig. 6). Additionally, the location of the vertebral compression fracture within the thoracic or lumbar spine and the type of deformity (wedge compression, crush or impaction deformity, and biconcave deformity) also influence the risk of a subsequent vertebral compression fracture.[41] Once correcting for the pre-existing vertebral fracture incidence in patients with osteoporosis, it has been consistently demonstrated that VA procedures do not increase adjacent level fracture rates when compared to non-surgically managed patients.[34] A controversial application of VA to prevent incident vertebral compression fractures in patients with osteoporosis is prophylactic VA, in which not only is the acute painful oVCF treated with VA but also the adjacent osteoporotic vertebra are prophylactically augmented with acrylic bone cement in order to prevent future oVCFs at these levels.[46] While this is not an indication for the procedure in the United States, prophylactic VA is performed in other countries. A meta-analysis of this intervention involving 6 randomized control trials that were either prospective or retrospective showed no difference in either adjacent or remote level fractures between patients who underwent prophylactic VA and those who did not.[46] In the absence of a clear-cut model that can be used

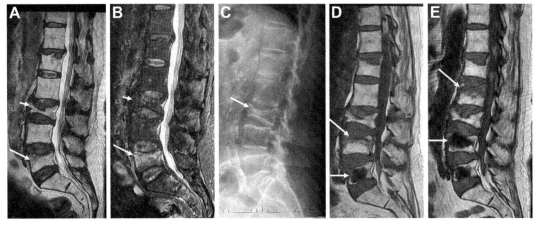

Fig. 6. 67F with osteoporosis presents with acute 7 out of 10 low back pain. T1 (*A*) and STIR (*B*) sagittal images show acute L5 oVCF (*large arrow*) and chronic L3 oVCF (*small arrow*). The L3 oVCF (*arrow*) was present on a lateral lumbar spine radiograph (*C*) performed 18 months earlier; note the marked osteopenia. The L5 fracture is treated with VA and 1 month later the patient presents with severe low back pain. T1 sagittal image (*D*) shows an acute L4 oVCF (*large arrow*) and a treated L5 fracture (*small arrow*). The L4 fracture is treated with VA and 3 months later the patient presents with acute 10 out of 10 low back pain. The T1 sagittal image (*E*) shows an acute L2 oVCF (*large arrow*) and a treated L4 fracture (*small arrow*).

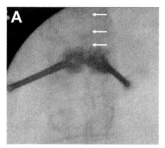 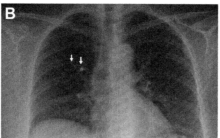 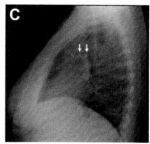

Fig. 7. Frontal fluoroscopic image (*A*) with patient prone shows linear cement extravasation coursing cephalad (*arrows*) in the expected location of the inferior vena cava. Frontal (*B*) and lateral (*C*) chest radiographs show radio-opaque acrylic cement within a proximal branching pulmonary artery segment (*arrows*) in this asymptomatic patient.

to identify osteoporotic vertebra at risk for fracture, the role of prophylactic intervention is not yet well defined.

Besides adjacent level fracture, another reported VA procedure-related complication that has been somewhat controversial is cement extravasation. This includes cement leakage into the spinal canal with the potential for spinal canal stenosis and spinal cord compromise and cement leakage into the anterior paraspinal veins with subsequent cement embolization into the lungs (**Fig. 7**). Given the relative hypoviscosity of the acrylic bone cement that was first used for VP procedures, it is understandable how this liquid-like polymer could extend beyond the confines of the vertebral body. Despite this challenge, the absolute numbers of serious adverse VP cement extravasation complications, even in the initial years of use, was low. Reported rates of cement extravasation range from 14.4% to 72% in the VP trials.[32] In the study with the highest extravasation rate, VERTOS II, all the cement extravasations were asymptomatic including 25% with silent pulmonary emboli.[31] KP, by creating a working cavity for subsequent cement injection, has been shown to have overall lower cement extravasation rates than VP, 4.5% to 33%, nearly all asymptomatic.[32] This must be compared to the risk of spinal cord compression from deteriorating oVCF or the risk of symptomatic pulmonary embolism in chronically bedridden elderly patients unable to ambulate because of their fracture pain and gait imbalance (see **Fig. 5**A, B). Indeed, in the VERTOS V trial, where a 70% cement leakage rate detected by computed tomography was reported, the only serious adverse event was seen in 1 patient from the sham group. This patient experienced spinal cord compression from progressive collapse of their untreated oVCF.[27] Further refinements, including the development and use of hyperviscous acrylic bone cements as well as combination use of the cement with other implants have decreased the risk of cement extravasation in what already are procedures with an excellent safety profile.[47]

CLINICS CARE POINTS

- Image-guided PVA procedures play an important role in the treatment of painful oVCFs.

- VA, being the subject of numerous randomized controlled studies and systemic reviews, has demonstrated efficacy in pain reduction, functional improvement, and improved quality of life.

- VA has also shown a clear benefit with respect to patient mortality, including a favorable "number-needed-to-treat in order to save one life in 1 year" profile.

DISCLOSURE

The authors have nothing to disclose.

REFERENCES

1. Jensen ME, Evans AJ, Mathis JM, et al. Percutaneous polymethylmethacrylate vertebroplasty in the treatment of osteoporotic vertebral body compression fractures: technical aspects. AJNR Am J Neuroradiol 1997;18:1897–904.

2. Mathis JM, Ortiz AO, Zoarski GH. Vertebroplasty versus kyphoplasty: a comparison and contrast. In: Mathis JM, Deramond H, Belkoff S, editors. Percutaneous vertebroplasty and kyphoplasty. 2nd edition. New York: Springer; 2006. p. 145–56.

3. Ortiz AO. Use and evaluation of a semi-permeable mesh implant in vertebral augmentation for the treatment of painful osteoporotic vertebral compression fractures. J NeuroIntervent Surg 2016;8:328–32.

4. Wang Q, Med M, Dong JF, et al. Application and modification of bone cement in vertebroplasty: a literature review. Jt Dis Relat Surg 2022;33:467–78.

5. Bae H, Hatten HP, Linovitz R, et al. A prospective randomized FDA-IDE trial comparing Cortoss to

PMMA for vertebroplasty: a comparative effectiveness research study with 24-months follow-up. Spine 2012;37:544–50.

6. Pumberger M, Schitz F, Burger J, et al. Kyphoplasty restores the global sagittal balance of the spine independently from pain reduction. Sci Rep 2020;10:8894.

7. Ortiz AO, Bordia R. Injury to the vertebral endplate-disk complex associated with osteoporotic vertebral compression fractures. AJNR Am J Neuroradiol 2011;32:115–20.

8. Tzermiadianos MN, Renner SM, Phillips FM, et al. Altered disc pressure profile after an osteoporotic vertebral fracture is a risk factor for adjacent vertebral body fracture. Eur Spine J 2008;17:1522–30.

9. Ortiz O, Mathis JM. Vertebral body reconstruction: techniques and tools. Neuroimaging Clin 2010;20: 145–58.

10. Tutton SM, Pflugmacher R, Davidian M, et al. KAST study: the Kiva system as a vertebral augmentation treatment – a safety and effectiveness trial: a randomized, non-inferiority trial comparing the Kiva system to balloon kyphoplasty in treatment of osteoporotic vertebral compression fractures. Spine 2015;40:865–75.

11. Noriega D, Marcia S, Theumann N, et al. A prospective, international, randomized, noninferiority study comparing an implantable titanium vertebral augmentation device versus balloon kyphoplasty in the reduction of vertebral compression fractures (SAKOS study). Spine 2019;19:1782–95.

12. Kortman KE, Ortiz AO, Miller T, et al. Multicenter study to assess the efficacy and safety of sacroplasty in patients with osteoporotic sacral insufficiency fractures or pathologic sacral lesions. J NeuroIntervent Surg 2013;5:461–6.

13. Barr JD, Jensen ME, Hirsch JA, et al, Society of Neurointerventional Surgery. Position statement on percutaneous vertebral augmentation: a consensus statement developed by the Society of Interventional Radiology (SIR), American Association of Neurological Surgeons (AANS) and the Congress of Neurological Surgeons (CNS), American College of Radiology (ACR), American Society of Neuroradiology (ASNR), American Society of Spine Radiology (ASSR), Canadian Interventional Radiology Association (CIRA), and the Society of NeuroInterventional Surgery (SNIS). J Vasc Intervent Radiol 2014;25: 171–81.

14. Tsoumakidou G, Too CW, Koch G, et al. CIRSE guidelines on percutaneous vertebral augmentation. Cardiovasc Intervent Radiol 2017;40:331–42.

15. Silverman SL. The clinical consequences of vertebral compression fracture. Bone 1992;13(Suppl 2): S27–31.

16. Kado DM, Duong T, Stone KL, et al. Incident vertebral fractures and mortality in older women: a prospective study. Osteoporos Int 2003;14:589–94.

17. Melton LJIII. Adverse outcomes of osteoporotic fractures in the general population. J Bone Miner Res 2003;18:1139–41.

18. Lau E, Ong K, Kurtz S, et al. Mortality following the diagnosis of a vertebral compression fracture in the Medicare population. J Bone Joint Surg Am 2008;90:1479–86.

19. Ponnusamy KE, Iyer S, Gupta G, et al. Instrumentation of the osteoporotic spine: biomechanical and clinical considerations. Spine J 2011;11:54–63.

20. Buchbinder R, Osborne RH, Ebeling PR, et al. A randomized trial of vertebroplasty for painful osteoporotic vertebral fractures. N Engl J Med 2009;361: 557–68.

21. Kallmes DF, Comstock BA, Heagerty PJ, et al. A randomized trial of vertebroplasty for osteoporotic spinal fractures. N Engl J Med 2009;361:569–79.

22. Rousing R, Anderson MO, Jespersen SM, et al. Percutaneous vertebroplasty compared to conservative treatment in patients with painful acute or subacute osteoporotic vertebral fractures: three months follow-up in a clinical randomized study. Spine 2009; 34:1349–54.

23. Wardlaw D, Cummings SR, Van Meirhaeghe J, et al. Efficacy and safety of balloon kyphoplasty compared with non-surgical care for vertebral compression fracture (FREE): a randomized controlled trial. Lancet 2009;373:1016–24.

24. Klazen CA, Lohle PN, De Vries J, et al. Vertebroplasty versus conservative treatment in acute osteoporotic vertebral compression fractures (Vertos II): an open-label randomized trial. Lancet 2010;376:1085–92.

25. Alvarez L, Alcaraz M, Perez-Higueras A, et al. Percutaneous vertebroplasty: functional improvement in patients with osteoporotic compression fractures. Spine 2006;31:1113–8.

26. Clark W, Bird B, Gonski P, et al. Safety and efficacy of vertebroplasty for acute painful osteoporotic fractures (VAPOUR): A multicenter, randomized, double-blind, placebo-controlled trial. Lancet 2016;388: 1408–16.

27. Carli D, Venmans A, Lodder P, et al. The Vertos V Randomized Controlled Trial. Radiology 2023; 308(1):e222535.

28. Hansen EJ, Simony A, Carreon L, et al. Vertebroplasty vs. sham for treating osteoporotic vertebral compression fractures: a double blind RCT (VOPE). Integr J Orthop Traumatol 2019;2:2–6.

29. Firanescu CE, de Vries J, Lodder P, et al. Vertebroplasty versus sham procedure for painful acute osteoporotic vertebral compression fractures (VERTOS IV): randomized sham controlled clinical trial. BMJ 2018;361:k1551.

30. Wilson D, Owen S, Corkill R. Facet injections as a means of reducing the need for vertebroplasty in insufficiency fractures of the spine. Eur Radiol 2011;21:1772–8.

31. Kamalian S, Bordia R, Ortiz AO. Post-vertebral augmentation back pain: Evaluation and management. AJNR Am J Neuroradiol 2012;33:370–5.

32. Papanastassiou ID, Phillips FM, Meirhaeghe JV, et al. Comparing effects of kyphoplasty, vertebroplasty, and non-surgical management in a systematic review of randomized and non-randomized controlled studies. Eur Spine J 2012;21:1826–43.

33. Beall D, Lorio MP, Min Yun B, et al. Review of vertebral augmentation: an updated meta-analysis of the effectiveness. Internet J Spine Surg 2018;12: 295–321.

34. Halvachizadeh S, Stalder AL, Bellut D, et al. Systematic review and meta-analysis of 3 treatment arms for vertebral compression fractures: a comparison of improvement in pain, adjacent-level fractures, and quality of life between vertebroplasty, kyphoplasty and nonoperative management. JBJS Rev 2021;9:e21.

35. Hirsch JA, Chiara Z, Giovanni C, et al. Vertebral augmentation: is it time to get past the pain? A consensus statement from the Sardinia Spine and Stroke Congress. Medicina 2022;58:1431.

36. Chen AT, Cohen DB, Skolasky RL. Impact of nonoperative treatment, vertebroplasty, and kyphoplasty on survival and morbidity after vertebral compression fracture in the Medicare population. J Bone Joint Surg Am 2013;95:1729–36.

37. Edidin AA, Ong K, Lau E, et al. Morbidity and mortality after vertebral fractures: comparison of vertebral augmentation and nonoperative management in the Medicare population. Spine 2015;40:1228–41.

38. Hinde K, Maingard J, Hirsch JA, et al. Mortality outcomes of vertebral augmentation (vertebroplasty and/or balloon kyphoplasty) for osteoporotic vertebral compression fractures: a systematic review and meta-analysis. Radiology 2020;295:96–103.

39. Hirsch JA, Chandra RV, Carter NS, et al. Number needed to treat with vertebral augmentation to save a life. AJNR Am J Neuroradiol 2020;41:178–82.

40. Liu JT, Li CS, Chang CS, et al. Long-term follow-up study of osteoporotic vertebral compression fracture treated using balloon kyphoplasty and vertebroplasty. J Neurosurg Spine 2015;23:94–8.

41. Lunt M, Oneill TW, Felsenberg D, et al. European prospective osteoporosis study group characteristics of a prevalent vertebral deformity predict subsequent vertebral fracture: results from the European prospective osteoporosis study (EPOS). Bone 2003;33:505–13.

42. Kanis JA, Johansson H, McCloskey EV, et al. Previous fracture and subsequent fracture risk: a meta-analysis to update FRAX. Osteoporos Int 2023;34: 2027–45.

43. Uppin AA, Hirsch JA, Centenera LV, et al. Occurrence of new vertebral body fracture after percutaneous vertebroplasty in patients with osteoporosis. Radiology 2003;226:119–24.

44. Gilula L, Persenaire M. Subsequent fractures post-vertebral augmentation: analysis of a prospective randomized trial in osteoporotic vertebral compression fractures. AJNR Am J Neuroradiol 2013;34: 221–7.

45. Lindsay R, Silverman SL, Cooper C, et al. Risk of new vertebral fracture in the year following a fracture. JAMA 2001;285:320–3.

46. Chen Z, Song C, Lin H, et al. Does prophylactic vertebral augmentation reduce the refracture rate in osteoporotic vertebral fracture patients: a meta-analysis. Eur Spine J 2021;30:2691–7.

47. Xiao H, Yang J, Feng X, et al. Comparing complications of vertebroplasty and kyphoplasty for treating osteoporotic vertebral compression fractures: a meta-analysis of the randomized and non-randomized controlled studies. Eur J Orthop Surg Traumatol 2015;25(Suppl 1):S77–85.

More than a Half Century of Misinformation About Breast Cancer Screening

Daniel B. Kopans, MD, FSBI*

KEYWORDS

- Breast • Breast cancer • Screening • Mammography • Breast imaging • Screening controversies

KEY POINTS

- Screening and early detection has been proven to save lives for women aged 40 to 74 years.
- Efforts have been made, over the past half century, to try to reduce access for women to screening.
- Misinformation has been promulgated about screening that has been refuted by science and evidence.

INTRODUCTION

The sad events of our times are an almost constant reminder of the now seemingly aphoristic observation by Spanish-American Philosopher George Santayana about the consequences of not recognizing that the errors of history repeat themselves. Unfortunately, and surprisingly, this is true in health care as well. The almost continuous "debates" about breast cancer screening are an example of how misinformation can have a life of its own and can be reinforced by unopposed repetition. Also unfortunately, as discussed later, the misinformation that has evolved and been the cause of the "debates" has been "validated" by respected medical journals that have had undisclosed publication biases against breast cancer screening and have been complicit in the promulgation of scientifically unsupported information. I wrote about this in 2005,[1] but, unfortunately, it continues today and has become even worse.[2]

Tragically, the coronavirus disease 2019 pandemic underscored the devastating consequences that result when information is corrupted, "alternative facts" are created, and science and evidence are ignored. Discussions about breast cancer screening have been complicated for decades by misinformation that has found its way into some of our most prestigious medical journals.[1–4] These have been repeated by major media outlets, which has caused a great deal of confusion among women and their physicians. My hope is to address several of the main concerns that have been raised and misreported about screening and to reference the scientific evidence that supports the recommendation that women begin annual screening starting at the age of 40 years.

There are legitimate concerns surrounding the diagnosis of ductal carcinoma in situ (DCIS) and how it should be treated. Consequently, the following is primarily related to invasive breast cancers.

I have also confined my comments to reducing deaths from breast cancer. There are clearly other benefits to early detection that include a reduction in the need for mastectomy, axillary dissection with its attendant risk of lymphedema, and less toxic systemic therapy.[5–7]

SCREENING GUIDELINES OVER TIME

In the 1960s, it was thought that breast cancer was systemic before it could be found. The randomized controlled trial (RCT) that was conducted within the Health Insurance Plan of New York (HIP) proved that deaths could be reduced by earlier detection.[8]

Department of Radiology, Harvard Medical School, Boston, MA 02115, USA
* 20 Manitoba Road, Waban, Massachusetts 02468.
E-mail address: dkopans@verizon.net

Radiol Clin N Am 62 (2024) 993–1002
https://doi.org/10.1016/j.rcl.2024.04.001

In the 1980s, there was neither agreement on the age at which to start screening nor was there agreement on the appropriate frequency for screening. In 1989, the major medical groups, including the National Cancer Institute (NCI), reached a consensus and advised that women aged 40 to 49 years be screened every 1 to 2 years, and that women aged 50 years and over to be screened every year.[9] In 1993, the NCI, using inappropriate statistical analysis,[10] dropped support for screening women aged 40 to 49 years and advised women aged 50 years and over to be screened every 2 years.[11] In 1997, when the benefit for women aged 40 to 49 years, analyzed separately, became statistically significant,[12] the NCI was initially and falsely told by a biased Consensus Development Conference Panel that there was no benefit for women aged 40 to 49 years, but this was reversed by a review of the data by the National Cancer Advisory Board,[13] and once again, NCI supported screening starting at the age of 40 years,[14] and then decided it would no longer issue guidelines. In 2007, the American College of Physicians (ACP) decided that women should wait until the age of 50 years and be screened every 2 years.[15,16] This position was adopted by the ACP's close ally, the United States Preventive Services Task Force (USPSTF) in 2009.[17]

Over the same time, the American Cancer Society (ACS) was a staunch defender of annual screening starting at the age of 40 years. However, political pressure prevailed, and in 2015, the ACS, explaining that "Women should have the opportunity to begin annual screening between the ages of 40 and 44 years (qualified recommendation)" developed a hybrid recommendation suggesting that women might want to delay screening until the age of 45 years, be screened annually until the age of 55 years, and then biennially after that.[18]

The USPSTF reaffirmed their position in 2016.[19]

Although the ACP agreed that lives are saved by screening starting at the age of 40 years: "Screening mammography has been shown to decrease the number of deaths from breast cancer in women ages 40 to 74.",[20] in their guidance document issued on April 8 of 2019, the ACP reaffirmed their support for the USPSTF and told women that they should wait until the age of 50 years and be screened every 2 years.[21] They advised delaying participation because of the "harms" of screening.

In the spring of 2023, the USPSTF finally agreed that women should begin screening at the age of 40 years, but they are still advising biennial and not annual screening.

The ACP and ACS recommendations are unchanged as of early 2024.

EXPERTS WERE EXCLUDED

What most do not realize is that the USPSTF, the ACS, and the ACP have all agreed that delaying screening will result in avoidable deaths.[18,19,22] Most are also unaware that the panels that made these decisions intentionally excluded experts in breast cancer screening. They did not even include anyone who provides care for women with breast cancer. They claim that they wanted to avoid anyone with conflicts of interest (COI). It is virtually impossible to be an expert in a field without some form of COI. You cannot become an expert without having it somehow connected to your livelihood. It is astonishing that experts were specifically excluded from these panels. Folks who have been deciding guidelines for breast cancer screening have not been involved in screening or caring for women with breast cancer. I have decades of experience in medicine and could review the literature, but *would you want me to set guidelines for neurosurgery?*! It is a major mistake to not include experts in a field to help set guidelines for that field. Their COIs can be made clear. Furthermore, there should also be a minority report for all these panels if there are major disagreements so that the medical community and the population can better understand the issues.

"EXPERTS" WITH NO EXPERTISE

Since the panel members had no actual expertise, they likely were swayed by advisers to these groups, many of whom were known opponents of screening. It also meant that the panel members brought their own personal biases into their decision. This is clear in the fact that although the RCTs of screening proved that it saves lives for women aged 40 to 74 years[12,23] (the ages of the women who participated), the ACP and the USPSTF argued that because of the "harms" of screening, women should delay their participation until the age of 50 years. The "harms" were "false positives," "overdiagnosis," and "overtreatment."

What has not been made clear by these panels is that of the 3, the only "harm" that is affected by delaying screening is the "false-positive rate" (see later discussion). This, itself, is a pejorative choice of words since women are not being, falsely, told that they have breast cancer. They are simply being recalled from screening for a few additional mammographic images, and perhaps an ultrasound. In fact, following recall, many are told that everything is fine.

If it even exists, "overdiagnosis" is not the fault of screening. The problem is that pathologists cannot accurately determine which cancers will be lethal and which women will die from some other cause and not from their cancers.

Of course, "overtreatment" is not the fault of screening. Treatment is decided by medical and surgical oncologists. Treating breast cancers is still an inexact science no matter how cancers are found. Most women who have adjuvant systemic treatment of breast cancer do not benefit from that treatment no matter how their cancers are found.[24]

There are major consequences of delaying screening. According to the Cancer Intervention Surveillance and Modeling Network known as CIS-NET (6 groups supported by the NCI whose models have been used by the major guidelines groups) if screening is delayed to age 45 or 50 years and the time between screens is lengthened, tens of thousands of women would die, unnecessarily, whose lives could be saved by annual screening starting at the age of 40 years.[25]

It should be noted that a better-informed US Preventive Services Task Force finally acknowledged what has been known for decades, namely, that screening saves lives for women starting at the age of 40 years. They have recently revised their recommendations to support screening women starting at the age of 40 years.[26] We are still trying to convince them to support annual screening discussed later.

FUNDAMENTAL FACT: THE RANDOMIZED CONTROLLED TRIALS PROVED THAT SCREENING SAVES LIVES FOR WOMEN AGED 40 TO 74 YEARS

RCTs eliminate lead-time bias, length bias sampling, selection bias, pseudo-disease bias, and so forth. If done correctly, they are the most rigorous science that we have. RCTs have proven that detecting breast cancers earlier by screening reduces deaths for women aged 40 to 74 years.[23,27] These are the ages of the women who participated in the trials, and it has been shown for all these women that there were, statistically significantly, fewer deaths among those allocated to screening compared to those assigned to the control arms *including women aged 40 to 49 years.*[12]

NONCOMPLIANCE AND CONTAMINATION

I suspect that most are unaware that RCTs, by their very design, underestimate the benefit. Since women cannot be forced to participate in a trial, they are "invited." A woman allocated to the screening arm may refuse the invitation ("noncompliance"). *If she dies from breast cancer, she is still counted as having been screened. Conversely, if a* woman is assigned to the control arm, she can still go out and get a mammogram on her own ("contamination"). If her life is saved by the mammogram, she is still counted as an unscreened control. Once a woman was allocated to one arm or the other, she was counted with that group no matter what her experience in order to avoid a possible self-selection bias.

There are opponents of screening who cite the percent of women who died from breast cancer in the RCTs, inferring that this is the best that can be expected, but they have ignored "noncompliance and contamination." There was "noncompliance" and "contamination" in all the trials. Consequently, the *RCTs can only underestimate the benefit.* The mortality reduction that is evident in the RCTs is almost certainly greater than what is often claimed. The RCTs proved the fundamental concept—earlier detection by screening saves lives. But it is a mistake to think that the RCTs provide an absolute measure of the benefit as has been suggested by some.

OBSERVATIONAL STUDIES CONFIRM THE BENEFIT IN GENERAL POPULATIONS

Having been proven in RCTs, the benefits of screening have been confirmed in numerous observational studies in which women in the general population, with access to screening, have much better survival than those who do not have access.[28–44] It is in these analyses of women ages 40 years and over, who participate in screening, that the data show a greater than 40% reduction in deaths.

"FROSTING ON THE CAKE"

A third way of evaluating benefit is in a "failure analysis." In a review of women who died from breast cancer in the Harvard teaching hospitals, 71% of the deaths were among the 20% of the women who were not participating in screening despite all the women having access to modern therapy.[45] Similar results were reported by Spencer and colleagues.[46]

More recently, in still another way to test the benefits from screening, a large study in Sweden showed that the incidence of death from breast cancer, in a population followed for decades, was 60% less at 10 years for women who participated in screening and 47% fewer at 20 years, despite everyone having access to therapy.[47] In a very large follow-up study of more than 500,000 women in Sweden, the risk of dying from breast cancer was reduced by 41% within 10 years for women who participated in screening compared to those who did not. Although some of this was due to a reduction in the rate of advanced cancers of 25%,[48] it suggests that some of the benefit was due to downsizing within stages. This is important to realize since studies such as the WISDOM (Women Informed to Screen Depending on Measures of Risk) trial and TMIST (Tomosynthesis Mammographic Imaging Screening Trial) are only evaluating decreases in the rate of advanced cancers. The Swedish data show that these trials may miss an important benefit.[49,50]

DEATH RATES FALL IN THE UNITED STATES SOON AFTER THE START OF SCREENING

In the United States, mammography screening began in the mid-1980s as evidenced by the sudden increase in breast cancer incidence at that time.[29] This signaled the beginning of a prolonged *prevalence peak* (clinically evident cancers + screened detected cancers detected in the first screen of a population) as more and more women began to participate in screening (had their first screen) over the next decade.[51] As expected, the death rate from breast cancer that had been unchanged for decades in the United States began to fall in 1990, soon after the start of screening. The death rate has continued to decline as more and more women have participated in screening, so that there are now more than 40% fewer women dying each year from breast cancer. It has been estimated that more than 600,000 lives have been saved since 1990.[52] Therapy has improved, but there is still no cure for advanced breast cancers. Therapy may extend lives, but breast cancer is cured when it is treated earlier. Unfortunately (and inexplicably), the Surveillance Epidemiology and End Results program of the NCI does not track how breast cancers are being detected, but certainly the 40,000 women who still die each year were not cured by therapy. The failure analyses[50,51] suggest that many of the women who have died were, likely, not participating in screening.

WHY DO WOMEN WITH BREAST CANCER DO BETTER THAN MEN?

The final piece of evidence that screening and treating breast cancers earlier is the main reason for the decline in breast cancer deaths is seen in the data for men with breast cancer. While the death rate for women with breast cancer has fallen markedly, the same has not been true for men with breast cancer. In 1990, as the death rate for women was beginning to fall, it increased for men with breast cancer. Staying elevated for several years, it returned to 1990 levels where it has remained,[53] unchanged, while deaths have continued to fall among women. The treatments of male breast cancer are the same as for women. Men present with more advanced cancers than women.[54] The difference is likely because women are being screened and men are not.

Therapy for breast cancer has improved, but many of the advances are toward delaying death. Cures result from treating breast cancers earlier.

"OVERDIAGNOSIS" HAS BEEN FALSELY BLAMED ON SCREENING

As noted above, it has been falsely claimed that there are thousands of breast cancers that, if left alone, will never be lethal. Finding them will lead to unnecessary concern and unnecessary treatment. Analysts have developed scientifically unsupportable arguments that there are tens of thousands of these "fake" cancers found by mammography screening, that if left alone, would disappear on their own. I suspect that there are some cancers that will never become lethal. This is likely true for all cancers, but no one has been able to safely determine which specific cancers these are prospectively. Furthermore, a woman may die in a car accident before her cancer might have been lethal. Her cancer would be considered having been "overdiagnosed" and "overtreated."

Regardless, it is pathologists who make the diagnosis, yet opponents claim that it is screening that has led to massive "overdiagnosis."[55–57] There are extremely rare reports of clinically evident cancers that have disappeared without treatment. The false claim is that screening finds numerous breast cancers that would disappear if left undetected.[58] Finding them leads to "overtreatment" for a cancer that would never become clinically evident.

The concept of "overdiagnosis" was initially based on a handful of reports of breast cancers that (miraculously) disappeared without treatment[59] (although at least 1 woman still died from her metastatic disease). The *extremely* rare (literally "miraculous") cases that have been reported have *all been clinically evident cancers*. Yet no one is suggesting that clinically evident cancers should be ignored. Opponents of screening are claiming that if screening is delayed until the age of 50 years, all of the "overdiagnosed" cancers that would be found among women in their forties, would disappear by the age of 50 years. *In fact, no one has ever seen a mammographically detected cancer disappear or even regress on its own.*[60] The "studies" making the claim that there are thousands of mammographically detected cancers that are "fake" have all been refuted and shown to be scientifically unsupportable.[61]

To understand how poor peer review has contributed to these false claims, you should review one often-cited article in the New England Journal of Medicine. *The authors claimed to have used the SEER database to show that, in 2008 alone, mammography revealed 70,000 cancers that were "overdiagnosed."*[55]

The inference was that screening should be delayed since these cancers would have disappeared if women waited until the age of 50 years and been screened every 2 years. Somehow the New England Journal of Medicine allowed the authors to use SEER data to claim that mammography was at fault when *SEER does not provide information on mammography nor on how cancers are detected.* Furthermore, you would think that with 70,000 "fake" cancers in 1 year, someone would have seen at least one disappear?! This article was shown by 3 separate and different analyses to be scientifically unsupportable,[51,62,63] yet the New England Journal of Medicine (NEJM) refused to withdraw the article and it is still quoted as if legitimate. This article had been based on the claim (the authors called it their "best guess") that, in the absence of screening, the incidence of breast cancer would have been almost a flat line (in a later article, one of the authors claimed, using the same data, that it was a flat line). In fact, the data show that the incidence of breast cancer had been increasing steadily by 1% to 2% per year since 1940,[64] long before there was any screening. If the facts are used instead of a "guess," the incidence of breast cancer is lower than the extrapolation. This indicates that there is no "overdiagnosis" of breast cancers.[65]

FALSE CLAIMS HAVE BEEN RAISED ABOUT THE "HARMS" OF SCREENING IN SUPPORT OF REDUCED SCREENING "RECALLS" FOR ADDITIONAL EVALUATION

There are some "risks" associated with screening. Inconvenience is one. To be efficient and keep costs down, screening studies are read in batches after women have left the center. If something is seen on the screening examination that warrants further attention, some women will be recalled for additional evaluation. "Recalls" for a few additional mammographic images or an ultrasound are considered by some to be a major "harm" ("risk") of screening. These have been called "false positives," which is another pejorative and misleading term. These are not women who have been falsely told that they have breast cancer. They are simply women who are "recalled" from screening for a

few additional images or an ultrasound. To keep costs down, screening examinations are interpreted in batches after women have left the screening center. If cost was of no importance, we could do these additional images at the time of screening, and there would be no "recalls."

Approximately 10% of screened women will be recalled. This is the same rate[66]as for cervical cancer screening (Pap testing).[67] "Recalls" are inconvenient and may cause anxiety, but most of these women will, ultimately, be reassured that everything is fine, and they *do not* have evidence of cancer. Opponents of screening who advise delaying until the age of 50 years and then screening every 2 years have suggested that the anxiety associated with screening "outweighs" the benefit (not dying from breast cancer), in women aged 40 to 49 years. Ironically, contradicting themselves, in their 2007 review of screening for women aged 40 to 49 years, the ACP stated "false-positive results have little effect on psychological health or subsequent mammography adherence."[15]

The argument for delaying screening is to avoid "overdiagnosis" and "overtreatment." This would require that the "fake" cancers that might be detected among women in their forties would disappear by the age of 50 years. Unless "overdiagnosed and overtreated breast cancers" disappear if left undetected, and since no one has ever seen this for mammographically detected cancers, it is important to understand that *"recalls" are the only major "harm" that is affected by delaying screening until the of age 50 years and delaying the time between screens. None of the groups that support delaying screening have explained: How many fewer recalls from screening "balance" allowing one woman to die, whose life could be saved by annual screening starting at the age of 40 years?*

Some, such as the ACP, are concerned that the "harms" of screening outweigh the benefits. The major "harms" that are cited are "false positives," "overdiagnosis," and "overtreatment." The term "harm" is, itself, pejorative. We all, periodically, experience some anxiety every day just driving in traffic, but we do not consider this a "harm." It is more accurately described as a "risk" of driving. There are certainly "risks" associated with breast cancer screening. It is claimed that the "harms" of screening have been weighed against the "benefits" of screening, yet the balance has never been provided. The major "harm" of screening, which can be affected by delaying the age to start screening and increasing the interval between screens, is "recalls" for additional evaluation. Unless "overdiagnosed" ("fake") cancers disappear, delaying screening until the age of 50 years and then screening every two years instead of annually, the "fake" cancers will still be there at the age of 50 years and every 2 years. Unless "overdiagnosed" cancers disappear, delaying screening will have no effect on "overdiagnosis" and "overtreatment." The question that remains unanswered by those who promote delaying screening is "How many fewer 'recalls' outweigh one avoidable death?"

THERE IS NO SCIENTIFIC SUPPORT FOR USING THE AGE OF 50 YEARS AS A THRESHOLD FOR SCREENING

To reduce the "harms," women are being advised to delay screening until the age of 50 years and then get screened every 2 years instead of annually. This advice is, actually, scientifically unsupportable. It also endangers tens of thousands of women. By grouping and averaging women by ages (the average for all women aged 40–49 years compared to the average for all women aged 50 years or older), you can (falsely) make it seem as if anything that changes with increasing age changes at that age.[4] *There are absolutely no data that have not been grouped and averaged (eg, by individual ages), to support using the age of 50 years as a threshold for screening.* None of the parameters of screening change, abruptly, at the age of 50 years or any other age.[67] The age of 50 years was chosen by one of the Principal Investigators of the HIP study as the average age of menopause with the expectation that screening benefit would change at menopause. In fact, none of the parameters of screening have been shown to be altered by menopause. The RCTs proved that screening saves lives for women aged *40* to 74 years, *period*.

Some groups have failed to tell women that the age of 40 years is the evidence-based threshold for screening. In the RCT, women aged 40 to 74 years participated in screening and deaths were averted. The groups that have advised delay have not directly informed women of the consequences of delaying screening. It has been clearly shown that women aged 40 to 49 years, analyzed separately, have a marked decline in breast cancer deaths.[12] The age of 40 years is the only science and evidence-based threshold for screening. Delaying screening will result in tens of thousands of deaths that could be avoided by annual screening starting at the age of 40 years.[25] Since delaying screening will only reduce "recalls" and will have no effect on "overdiagnosis" and "overtreatment," delaying screening will result in tens of thousands of avoidable deaths[25] just to reduce the inconvenience and anxiety of being recalled!

IT IS FALSELY CLAIMED THAT SCREENING DOES NOT REDUCE "ALL-CAUSE MORTALITY"

This is simply ignoring science. Those who disparage screening for this reason should be embarrassed. It is a false claim that arose because those analyzing the data, with no screening expertise, lacked a fundamental understanding of the data and its analysis.[68] Reducing all-cause mortality is evaluated in treatment trials where all the women have breast cancer and most deaths (all causes) are due to breast cancer. Critics ignore the fact that, in the general population, breast cancer only accounts for 3% of total deaths each year ("all causes"). Most deaths in the screening trials are due to causes other than breast cancer. It would take a trial of more than 2.5 million women to show that reducing breast cancer deaths, in the general population, by 30% (1% of "all-cause" deaths) would, significantly, reduce "all-cause" mortality.[69] The RCTs showed that screening does reduce "all-cause" mortality among women with breast cancer.[69]

IT IS FALSELY CLAIMED THAT SCREENING IS INEFFECTIVE BECAUSE IT DOES NOT REDUCE THE RATE OF ADVANCED CANCERS

This is another, fundamentally, false claim on several levels. Screening does not have to reduce the rate of advanced cancers to reduce deaths. The probability of successful metastatic spread (the key step in lethality) is directly related to the number of cells in a cancer, and this is directly related to its size.[70,71] Lives are saved by reducing the size of cancers within stages.[72–76] This is clearly evident in the Swedish data where the rate of advanced cancers was reduced by 25%, while the risk of dying was reduced by 41%.[47]

The claim is also false because it has been clearly shown that *screening does reduce the rate of advanced cancers.* This has been shown in the RCTs,[23,27] as well as when screening is introduced into the population.[27,44,62,64,77–79]

IT IS CLAIMED THAT WE SHOULD ONLY SCREEN WOMEN WHO ARE AT ELEVATED RISK OF DEVELOPING BREAST CANCER

It would be wonderful if we only had to screen women who will develop breast cancer and not bother (and have the expense of) screening everyone else, but we are not even close to being able to identify these women. We cannot even identify women who will not develop breast cancer so they would not need to participate in screening. The panels that have issued guidelines have required RCTs as proof of benefit. The RCTs have shown a clear benefit for screening women in the general population with a, statistically significant, mortality reduction for these women. However, *none of the RCTs were stratified by risk,* so *there is no proof that screening only high-risk women will save any lives.* Perhaps, of greater importance is the fact that the highest risk women (BRCA1 and 2 mutation carriers) only account for, at most, 10% of breast cancers diagnosed each year. If we add women with a family history and other risk factors, these account for another 15% of breast cancers. In fact, *the majority of women diagnosed each year with breast cancer* are *not at elevated risk*. This means that if we were to only screen high-risk women, approximately, 75% of those who develop breast cancer each year would not have the advantage of early detection.[80,81]

SCREENING EVERY 2 YEARS MEANS THAT WOMEN WILL DIE WHOSE LIVES COULD BE SAVED BY ANNUAL SCREENING

Unfortunately, there has never been an RCT to test the difference between annual screening and biennial, but since cancers do not stop growing, and the risk of metastatic spread increases with increasing tumor size,[82] it makes sense that more frequent screening saves more lives,[83] and this is supported by the data.[81] Data confirm the benefit of annual screening.[84]

The CISNET models all show that the most lives are saved by annual screening starting at the age of 40 years.[19] The consequences of the various guidelines have been analyzed.[66] They show that annual screening starting at the age of 40 years reduces deaths by 40%. Waiting until the age of 45 years, then screening annually until the age of 55 years, and then biennially after that (ACS) reduces deaths by 31%, while biennial after the age of 50 years (old USPSTF and current ACP) only reduces deaths by 23%. In actual numbers, for women who are aged 40 years today, annual screening starting at the age of 40 years saves 29,369 lives, while the ACS approach will save 22,829 with the ACP saving only 17,153. Annual screening starting at the age of 40 years saves 70% more lives than waiting until the age of 50 years and screening biennially. The ACP and the previous USPSTF forgot to tell this to women.

THE BOTTOM LINE

Mammography screening is not the ultimate answer to breast cancer, but a universal cure is not even on the horizon. Currently, earlier detection is the best way to save the most lives. The most lives are saved by annual screening starting at the age of 40 years. Ignoring the fact that there is no scientific support for using the age of 50 years as a threshold for screening, delaying screening until the age of 50 years and then screening every 2 years will have no effect on "overdiagnosis" and "overtreatment," but it will result in tens of thousands of deaths that could be saved by annual screening starting at the age of 40 years.

"Informed decision-making" does not stop at the age of 50 years. All women should be provided with accurate information. Women should decide for themselves whether to participate or not in screening. The decision should not be made for them.

DISCLOSURE

Royalties from IZI Medical for Kopans localization system. Advisor to DART Imaging in China. Advisor to Malcova Imaging developing CT for the breast.

REFERENCES

1. Kopans DB. Bias in the medical journals: a commentary. AJR Am J Roentgenol 2005;185(1):176–7.
2. Kopans DB. More misinformation on breast cancer screening. Gland Surg 2017;6(1):125–9.
3. Kopans DB. Breast cancer screening panels continue to confuse the facts and inject their own biases. Curr Oncol 2015;22(5):e376–9.
4. Kopans DB. Informed decision making: The age of 50 is arbitrary and has no demonstrated influence on breast cancer screening in women. Am J Roentgenol 2005;185:177–82.
5. Ahn S, Wooster M, Valente C, et al. Impact of screening mammography on treatment in women diagnosed with breast cancer. Ann Surg Oncol 2018;25(10):2979–86.
6. Coldman AJ, Phillips N, Speers C. A retrospective study of the effect of participation in screening mammography on the use of chemotherapy and breast conserving surgery. Int J Cancer 2007; 120(10):2185–90.
7. Yaffe MJ, Jong RA, Pritchard KI. Breast cancer screening: beyond mortality. J Breast Imag 2019; 1(3):161–5.
8. Shapiro S. Evidence on screening for breast cancer from a randomized trial. Cancer 1977;39:2772–3278.
9. Vanchieri C. Press release from the National Medical Roundtable on Mammography Screening Guidelines. June 27, 1989, Medical Groups' Message to Women: If 40 or Older, Get Regular Mammograms JNCI Vol. 81, No. 15, 1989 -1128.
10. Kopans DB, Halpern E, Hulka CA. Statistical power in breast cancer screening trials and mortality reduction among women 40-49 with particular

emphasis on The National Breast Screening Study of Canada. Cancer 1994;74:1196–203.

11. House Committee on Government Operations. Misused Science: The National Cancer Institutes Elimination of Mammography Guidelines for Women in Their Forties. Union Calendar No. 480. House Report 103-863. October 20, 1994.

12. Hendrick RE, Smith RA, Rutledge JH, et al. Benefit of screening mammography in women ages 40-49: a new meta- analysis of randomized controlled trials. J Natl Cancer Inst Monogr 1997;22:87–92.

13. Kopans DB. The breast cancer screening controversy and the national institutes of health consensus development conference on breast cancer screening for women ages 40-49. Radiology 1999;210:4–9.

14. Available at: https://academic.oup.com/jnci/article-lookup/doi/10.1093/jnci/89.8.538 Last accessed December/27/2023

15. Armstrong K, Moye E, Williams S, et al. Screening mammography in women 40 to 49 years of age: a systematic review for the American College of Physicians. Ann Intern Med 2007;146(7):516–26.

16. Qaseem A, Fontham ET, Sherif K, et al. Clinical Efficacy Assessment Subcommittee of the American College of Physicians. Screening mammography for women 40 to 49 years of age: a clinical practice guideline from the American College of Physicians. Ann Intern Med 2007;146(7):511–5.

17. US Preventive Services Task Force. Screening for breast cancer: U.S. Preventive Services Task Force recommendation statement. Ann Intern Med 2009;151(10):716–26.

18. Oeffinger KC, Fontham ET, Etzioni R, et al. Breast cancer screening for women at average risk: 2015 guideline update From the American Cancer Society. JAMA 2015;314(15):1599–614.

19. Siu AL, U.S. Preventive Services Task Force. Screening for Breast Cancer: U.S. Preventive Services Task Force Recommendation Statement. Ann Intern Med 2016;164(4):279–96.

20. Available at: http://www.acpinternist.org/archives/2012/05/policy.htm. [Accessed 29 December 2020].

21. Qaseem A, Lin JS, Mustafa RA, et al, Clinical Guidelines Committee of the American College of Physicians. Screening for breast cancer in average-risk women: A Guidance Statement From the American College of Physicians. Ann Intern Med 2019. https://doi.org/10.7326/M18-2147. [Epub ahead of print].

22. Available at: http://www.acpinternist.org/archives/2012/05/policy.htm. [Accessed 9 December 2019].

23. Smith RA, Duffy SW, Gabe R, et al. The randomized trials of breast cancer screening: what have we learned? Radiol Clin North Am 2004;42(5):793–806.

24. Early Breast Cancer Trialists' Collaborative Group (EBCTCG). Effects of chemotherapy and hormonal therapy for early breast cancer on recurrence and 15-year survival: an overview of the randomised trials. Lancet 2005;365(9472):1687–717.

25. Hendrick RE, Helvie MA. USPSTF Guidelines on Screening Mammography Recommendations: Science Ignored. Am J Roentgenol 2011;196:W112–6.

26. Available at: https://uspreventiveservicestaskforce.org/uspstf/draft-recommendation/breast-cancer-screening-adults. [Accessed 24 June 2023].

27. Tabár L, Yen AM, Wu WY, et al. Insights from the breast cancer screening trials: how screening affects the natural history of breast cancer and implications for evaluating service screening programs. Breast J 2015-Feb;21(1):13–20.

28. Tabar L, Vitak B, Tony HH, et al. Beyond randomized controlled trials: organized mammographic screening substantially reduces breast carcinoma mortality. Cancer 2001;91:1724–31.

29. Kopans DB. Beyond randomized, controlled trials: organized mammographic screening substantially reduces breast cancer mortality. Cancer 2002;94:580–1.

30. Duffy SW, Tabar L, Chen H, et al. The impact of organized mammography service screening on breast carcinoma mortality in seven Swedish Counties. Cancer 2002;95:458–69.

31. Otto SJ, Fracheboud J, Looman CWN, et al. the National Evaluation Team for Breast Cancer Screening* Initiation of population-based mammography screening in Dutch municipalities and effect on breast-cancer mortality: a systematic review. Lancet 2003;361:411–7.

32. Swedish Organised Service Screening Evaluation Group. Reduction in breast cancer mortality from organized service screening with mammography: 1. Further confirmation with extended data. Cancer Epidemiol Biomarkers Prev 2006;15:45–51.

33. Coldman A, Phillips N, Warren L, et al. Breast cancer mortality after screening mammography in British Columbia women. Int J Cancer 2007;120(5):1076–80.

34. Jonsson H, Bordás P, Wallin H, et al. Service screening with mammography in Northern Sweden: effects on breast cancer mortality - an update. J Med Screen 2007;14(2):87–93.

35. Paap E, Holland R, den Heeten GJ, et al. A remarkable reduction of breast cancer deaths in screened versus unscreened women: a case-referent study. Cancer Causes Control 2010;21:1569–73.

36. Otto SJ, Fracheboud J, Verbeek ALM, et al, for the National Evaluation Team for Breast Cancer Screening. Mammography screening and risk of breast cancer death: a population-based case–control study. Cancer Epidemiol Biomarkers Prev 2011. https://doi.org/10.1158/1055-9965.EPI-11-0476.

37. van Schoor G, Moss SM, Otten JD, et al. Increasingly strong reduction in breast cancer mortality

due to screening. Br J Cancer 2011. [Epub ahead of print].

38. Mandelblatt JS, Cronin KA, Bailey S, et al. Effects of mammography screening under different screening schedules: model estimates of potential benefits and harms. Ann Intern Med 2009;151:738–47. Available at: http://cisnet.cancer.gov. [Accessed 16 April 2011].

39. Hellquist BN, Duffy SW, Abdsaleh S, et al. Effectiveness of population-based service screening with mammography for women ages 40 to 49 years: evaluation of the Swedish Mammography Screening in Young Women (SCRY) cohort. Cancer 2011;117(4):714–22.

40. Broeders M, Moss S, Nyström L, et al, EUROSCREEN Working Group. The impact of mammographic screening on breast cancer mortality in Europe: a review of observational studies. J Med Screen 2012;19(Suppl 1):14–25.

41. Hofvind S, Ursin G, Tretli S, et al. Breast cancer mortality in participants of the Norwegian Breast Cancer Screening Program. Cancer 2013;119(17):3106–12.

42. Sigurdsson K, Olafsdóttir EJ. Population-based service mammography screening: the Icelandic experience. Breast Cancer (Dove Med Press) 2013;5:17–25.

43. Coldman A, Phillips N, Wilson C, et al. Pan-canadian study of mammography screening and mortality from breast cancer. J Natl Cancer Inst 2014;106(11).

44. Puliti D, Bucchi L, Mancini S, et al, IMPACT COHORT Working Group. Advanced breast cancer rates in the epoch of service screening: The 400,000 women cohort study from Italy. Eur J Cancer 2017;75:109–16.

45. Webb ML, Cady B, Michaelson JS, et al. A failure analysis of invasive breast cancer: most deaths from disease occur in women not regularly screened. Cancer 2014;120(18):2839–46.

46. Spencer DB, Potter JE, Chung MA, et al. Mammographic screening and disease presentation of breast cancer patients who die of disease. Breast J 2004;10(4):298–303.

47. Tabár L, Dean PB, Chen TH, et al. The incidence of fatal breast cancer measures the increased effectiveness of therapy in women participating in mammography screening. Cancer 2019;125(4):515–23.

48. Duffy SW, Tabár L, Yen AM, et al. Mammography screening reduces rates of advanced and fatal breast cancers: Results in 549,091 women. Cancer 2020;126(13):2971–9. Epub 2020 May 11. PMID: 32390151; PMCID: PMC7318598.

49. Kopans DB. The wisdom trial is based on faulty reasoning and has major design and execution problems. Breast Cancer Res Treat 2021;185(3):549–56. Epub 2020 Nov 25. PMID: 33237397.

50. Kopans DB. Design, implementation, and pitfalls of TMIST. Clin Imag 2021;78:304–7. Epub 2021 Jun 24. PMID: 34218941.

51. Kopans DB. Arguments Against Mammography Screening Continue to be Based on Faulty Science. Oncol 2014;19:107–12.

52. Hendrick RE, Baker JA, Helvie MA. Breast cancer deaths averted over 3 decades. Cancer 2019. https://doi.org/10.1002/cncr.31954 [Epub ahead of print] PubMed PMID: 30740647.

53. Available at: http://seer.cancer.gov/csr/1975_2010/results_merged/sect_04_breast.pdf. [Accessed 30 December 2020].

54. Giordano SH, Cohen DS, Buzdar AU, et al. Breast carcinoma in men: a population-based study. Cancer 2004;101(1):51–7. PMID: 15221988.

55. Bleyer A, Welch HG. Effect of three decades of screening mammography on breast-cancer incidence. N Engl J Med 2012;367(21):1998–2005.

56. Welch HG, Gorski DH, Albertsen PC. Trends in metastatic breast and prostate cancer. N Engl J Med 2016;374(6):596.

57. Welch HG, Prorok PC, O'Malley AJ, et al. Breast-cancer tumor size, overdiagnosis, and mammography screening effectiveness. N Engl J Med 2016;375(15):1438–47.

58. Zahl PH, Mæhlen J, Welch HG. The natural history of invasive breast cancers detected by screening mammography. Arch Intern Med 2008;168(21):2311–6.

59. Larsen SU, Rose C. [Spontaneous remission of breast cancer. A literature review]. Ugeskr Laeger 1999;161(26):4001–4. Review. Danish. PubMed PMID: 10402936.

60. Arleo EK, Monticciolo DL, Monsees B, et al. Persistent untreated screening-detected breast cancer: an argument against delaying screening or increasing the interval between screenings. J Am Coll Radiol 2017;14:863–7.

61. Puliti D, Duffy SW, Miccinesi G, et al, EUROSCREEN Working Group. Overdiagnosis in mammographic screening for breast cancer in Europe: a literature review. J Med Screen 2012;19(Suppl 1):42–56.

62. Helvie MA, Chang JT, Hendrick RE, et al. Reduction in late-stage breast cancer incidence in the mammography era: Implications for overdiagnosis of invasive cancer. Cancer 2014;120(17):2649–56.

63. Etzioni R, Xia J, Hubbard R, et al. A reality check for overdiagnosis estimates associated with breast cancer screening. J Natl Cancer Inst 2014;106(12).

64. Anderson WF, Jatoi I, Devesa SS. Assessing the impact of screening mammography: Breast cancer incidence and mortality rates in Connecticut (1943-2002). Breast Cancer Res Treat 2006;99(3):333–40.

65. Kopans DB, Moore RH, McCarthy KA, et al. Biasing the Interpretation of Mammography Screening Data By Age Grouping: Nothing Changes Abruptly at Age 50. Breast J 1998;4:139–45.

66. Arleo EK, Hendrick RE, Helvie MA, et al. Comparison of recommendations for screening mammography using CISNET models. Cancer 2017;123(19): 3673–80.

67. Saraiya M, Irwin KL, Carlin L, et al. Cervical cancer screening and management practices among providers in the National Breast and Cervical Cancer Early Detection Program (NBCCEDP). Cancer 2007;110(5):1024–32.

68. Kopans DB, Halpern E. Re: All-cause mortality in randomized trials of cancer screening. J Natl Cancer Inst 2002;94(11):863.

69. Tabar L, Duffy SW, Yen MF, et al. All-cause mortality among breast cancer patients in a screening trial: support for breast cancer mortality as an end point. J Med Screen 2002;9(4):159–62.

70. Michaelson JS, Halpern E, Kopans DB. Breast Cancer: Computer Simulation Method for Estimating Optimal Intervals for Screening. Radiology 1999; 21:551–60.

71. Michaelson JS, Silverstein M, Wyatt J, et al. Predicting the survival of patients with breast carcinoma using tumor size. Cancer 2002;95(4):713–23.

72. Quiet CA, Ferguson DJ, Weichselbaum RR, et al. Natural history of node-negative breast cancer: a study of 826 patients with long-term follow-up. J Clin Oncol 1995;13(5):1144–51.

73. Saadatmand S, Bretveld R, Siesling S, et al. Influence of tumour stage at breast cancer detection on survival in modern times: population based study in 173,797 patients. BMJ 2015;351:h4901. PubMed PMID: 26442924.

74. Elkin EB, Hudis C, Begg CB, et al. The effect of changes in tumor size on breast carcinoma survival in the U.S.: 1975-1999. Cancer 2005;104(6): 1149–57.

75. Rosen PP, Groshen S, Saigo PE, et al. A long-term follow-up study of survival in stage I (T1 N0 M0) and stage II (T1 N1M0) breast carcinoma. J Clin Oncol 1989;7:355–66.

76. Chu KC, Smart CR, Tarone RE. Analysis of breast cancer mortality and stage distribution by age for the Health Insurance Plan clinical trial. J Natl Cancer Inst 1988;80(14):1125–32.

77. Swedish Organised Service Screening Evaluation Group. Effect of mammographic service screening on stage at presentation of breast cancers in Sweden. Cancer 2007;109(11):2205–12.

78. Oberaigner W, Geiger-Gritsch S, Edlinger M, et al. Reduction in advanced breast cancer after introduction of a mammography screening program in Tyrol/ Austria. Breast 2017;33:178–82.

79. Malmgren JA, Parikh J, Atwood MK, et al. Impact of mammography detection on the course of breast cancer in women aged 40-49 years. Radiology 2012;262(3):797–806.

80. Destounis SV, Arieno AL, Morgan RC, et al. Comparison of breast cancers diagnosed in screening patients in their 40s with and without family history of breast cancer in a community outpatient facility. Am Journal Rev 2014;202:928–32.

81. Price ER, Keedy AW, Gidwaney R, et al. The Potential Impact of Risk-Based Screening Mammography in Women 40-49 Years Old. AJR Am J Roentgenol 2015;205(6):1360–4.

82. Michaelson J, Satlja S, Kopans D, et al. Gauging the Impact of Breast Carcinoma Screening in Terms of Tumor Size and Death Rate. Cancer 2003;98: 2114–24.

83. Michaelson JS, Halpern E, Kopans DB. Breast cancer: computer simulation method for estimating optimal intervals for screening. Radiology 1999; 212(2):551–60.

84. Available at: https://press.rsna.org/timssnet/media/ pressreleases/14_pr_target.cfm?ID=2123 last accessed December/27/2023

Venous Interventions
Controversies in the Management of Acute Deep Venous Thrombosis and the Role of the Interventional Radiologist

Rocío G. Márquez, MD, Kush R. Desai, MD*

KEYWORDS

• Deep venous thrombosis • Pulmonary embolism • Post-thrombotic syndrome

KEY POINTS

- Anticoagulation remains the reference standard treatment of acute deep venous thrombosis (DVT).
- Up to 50% of patients with DVT develop post-thrombotic syndrome (PTS)—a major determinant of morbidity and health-related quality of life. Endovascular therapies (ETs) have become of interest in resolving venous obstruction as a means of mitigating the symptoms of PTS.
- Results of early comparative studies and multicenter randomized trials have demonstrated the ability of endovascular treatments to reduce disease severity in patients with iliofemoral venous involvement—a phenotypically distinct entity from DVT isolated to more caudal distributions.
- Additional studies evaluating new devices, including those that are lytic-free, are needed.
- At this time, treatment and prevention of PTS should be a multidisciplinary effort to identify the cohort of patients most likely to benefit from ET through an individualized, patient-centered approach.

ACUTE LOWER EXTREMITY DEEP VEIN THROMBOSIS AND POST-THROMBOTIC SYNDROME: SCOPE OF THE PROBLEM

Lower extremity deep venous thrombosis (DVT) is a highly prevalent disease, occurring in an estimated 1 in 1000 persons per year; along with pulmonary embolism (PE), it is the third most common cause of cardiovascular morbidity and mortality after coronary artery disease (CAD) and stroke in Western populations.[1,2] The term *acute* DVT has variable definitions, with pivotal trials referring to thrombosis identified from 14 to 21 days of symptom onset, while the term *chronic* DVT is often used colloquially to reflect post-thrombotic obstruction with organized, collagenous material.[2]

Proximal DVT involves the iliofemoral or femoropopliteal distribution, whereas *distal* DVT is isolated to the deep veins of the calf without involvement of the popliteal vein. DVT typically mandates medical and possibly interventional management when it involves the popliteal veins or above. Infrapopliteal DVT without severe symptoms or risk factors for extension can instead be followed with serial imaging for 2 weeks to verify for proximal extension of thrombus[3]; most observational studies have shown that distal DVT will resolve spontaneously without medical treatment and embolization is unlikely unless there is extension into proximal veins.

Anticoagulation remains the mainstay of DVT treatment, through the reduction of PE risk,

Division of Vascular and Interventional Radiology, Department of Radiology, Northwestern University Feinberg School of Medicine, Chicago, IL, USA
* Corresponding author. Department of Radiology, Northwestern University, Feinberg School of Medicine, 676 North St. Clair Street, Suite 800, Chicago, IL 60611.
E-mail address: Kdesai007@northwestern.edu

Radiol Clin N Am 62 (2024) 1003–1011
https://doi.org/10.1016/j.rcl.2024.04.006
0033-8389/24/© 2024 Elsevier Inc. All rights reserved.

thrombus propagation, and thrombus recurrence; however, many patients go on to develop manifestations of post-thrombotic syndrome (PTS). PTS develops in up to 50% of patients after DVT and is a major determinant of morbidity and health-related quality of life (HRQOL), associated with major socioeconomic costs.[4] A study conducted in the United States in 2001 estimated that the annual direct cost of PTS is at least 200 million dollars.[5] It is also estimated that approximately 2 million workdays are lost annually in the United States because of venolymphatic lower extremity ulceration.[6] An analysis of a Swedish cohort demonstrated that the additional long-term health care costs of post-thrombotic complications are approximately 75% the cost of primary DVT.[7]

A retrospective study followed a cohort of 387 patients of which 60% had proximal DVT and determined that the presence of PTS alone independently predicted 2 year Venous Disease-specific Venous Insufficiency Epidemiologic and Economic Study Quality of Life (VEINES-QOL) and VEINES-Symptoms VEINES-Sym questionnaire scores.[8]

POST-THROMBOTIC SYNDROME: PATHOPHYSIOLOGY AND THE "OPEN VEIN HYPOTHESIS"

PTS refers to a symptom complex characterized by limb edema, heaviness, pain, venous claudication (progressive pain/heaviness with standing/walking), limb hyperpigmentation, and the most severe manifestation, venous stasis ulceration.[9] Several scoring systems have been developed to both diagnose the condition and classify its severity, most notably the Villalta score and the Venous Clinical Severity Score (VCSS). These scores also serve as a continuous measurement for longer term follow-up to grade disease progression and assess the effectiveness of treatments.[10] Adjunctive scoring with the VCSS has been proposed, with some suggesting greater objectivity, along with increased sensitivity of this metric at the severe end of the disease spectrum.[10]

The development of PTS is a result of 2 major processes[11]: venous outflow obstruction and an incited inflammatory response that directly damages venous valves, alters the composition of the vein wall, and leads to valvular reflux. This interplay of venous obstruction and insufficiency leads to ambulatory venous hypertension. The "open vein hypothesis" suggests that the quantity of residual thrombus predicts the development of PTS; therefore, thrombus elimination and restoration of deep venous flow may yield benefit in PTS severity reduction. A systematic meta-analysis of 11

randomized DVT trials[12] suggested a predictive correlation for thrombus burden change and the development of recurrent venous thromboembolism (VTE; relative risk 0.56; 95% CI 0.42–0.76).

While numerous studies have addressed the risk of recurrent VTE following DVT, few to our knowledge have provided longitudinal data on the risks for developing PTS. A prospective multicenter study of long-term outcomes after DVT aimed to identify potential predictors of PTS, demonstrating that patients who developed PTS were more likely to be older, have atherosclerotic risk factors (such as hypertension and hypercholesterolemia), higher.

Body Mass Index and Longer Duration of Deep Venous Thrombosis Symptoms Before Diagnosis

A subsequent prospective multicohort study of 387 outpatients[13] reported that greater PTS severity category at the 1 month visit strongly predicted higher PTS scores throughout the 24 month follow-up. Additional predictors of higher scores over time were venous thrombosis of the common femoral or iliac vein (2.23 increase in score vs distal calf venous thrombosis), previous ipsilateral venous thrombosis (1.78 increase in score), older age (0.30 increase in score per 10 year age increase), and female sex (0.79 increase in score).

Quality and adherence to anticoagulation therapy also influences later development of PTS. It is estimated that patients treated with vitamin K antagonists (VKAs) spend only 60% of time between a therapeutic international normalized ratio (INR). A prospective cohort study followed 244 patients with symptomatic episode of proximal DVT who were treated with VKA for at least 3 months and conducted follow-up assessments for a maximum of 5 years. Multivariate model showed that patients who spend more than 50% of time beneath an INR level of 2.0 are at over 2 fold higher risk of PTS.[14] Fortunately, the development of direct oral anticoagulants, which do not require active monitoring, has reduced the risk of patients being subtherapeutic.

ANTICOAGULATION AS FIRST-LINE THERAPY

The national DVT registry (1999) emphasized that the therapeutic goals for treating patients with acute DVT should encompass "prevention of pulmonary embolism, restoration of unobstructed blood flow through the thrombosed segment and preservation of venous valve function." Systemic anticoagulants have thus been the cornerstone of DVT therapy since as early as the 1960s,[15] with current evidence suggesting that anticoagulant therapy changes clot burden and long term influences the frequency of recurrent VTE.

Most recent anticoagulation guidelines suggest that selection of an anticoagulant agent should be made in the context of understanding patient's overall clinical condition, patient comorbidities (eg, cancer, pregnancy, renal failure), risk of bleeding, and patient preference. In most patients with DVT who hemodynamically stable, initial anticoagulation consists of administration of anticoagulant drug, preferably subcutaneous low molecular weight heparin (LMWH), fondaparinux, or the oral factor Xa inhibitors, such as rivaroxaban or apixaban, immediately following the diagnosis of DVT to decrease risk for potential life-threatening embolization. Duration of therapy should be determined based on the presence or absence of risk factors for recurrence, whether the DVT was provoked or unprovoked, and if there is a history of active cancer, though in general should be maintained for a minimum of 3 months. In patients with unprovoked DVT, length of therapy should be extended and reevaluated at least on an annual basis, and at times of significant change in health status.[3]

While studies show that anticoagulation alone serves to prevent thrombus extension and embolization to the pulmonary arteries, it is not protective against PTS as it does not directly lyse the thrombus that is already present. However, endovascular therapy (ET), including catheter-directed thrombolysis (CDT), and more recently mechanical thrombectomy, allows for active thrombus dissolution or removal (Fig. 1). Numerous clinical studies have observed a reduction in PTS burden in patients who have undergone ET.[12,16–18] A Cochrane database systematic meta-analysis noted an estimated risk reduction of 0.64 for developing PTS after undergoing CDT when compared to anticoagulation alone.[19]

Interventional strategies to achieve early thrombus removal and restoration of unobstructed deep venous flow have thus become the subject of several studies comparing these to standard anticoagulation therapy alone,[12] predominantly for their role in limiting PTS.

EVIDENCE-BASED ROLE OF CATHETER-DIRECTED THROMBOLYSIS AND PHARMACOMECHANICAL THROMBECTOMY IN PREVENTION OF POST-THROMBOTIC SYNDROME: EARLY SUPPORTIVE STUDIES

The most substantive data evaluating CDT in limiting PTS stem from two large multicenter randomized trials comparing the use of CDT or pharmachomechanical CDT (PCDT) combined with standard anticoagulation against standard anticoagulation alone for DVT in predicting the occurrence of PTS as determined by the Villalta score. However, earlier and smaller comparative studies demonstrated some benefit to CDT in prevention of PTS, albeit with several methodologic limitations (Fig. 2).

As early as 1999, the organized multicenter national DVT registry assessed the impact of CDT in patients with symptomatic DVT by means of venography in patients who had undergone urokinase infusions.[20] Patients with iliofemoral DVT were demonstrated to have greater impact following thrombolysis than those with femoropopliteal DVT, acute DVT better than chronic DVT, and catheter-directed therapy better than systemic infusions. The degree of lysis was found to be a significant predictor of early and continued patency, as approximately 75% of limbs in which complete lysis was achieved remained patent at 1 year compared with 32% of limbs in which less than 50% lysis was achieved. No infusion achieved complete lysis when isolated femoropopliteal DVT was present for more than 10 days, suggesting a contributing factor of time-to-lysis in its success.

Comerota and colleagues [21] conducted a retrospective study to evaluate the potential benefit of CDT in improving HRQOL for patients with iliofemoral DVT when compared with patients treated with standard anticoagulation alone. Questionnaires were administered to 98 retrospectively identified patients with iliofemoral DVT within the last 6 months, all of whom were candidates for both anticoagulation and CDT. Results demonstrated that patients who underwent CDT had better functioning and well-being when compared with those patients treated with anticoagulation alone. They reported overall improved physical function and fewer sequelae of PTS. Furthermore, venographically successful lysis correlated with improved HRQOL.

THE CATHETER-DIRECTED VENOUS THROMBOLYSIS TRIAL

The Catheter-directed Venous Thrombolysis (CAVENT) trial was the first randomized-controlled trial to evaluate the clinically relevant effect of adding CDT for patients with acute proximal DVT above the level of the mid-thigh in reducing the development of PTS compared to conventional treatment alone. A total of 209 patients, aged 18 to 75 years, with a first-time acute DVT (<21 days from symptom onset) were included across 20 hospitals from the Norwegian southeastern health region.[22] The 2 primary endpoints were iliofemoral patency after 6 months and frequency of PTS after 24 months

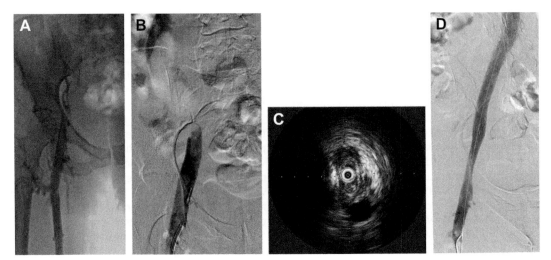

Fig. 1. Mechanical thrombectomy of left lower extremity iliofemoral thrombosis. (*A*) Prone spot image during left common femoral (LCF) venography demonstrates partial thrombosis of the proximal left common femoral vein (LCFV) and subtotal thrombosis of the left external iliac (LEI) and common iliac (CI) veins. (*B*) Mechanical (aspiration) thrombectomy performed, resulting in subtotal resolution of acute thrombus. (*C*) Intravascular ultrasound (IVUS) catheter demonstrates thrombotic expansion of the left external iliac vein (LEIV). (*D*) Completion venography demonstrates subtotal luminal restoration after 16 × 120 mm (Venovo) self-expanding stent deployment within an underlying segment of LCIV stenosis due to an overriding RCIA.

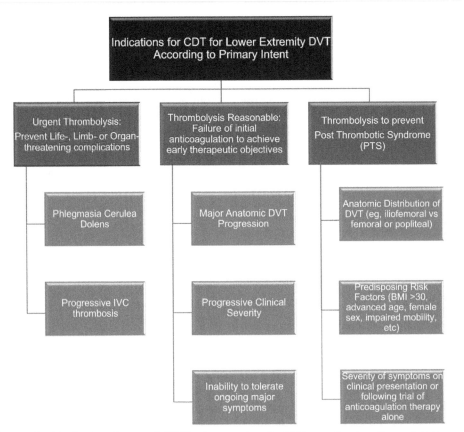

Fig. 2. Summarized indications for use of CDT for lower extremity DVT according to primary intent.

as measured by a Villalta score ($\geq$5), with secondary effect variables including recurrent VTE during follow-up, bleeding related to CDT, and others. All patients were initiated on anticoagulation on the day of diagnosis in accordance with international guidelines, consisting of LMWH in combination with oral warfarin for at least 5 days until reaching an INR between 2 to 3. The mean duration of CDT was 2.4 days, but recombinant tissue plasminogen activity (rTPA) infusions could be continued up to 4 days. Thrombectomy devices were not used, and thrombus burden was assessed with venography. In the 2 year results, patients in the treatment group demonstrated an absolute reduced frequency of PTS of 14.4% (95%CI 0.2–27.9). Of note, most cases of PTS were reported as mild severity, and there was no statistically significant effect on long-term quality of life. Subsequent sub-analyses allowed review of their venography data and quantification of thrombus load to calculate scores (14 point scale), revealing statistically significant correlation of thrombus score after CDT with increased vessel patency at 24 months.[23]

Results of a 5 year follow-up were reported in 2016,[4] with data available for 84% of patients originally randomized. The absolute risk reduction of 14% after 2 years increased to 28% (95% CI 14–42) in the treatment group, and the number needed to treat decreased from 7 to 4 (95% CI 2–7), supporting the hypothesis that early thrombus elimination and restoration of flow may prevent PTS. Again, however, this reduction in the occurrence of PTS did not result in better quality of life. While results of this study suggested a promising role for CDT, several limitations include modest recruitment size, the fact that an only infusion CDT technique was used relative to the modern US practice featuring thrombectomy devices,[24] and the inherent possibility of bias from an open-label design. Further, overall treatment efficacy may have also been reduced by the limited use of angioplasty and stent placement within the pelvic veins, which may have failed to correct underlying venous stenosis.

THE ACUTE VENOUS THROMBOSIS: THROMBUS REMOVAL WITH ADJUNCTIVE CATHETER-DIRECTED THROMBOLYSIS TRIAL

The ATTRACT trial is the largest multicenter randomized open-label-controlled clinical trial to date of relevance to this topic, to our knowledge. The trial involved a larger cohort of 692 patients from 56 clinical centers in the United States. Patients selected were diagnosed with acute proximal DVT extending above the level of the popliteal vein and randomized to receive or not receive PCDT with rTPA delivery using several methods, which involved additional mechanical thrombectomy devices. Unlike the CAVENT trial, rTPA infusions were limited to no more than 30 hours and dose did not exceed 35 mg. Primary efficacy outcomes were the development of PTS (Villalta score of $\geq$5) at 6 and 24 months of follow-up. The clinical severity of PTS was also evaluated at 6, 12, 18, and 24 months using the Villalta and VCSS. Secondary outcomes included HRQOL at baseline and at 24 months, assessed with the VEINES-QOL questionnaire. There was no significant reduction of PTS over 2 years (49% PCDT vs 51% control; RR 0.95, 95%CI 0.78–1.15), seemingly contradicting results of the previous CAVENT trial. The PCDT treatment group, however, did have a greater improvement in early leg pain and swelling within 30 days and reduced occurrence of moderate to severe PTS over 2 years (18% PCDT vs 28% control; RR 0.65, 95%CI 0.45–0.94). PCDT also lead to a measurable QOL benefit within the first 6 months (9 points on the VEINES-QOL scale). Major bleeding occurring within 10 days occurred in 6 patients (1.7%) assigned to the PCDT group, as compared with 1 patient in the control group.

Given the larger size of this trial and wider geographic and demographic scope, results served to question previous literature supporting adjunctive CDT in patients with proximal acute DVT. However, several limitations from the ATTRACT trial and differences in tested cohorts must be acknowledged. It is known that the design of prospective trails that aim for statistical significance require "careful selection of a highly defined, and very specific patient population that can be compared, sacrificing some generalizability to the heterogeneity of patients that are encountered in real clinical practice."[25] The cohort of patients studied in the ATTRACT trial included those with involvement of the femoropopliteal segments alone, in part to ensure statistical purity and meet recruitment goals to power the study in a reasonable timeframe. It is known that there is a 2 fold higher risk of PTS in patients with iliofemoral thrombosis, but limiting enrollment to these cases may have impeded recruitment. Thus, it should be noted that the study was powered to answer whether "the entire group, both iliofemoral and more distal femoropopliteal DVT combined, experienced improved outcomes with PCDT."[25] Recent guidelines acknowledge that patients with iliofemoral DVT are phenotypically distinct from patients with calf or femoropopliteal DVT based on more frequent recurrence of thromboembolism, higher risk of PTS, and more severe presentation of PTS.[26] This may relate to the observation that venous recanalization occurs less often in patients with iliofemoral thrombosis.

A subanalysis of the ATTRACT trial stratified patients by most proximal extent of their DVT (iliofemoral vs femoropopliteal) before randomization, allowing for an exploratory analysis on these two distinct phenotypical entities.[26] Their data collectively suggested that PCDT improved short-term recovery from DVT and reduced long-term progression of PTS severity in patients with iliofemoral DVT. In this specific cohort of patients, there was greater reduction in leg pain and swelling through 30 days and even greater improvement in venous disease-specific QOL from baseline to 24 months (5.6 points on VEINES-QOL scale). Logically, definitive conclusions cannot be drawn from these analyses as only 57% of patients had iliofemoral DVT, limiting the power of this analysis.

Another subanalysis of the ATTTRACT trial[27] aimed to investigate known and newer predictors of the development of PTS in the population of patients from the ATTRACT trial "using multi-variable logistic regression to identify baseline and postbaseline factors predictive of PTS during study follow-up." Results suggest that age, sex, and BMI were predictors of PTS development in this cohort. The use of rivaroxaban at day 10 was found to have a more pronounced protective effect for moderate-to-severe PTS (odds ratio [OR] 0.53), suggesting that the choice of anticoagulant may also play a small role in development of PTS.

Despite its widespread use in clinical practice, there remain a lack of data that compare specific mechanical thrombectomy strategies, devices, or adjunctive therapies, to our knowledge. An additional subanalysis of the ATTRACT trial[28] by Vedantham and colleagues identified 33 sites where physicians had designated use of rheolytic thrombectomy (AngioJet, Boston Scientific, Marlborough, MA) as their preferred instrument for PCDT. These patients were randomized to a strategy of PCDT that incorporated either rhizolysis with anticoagulation compared with anticoagulation alone to evaluate PTS, QOL, and safety over 24 months of follow-up. Results suggested that use of AngioJet-PCDT reduced PTS at 6 months (24% with AngioJet-PCDT vs 40% with control), but did not influence PTS nor QOL between 12 and 24 months. Complications such as major bleeding or PE were infrequent with AngioJet PCDT (<2% each; **Table 1**).

SUMMARY AND FUTURE DIRECTIONS

National health organizations and medical specialty societies have developed specific recommendations on endovascular management for patients with acute DVT. For example, per the American College of Chest Physicians (2021), anticoagulant therapy alone is suggested over interventional therapy for patients with acute DVT of the leg, unless there is very severe, limb-threatening DVT, when benefit of rapid thrombus resolution may outweigh risk of harm. The European Society of Vascular Surgery, on the other hand, suggests considering early thrombus removal strategies in select patients with symptomatic iliofemoral DVT, but not for patients with DVT limited to femoral, popliteal, or calf veins.

In essence, treatment and prevention of PTS in patients with DVT should be a multimodal and interdisciplinary effort to identify the population of patients most likely to benefit from ETs through a selective, individualized, patient-centered approach. Several of the subanalyses of the ATTRACT trial serve to underscore the importance of addressing varying anatomic distributions of DVT as distinct phenotypical entities, and this should be considered when devising a treatment strategy. Acknowledging the distinct populations of patients with acute iliofemoral versus femoral DVT, popliteal or calf DVT, recent guidelines encourage "judicious use of ET in a manner that optimizes benefit and minimizes harm" by carefully considering patient-specific variables including projected risk of bleeding, clinical severity of DVT, anatomic extent of DVT and baseline ambulatory capacity and comorbidities, and others. ET should not be routinely performed in pregnant patients, children, or younger adolescents, unless there are compelling clinical indications (ie, acute limb ischemia or unacceptably high risk from progression despite anticoagulation). Overall, the decision to intervene should be based on the primary intent of treatment.[24]

While compelling benefit of large-scale use of thrombolytic therapy has yet to be demonstrated given the increased risk of bleeding, endovascular treatments have shown the ability to reduce disease severity in patients with iliofemoral venous involvement. Additional investigative studies to find alternate ways to eliminate thrombus and open veins without increased risk of bleeding are needed to consolidate the management of acute DVT. Furthermore, data from the CAVENT and ATTRACT trial noted development of PTS in 44% patients who did undergo CDT, suggesting that alternate underlying mechanisms not influenced by the thromboreductive effect of fibrinolytics or thrombectomy are at physiologically at play; further understanding of these mechanisms is necessary to direct focused investigations on therapeutic targets.[29,30] Few recent studies have turned attention to investigating the safety and efficacy of venous-specific thrombectomy devices that would result in rapid thrombus elimination and immediate

Table 1
Key differences between the Catheter-directed Venous Thrombolysis and ATTRACT trial

	CAVENT	ATTRACT
Overview	Open-label, randomized controlled trial involving 209 patients with a first-time acute *iliofemoral DVT*, randomly allocated to treatment groups: conventional treatment alone or additional CDT.	Multicenter, randomized, open-label assessor-blinded, controlled clinical trial involving 692 patients with acute DVT *extending above the popliteal vein*, randomized to receive single session PCDT plus anticoagulation or anticoagulation alone.
Primary outcomes	• Frequency of PTS as assessed by Villalta score at 24 mo • Iliofemoral patency after 6 mo	• Development of post-thrombotic syndrome between 6 and 24 mo of follow-up
Demographics	• Patients aged 18–75 y from across *20* hospitals across the *Norwegian* southeastern health region.	• Patients aged 16–75 y from across *56* clinical centers in the *United States*.
Results	• At 24 mo, 41% (95% CI 31.5–51.4) patients allocated to receive CDT presented with PTS vs 55.6% (95% CI 45.7–65.0) in the control group (*P* = .047). • This difference represents an absolute risk reduction of 14% (95% CI 0.2–27.9). • Iliofemoral patency at 6 mo was reported in 65.9% (95% CI 55.5–75.0) in CDT group vs 47.4% (95% a 37.6–57.3) on control(*P* = .012).	• Between 6–24 mo, there was no significant difference in the development of PTS between groups. • Subgroup analyses demonstrated reduced PTS severity in select patients with isolated acute iliofemoral DVT. • At 24 mo, there was no significant difference in recurrence of venous thromboembolism between groups. • Severity scores for those who had PTS were lower in the PCDT group than in control *P* < .01.
Complications	20 bleeding complications related to CDT were reported (3 were classified as "major" and 5 as "clinically relevant").	PCDT led to increased "major" bleeding events within 10 d (1.7% vs 0.3%, *P* = .049).
Limitations	• Inherent potential for bias from an open-label design • Modest sample size • Use of older drug-only infusion CDT technique relative to current US practice including adjunctive mechanical devices	• Inherent potential for bias from an open-label design • Analyses did not acknowledge the phenotypically distinct entities of iliofemoral DVT and those with femoropopliteal or popliteal segments alone upon drawing conclusions • Substantial number of loss to follow-up and missing assessments of post-thrombotic syndrome

re-establishment of venous flow. For example, aspiration devices (Indigo Lightning/FLASH, Penumbra, Alameda, CA) use pressure sensors to optimize continuous or intermittent thrombus aspiration. Rheolytic devices (Angioget ZelanteDVT, Boston Scientific, MN) inject pressurized saline so that through Bernoulli effect, thrombus is drawn into the catheter. The multicenter prospective CLOUT registry seeks to assess the safety and effectiveness of the ClotTriever System (Inari Medical, Irvine, CA) for the treatment of acute and nonacute lower extremity DVT in all-comer patients. Effectiveness end point was defined as complete or near-complete (≥75%) thrombus removal determined by independent core laboratory-adjudicated Marder scores. Of the first enrolled 250 patients, the primary effectiveness end point was achieved in 86% of limbs treated in a single session without thrombolytics. At 6 months follow-up, 24% of patients had PTS.[31] While promising results thus far, the lack of a comparator arm limits the validity of these results. Future investigations should include valid comparator arms and uniform treatment arms to minimize bias.

CLINICS CARE POINTS

- Patients with acute iliofemoral deep vein thrombosis are the most likely to benefit from an endovascular intervention through reduction of future severity of post-thrombotic syndrome.
- Patients with isolated femoropopliteal deeo vein thrombosis are not likely to benefit from an endovascular intervention, in most cases.

FUNDING

No funding sources.

REFERENCES

1. Lin M, Hsieh JCF, Hanif M, et al. Evaluation of thrombolysis using tissue plasminogen activator in lower extremity deep venous thrombosis with concomitant femoral-popliteal venous segment involvement. J Vasc Surg Venous Lymphat Disord 2017;5(5): 613–20.
2. Sista AK, Vedantham S, Kaufman JA, et al. Endovascular Interventions for Acute and Chronic Lower Extremity Deep Venous Disease: State of the Art. Radiology 2015;276(1):31–53.
3. Stevens SM, Woller SC, Kreuziger LB, et al. Antithrombotic Therapy for VTE Disease: Second Update of the CHEST Guideline and Expert Panel Report. Chest 2021;160(6):e545–608.
4. Haig Y, Enden T, Grøtta O, et al. Post-thrombotic syndrome after catheter-directed thrombolysis for deep vein thrombosis (CaVenT): 5-year follow-up results of an open-label, randomised controlled trial. Lancet Haematol 2016;3(2):e64–71.
5. Heit JA, Rooke TW, Silverstein MD, et al. Trends in the incidence of venous stasis syndrome and venous ulcer: a 25-year population-based study. J Vasc Surg 2001;33(5):1022–7.
6. Phillips T, Stanton B, Provan A, et al. A study of the impact of leg ulcers on quality of life: financial, social, and psychologic implications. J Am Acad Dermatol 1994;31(1):49–53.
7. Bergqvist D, Jendteg S, Johansen L, et al. Cost of long-term complications of deep venous thrombosis of the lower extremities: an analysis of a defined patient population in Sweden. Ann Intern Med 1997; 126(6):454–7.
8. Kahn SR, Shbaklo H, Lamping DL, et al. Determinants of health-related quality of life during the 2 years following deep vein thrombosis. J Thromb Haemostasis 2008;6(7):1105–12.
9. Vedantham S, Thorpe PE, Cardella JF, et al. Quality improvement guidelines for the treatment of lower extremity deep vein thrombosis with use of endovascular thrombus removal. J Vasc Intervent Radiol 2009;20(7 Suppl):S227–39.
10. Soosainathan A, Moore HM, Gohel MS, et al. Scoring systems for the post-thrombotic syndrome. J Vasc Surg 2013;57(1):254–61.
11. Kahn SR. The post-thrombotic syndrome: progress and pitfalls. Br J Haematol 2006;134(4):357–65.
12. Hull RD, Marder VJ, Mah AF, et al. Quantitative assessment of thrombus burden predicts the outcome of treatment for venous thrombosis: a systematic review. Am J Med 2005;118(5):456–64.
13. Kahn SR, Shrier I, Julian JA, et al. Determinants and time course of the postthrombotic syndrome after acute deep venous thrombosis. Ann Intern Med 2008;149(10):698–707.
14. van Dongen CJ, Prandoni P, Frulla M, et al. Relation between quality of anticoagulant treatment and the development of the postthrombotic syndrome. J Thromb Haemostasis 2005;3(5):939–42.
15. Elsharawy M, Elzayat E. Early results of thrombolysis vs anticoagulation in iliofemoral venous thrombosis. A randomised clinical trial. Eur J Vasc Endovasc Surg 2002;24(3):209–14.
16. Roumen-Klappe EM, den Heijer M, Janssen MCH, et al. The post-thrombotic syndrome: incidence and prognostic value of non-invasive venous examinations in a six-year follow-up study. Thromb Haemostasis 2005;94(4):825–30.
17. Plate G, Akesson H, Einarsson E, et al. Long-term results of venous thrombectomy combined with a temporary arterio-venous fistula. Eur J Vasc Surg 1990;4(5):483–9.
18. Meissner MH, Manzo RA, Bergelin RO, et al. Deep venous insufficiency: the relationship between lysis and subsequent reflux. J Vasc Surg 1993;18(4): 596–605 [discussion 606-8].
19. Watson L, Broderick C, Armon MP. Thrombolysis for acute deep vein thrombosis. Cochrane Database Syst Rev 2014;(1):Cd002783.
20. Mewissen MW, Seabrook GR, Meissner MH, et al. Catheter-directed thrombolysis for lower extremity deep venous thrombosis: report of a national multicenter registry. Radiology 1999;211(1):39–49.
21. Comerota AJ, Throm RC, Mathias SD, et al. Catheter-directed thrombolysis for iliofemoral deep venous thrombosis improves health-related quality of life. J Vasc Surg 2000;32(1):130–7.
22. Enden T, Haig Y, Kløw NE, et al. Long-term outcome after additional catheter-directed thrombolysis versus standard treatment for acute iliofemoral deep vein thrombosis (the CaVenT study): a randomised controlled trial. Lancet 2012;379(9810):31–8.
23. Kuo WT. Optimizing catheter-directed thrombolysis for acute deep vein thrombosis: validating the open

vein hypothesis. J Vasc Intervent Radiol 2013;24(1): 24–6.

24. Vedantham S, Desai KR, Weinberg I, et al. Society of interventional radiology position statement on the endovascular management of acute iliofemoral deep vein thrombosis. J Vasc Intervent Radiol 2023;34(2):284–99.e7.

25. Das M. Does ATTRACT change our DVT management practice? Br J Radiol 2021;94(1120):20200939.

26. Comerota AJ, Kearon C, Gu CS, et al. Endovascular thrombus removal for acute iliofemoral deep vein thrombosis. Circulation 2019;139(9):1162–73.

27. Rinfret F, Gu CS, Vedantham S, et al. New and known predictors of the postthrombotic syndrome: A subanalysis of the ATTRACT trial. Res Pract Thromb Haemost 2022;6(6):e12796.

28. Vedantham S, Salter A, Lancia S, et al. Clinical outcomes of a pharmacomechanical catheter-directed venous thrombolysis strategy that included rheolytic thrombectomy in a multicenter randomized trial. J Vasc Intervent Radiol 2021;32(9):1296–309.e7.

29. Huang MH, Benishay ET, Desai KR. Endovascular management of acute iliofemoral deep vein thrombosis. Semin Intervent Radiol 2022;39(5):459–63.

30. Desai KR, Grewal S, Shah R, et al. Endovascular management of acute lower extremity deep vein thrombosis: rationale for use and lessons learned from emerging clinical trials. Advances in Clinical Radiology 2019;1:251–7.

31. Dexter DJ, Kado H, Schor J, et al. Interim outcomes of mechanical thrombectomy for deep vein thrombosis from the All-Comer CLOUT Registry. J Vasc Surg Venous Lymphat Disord 2022;10(4):832–40.e2.

Imaging of Cirrhosis and Hepatocellular Carcinoma
Current Evidence

Krishna Shanbhogue, MD*, Hersh Chandarana, MD

KEYWORDS

- Cirrhosis • Hepatocellular carcinoma • Liver Imaging Reporting and Data System

KEY POINTS

- Imaging plays an important role in screening and diagnosis of hepatocellular carcinoma (HCC) in at risk populations and enables individualized management.
- Current HCC surveillance strategies (ultrasound ± serum alpha fetoprotein) have suboptimal sensitivity for detection of HCC. Role of newer serum markers and abbreviated MRI are evolving.
- MRI outperforms computed tomography for the diagnosis of early HCCs; the choice of MRI contrast agent (extracellular agent vs hepatobiliary specific agent) is determined by the intended sensitivity and specificity for HCC diagnosis.

INTRODUCTION

Worldwide, liver cancer is the sixth most common cancer and the third most common cause of cancer-related death.[1] With the current rate of newly diagnosed cancers, the number of new cases and deaths from liver cancer are predicted to increase by 50% over the next 2 decades.[2] Hepatocellular carcinoma (HCC) accounts for over three-fourths of all primary liver malignancies and majority of HCCs (90%) arise in patients with cirrhosis or chronic liver disease secondary to hepatitis B, alcohol abuse, or non-alcoholic liver disease.[3,4] In this article, the authors aim to provide a current update on imaging diagnosis of cirrhosis and HCC.

DIAGNOSIS OF CIRRHOSIS

Cirrhosis is diagnosed by a combination of clinical history, physical examination, laboratory findings, and imaging findings[5] (Fig. 1). Early and accurate diagnosis of hepatic fibrosis has several implications. The stage of hepatic fibrosis at initial diagnosis has been shown to predict the 5-year risk of disease progression, death, and development of hepatocellular carcinoma.[6] Laboratory findings of cirrhosis include abnormal liver function tests (elevated aspartate aminotransferase [AST] and alanine transaminase for over 6 m) with or without low platelets and elevated international normalised ratio [INR].[5] However, laboratory results can be normal in compensated cirrhosis raising the need for accurate biomarkers to detect earlier stages of liver fibrosis and compensated cirrhosis. Conventional imaging modalities that assess the morphologic changes of cirrhosis including surface nodularity and lobar redistribution (atrophy of the posterior right lobe and medial left lobe, hypertrophy of the caudate lobe and lateral left lobe) are limited by poor sensitivity and specificity for the detection of hepatic fibrosis, with reported area under the curve (AUC) of 0.54 to 0.80[7] (Fig. 2). Elastography-based techniques are increasingly used to detect and stage hepatic fibrosis with high diagnostic accuracy (AUC of >0.90) for detection of advanced fibrosis.[8,9] Several laboratory indices including Fibrosis-4 (FIB-4) index, enhanced liver fibrosis score (ELF score), and AST to platelet ratio index score

Department of Radiology, NYU Langone Health, 660 1st Avenue, 3rd Floor, New York, NY 10016, USA
* Corresponding author.
E-mail address: Krishna.shanbhogue@nyulangone.org

Radiol Clin N Am 62 (2024) 1013–1023
https://doi.org/10.1016/j.rcl.2024.04.004
0033-8389/24/© 2024 Elsevier Inc. All rights reserved.

radiologic.theclinics.com

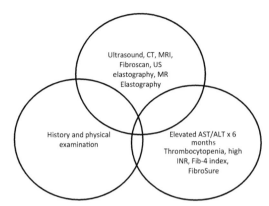

Fig. 1. Schematic representation of diagnosis of cirrhosis. Cirrhosis is diagnosed by a combination of clinical history, physical examination, laboratory findings, and imaging findings. Liver biopsy remains the gold standard for the diagnosis of cirrhosis and staging hepatic fibrosis.

(APRI) have emerged in the last decade, with reported AUC of up to 0.89 for detection of advanced fibrosis.[10] Consequently, combination of imaging and laboratory-based biomarkers have evolved recently, including MAST index (Magnetic resonance elastography [MRE], proton density fat fraction [PDFF], and AST) and MEFIB Index (MRE and FIB-4), which have shown high performance for the detection of fibrosis.[11] Although MRE has been reported to be as accurate as liver biopsy,[12] biopsy remains the reference standard for detection and staging of liver fibrosis.[13] Liver biopsies are, however, invasive, prone to sampling error, as well as inter- and intra-observer variability.[13]

SCREENING OF HEPATOCELLULAR CARCINOMA
Current Screening Guidelines

HCC screening is typically performed by bi-annual ultrasound with or without serum alpha fetoprotein (AFP) testing in at-risk individuals. A large population-based study on 9000 patients with hepatitis B infection in China revealed that 6 monthly surveillance ultrasound with AFP resulted in 37% reduction in mortality compared with the unscreened group.[14] A meta-analysis of 47 studies (15,158 patients) revealed statistically significantly higher pooled 3-year survival in patients who underwent surveillance (50.8%) compared with the control group (27.9%).[15] Surveillance in patients at high-risk for developing HCC is therefore no longer controversial because it enables early detection and curative therapies including liver resection and transplantation, improving the overall survival. The target population, optimal surveillance interval,

and techniques used in surveillance may vary amongst various current screening guidelines. The current eastern guidelines including the Asia-Pacific Association for the Study of the Liver (APASL 2017), the Korean Liver Cancer Association-National Cancer Center Korea (KLCA-NCC 2018), the Japan Society of Hepatology (JSH 2021), and the China Liver Cancer national guidelines (CNLC 2019) recommend 6-monthly surveillance ultrasound with serum AFP. The current American Association for the Study of Liver Diseases (AASLD) and European Association for the Study of the Liver (EASL) guidelines recommend 6-month surveillance with ultrasound with or without serum AFP testing. The target population for screening includes any patient with cirrhosis (Child-Pugh A and B, Child-Pugh C awaiting liver transplant, with an estimated HCC risk of >1.5%/ y), and select patients with chronic hepatitis B with HCC risk of greater than 0.2% per year.[16] The most widely accepted interval for screening is 6 months, which is based on doubling time of HCC, rather than risk of developing HCC.[17]

Limitations of Current Surveillance Strategies

In spite of availability of several elaborate screening guidelines, fewer than 50% of patients who are diagnosed with HCC meet Milan criteria for liver transplant allocation,[18] and survival rates for HCC are dismally low, with fewer than a third of the patients surviving 5 years after the diagnosis.[19] Delayed diagnosis is a major factor contributing to the poor survival rates in HCC. The 5-year survival rate for HCC drops from 70% for early-stage HCC, to less than 10% for advanced stage. Two most common factors leading to delayed diagnosis

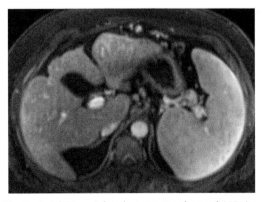

Fig. 2. Axial T1-weighted contrast enhanced MRI image demonstrates conventional imaging features of cirrhosis including atrophy of posterior right lobe and segment 4 with surface nodularity. Splenomegaly and upper abdominal varices are also seen, compatible with portal hypertension.

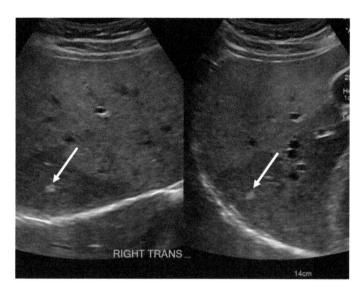

Fig. 3. Screening ultrasound showing a 6 mm hyperechoic lesion in the posterior right lobe. Subsequent MRI did not reveal any suspicious focal lesion. The lesion was stable for over 5 years. Small hyperechoic lesions are not uncommon in cirrhosis. Note geographic wedge shaped area of fatty sparing in segment 7.

of HCC are poor adherence to the screening guidelines and limited sensitivity of the current screening tests. Fewer than 25% of the patients with cirrhosis undergo surveillance.[20] Pooled sensitivity of ultrasound for detection of early HCC ranges from 45% to 63%,[21–23] which is suboptimal for a modality intended to be a screening technique. Although only few of early HCCs are detected by ultrasound screening, routine ultrasound surveillance in cirrhotic patients has shown to be associated with increased early tumor detection, higher rate of curative treatment, and improved survival.[24]

Interpretation of Screening Ultrasound and Ultrasound-Liver imaging and Reporting Data System

When interpreting screening ultrasound, it is imperative to know that small hyperechoic foci are common in cirrhosis (**Fig. 3**). These may represent regenerative nodules or altered echotexture because of hepatic fibrosis. The Liver imaging and Reporting Data System (LI-RADS) classifies lesions visualized on screening ultrasound into 3 categories (**Fig. 4**).[25] Ultrasound LI-RADS (US-LI-RADS) 1 refers to a normal examination with no focal lesions lesion detected and can be surveilled with 6-month interval ultrasound. A new subcentimeter lesion spotted on surveillance ultrasound warrants short-term follow-up imaging in 3 to 6 months (US-LI-RADS category 2). A new focal lesion larger than 1 cm warrants further evaluation with multidetector computed tomography (MDCT) or MRI (US-LI-RADS category 3) (**Fig. 5**). Incidence of malignancy in an ultrasound LI-RADS 3 observation is reported to range from 18.8% to 34%.[26–29] Positive predictive value of ultrasound LI-RADS 3 observation is reported to be much lower at 4% in patients without cirrhosis.[27] LI-RADS also recommend use of ultrasound visualization score to assess the quality and adequacy of the examination, by using the following classifications: score A, no, or minimal limitations (limitations unlikely to meaningfully affect sensitivity); score B, moderate limitations (limitations that may obscure small masses); and score C, severe

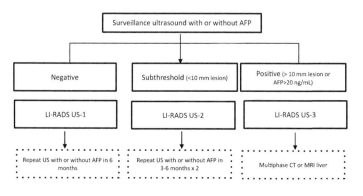

Fig. 4. Current American Association for the Study of Liver Diseases (AASLD) guidelines for Hepatocellular carcinoma (HCC) screening at-risk population with corresponding Liver imaging and reporting data system (LI-RADS) Ultrasound scores.

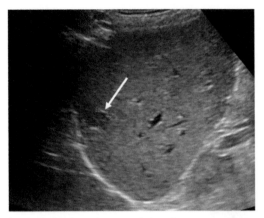

Fig. 5. Screening ultrasound showing a new hypoechoic lesion which measured 1.5 cm compatible with a Liver imaging and reporting data system (LI-RADS) US 3 observation. Subsequent MRI confirmed the diagnosis of Hepatocellular carcinoma (HCC).

limitations (limitations substantially lowering the sensitivity for focal liver lesions).[25] Studies have shown that visualization score of C accounts for up to 86% false-negative rate for diagnosing HCC on surveillance ultrasound.[28]

Serum Tumor Markers in Hepatocellular Carcinoma Surveillance

Addition of serum AFP levels to screening ultrasound has been shown to improve sensitivity for detection of early HCC from 45% (ultrasound alone) to 63% (ultrasound + AFP).[21] Although elevated AFP (>20 ng/mL) can be detected in up to 80% of patients with HCC, the overall reported sensitivity of AFP can be as low as 41% when using 20 ng/mL cut-off value.[17] Reported specificity of AFP ranges from 80% to 94% (cutoff of 20 ng/mL). Elevated AFP, however, indicates poor prognosis and has been associated with poor survival and increased risk of recurrence serum AFP has also been found to be useful in assessing treatment response. Several newer biomarkers have shown promising results as screening tools for detection of early HCC. These include AFP-L3, DCP (Des-gamma-carboxy prothrombin, also known as prothrombin induced by vitamin K absence or antagonist-II/prothrombin induced by vitamin K absence [PIVKA]-II), glycoproteins, and circulating tumor deoxyribonucleic acid.[17,30] AFP-L3 has a relatively low sensitivity of 48% to 56% with specificity of 90% to 92%.[30] When used in isolation, PIVKA-II has a reported sensitivity of 66% to 74% with specificity of 84% to 92%.[17,30] Recently, GALAD Model (incorporating the age, sex, AFP, PIVKA II and AFP-L3) has been proposed to be an effective screening tool for early HCC, with

reported sensitivity of up to 87%, outperforming AFP and other tumors markers.[31]

Other Imaging Modalities in Hepatocellular Carcinoma Surveillance

MDCT is second-line imaging modality for HCC screening with reported sensitivity of 40% to 68% for early HCC (<2 cm),[32,33] superior to ultrasound. MDCT is, however, currently not routinely used for HCC surveillance because of its high cost and ionizing radiation. A recent cost-effectiveness analysis also concluded that assuming 100% patient compliance to surveillance guidelines, surveillance with CT followed by MRI for inadequate surveillance is the most cost-effective imaging strategy for surveillance of patients at risk for HCC.[34] Assuming a more conservative scenario with limited compliance, this study concluded that abbreviated MRI is the most cost-effective screening tool. Abbreviated MRI (AMRI) using hepatobiliary contrast agent (hepatobiliary phase [HBP]-AMRI) has shown to be a sensitive technique for detection of early HCC, with sensitivity of 81% to 92% based on simulated studies performed retrospectively.[35] AMRI can also be performed with unenhanced MRI alone or extracellular contrast agent alone (ECA-AMRI). Head-to-head comparison between various AMRI protocols has not been reported in the literature. Per-patient sensitivity for unenhanced AMRI is reported to be lower than ECA-AMRI and HBP-AMRI,[36] although a recent meta-analyses found no significant difference in sensitivity between unenhanced AMRI and ECA-AMRI protocols.[37] This meta-analyses revealed that the AMRI techniques outperform ultrasound with reported pooled per-patient sensitivity and specificity of 86% and 94%, respectively.[37,38] As expected, sensitivity of AMRI protocols for HCC detection decreases with lesion size, with reported sensitivity drop from 86% (for >2 cm lesions) to 69% (for lesions < 2 cm).[37,38] A recent cost-effectiveness analysis has also shown that semi-annual abbreviated MRI is cost-effective and may outperform surveillance ultrasound, in patients at high risk for developing HCC.[39] Aside from cost-effectiveness, potential harm from false positive results should also be considered when adopting various HCC surveillance strategies. Biannual surveillance with ultrasound and AFP has been reported to result in false positive or indeterminate diagnosis resulting in unnecessary imaging follow-up or rarely biopsy, in up to 20% of patients,[40,41] potentially increasing the true cost per true HCC detected. AMRI can potentially mitigate this problem, by being more specific than ultrasound. AMRI techniques are

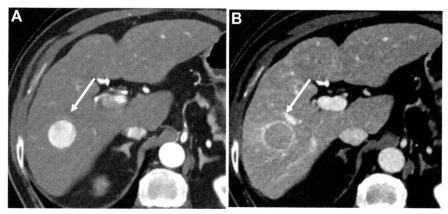

Fig. 6. Dynamic contrast enhanced computed tomography (CT) in the hepatic arterial phase (*A*) and 3 minute delayed phase (*B*) demonstrating a homogeneous arterially enhancing lesion within hepatic segments 7/8 with delayed washout and pseudocapsule (LI-RADS 5, Definitely HCC).

also likely to be technically adequate more often than ultrasound.[35]

DIAGNOSIS OF HEPATOCELLULAR CARCINOMA
Liver Imaging Reporting and Data System

Current imaging guidelines allow hepatocellular carcinoma to be non-invasively diagnosed solely based on imaging criteria in patients at high risk for development of HCC (cirrhosis and chronic hepatitis B).[16] A lesion that measures greater than 1 cm in size, with arterial phase hyperenhancement (APHE) and venous or delayed phase washout, with or without pseudocapsule on contrast-enhanced CT or MRI can be confidently diagnosed as a hepatocellular carcinoma without the need for tissue sampling[16,42] (**Figs. 6** and **7**). The American College of Radiology (ACR) Liver Imaging Reporting And Data System (LI-RADS) guidelines for the use of multi-phase CT and MR examinations in diagnosis of HCC were first introduced in 2011, and were incorporated in to the AASLD guidelines for diagnosis and management of HCC in the year 2018[16] (**Tables 1** and **2**). LI-RADS guidelines have shown to improve communication with referring physicians and patients and convey an unambiguous estimate of HCC risk.[43] Current CT/MRI LI-RADS guidelines are highlighted in the table. LI-RADS is applicable to adult patients (>18 years of age) with cirrhosis, chronic hepatitis B, or current or prior HCC, and uses a scale ranging from LI-RADS 1 (benign) to LI-RADS 5 (HCC) to characterize liver lesions in these patient population. Major imaging features used in LI-RADS guidelines for the diagnosis of HCC include APHE, portal venous or delayed phase washout, pseudo-capsule, and threshold growth.

Major Imaging Features for Hepatocellular Carcinoma Diagnosis

APHE reflects angiogenesis and formation of unpaired neo-arteries, an important early step during hepatocarcinogenesis[44] and refers to non-rim like enhancement within a lesion, unequivocally greater than the background liver in the hepatic arterial phase of imaging (CT or MRI).[45] A recent meta-analysis of 18 studies reported sensitivity of APHE in the diagnosis of HCC to range from 65% to 96%, with a reported sensitivity of 74% when using studies with explant pathology.[42] APHE is not unique to HCC, with reported positive predictive value of 65% to 81%.[42]

'Washout' appearance of a lesion assessed in the portal venous phase, or 3 to 5 minute delayed phase refers to hypo-enhancement of the lesion relative to background liver.[45] Washout reflects diminished portal venous supply, high tumor cellularity, and decreased extracellular volume of the tumor.[42] Washout is assessed subjectively, although attempts have been made to quantify the lesion to liver signal intensity ratios to better define this feature quantitatively. A meta-analysis of 25 studies reported that per nodule sensitivity of washout appearance for detection of HCC ranges from 50% to 79% with a specificity of 50% to 100%. A combination of APHE and washout results in significantly improved specificity (81%-100%) and positive predictive value (81%-100%), with sensitivity of 43% to 98%.[42]

A pseudo-capsule, or capsule appearance (preferred terminology per ACR LI-RADS guidelines) is a smooth, sharp enhancing rim around an observation, unequivocally more conspicuous than fibrotic tissue, and detectable in portal venous delayed phase of enhancement.[45] A capsule

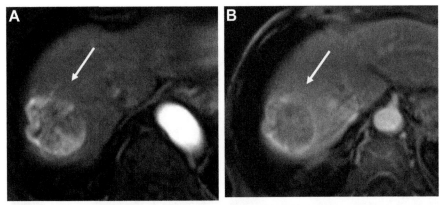

Fig. 7. Dynamic contrast enhanced MRI in the hepatic arterial phase (*A*) and 3 minute delayed phase (*B*) demonstrating a homogeneous arterially enhancing lesion within hepatic segment 7 with delayed washout and pseudocapsule (LI-RADS 5, Definitely HCC).

appearance can be secondary to a true fibrous capsule, or a mix of fibrous tissue and prominent sinusoids, or may represent a pseudo-capsule from compressed liver parenchyma, a differentiation that can only be made at histopathology.[46,47] A capsule appearance has a reported sensitivity of 42% to 64% with a relatively high specificity of 86% to 96% for the diagnosis of HCC.[42]

The lesion size is an important factor, which should be accounted for when characterizing focal hepatic lesions in an at risk population. Several studies have shown that likelihood of HCC increases with nodule diameter, with pre-malignant nodules rarely exceeding 20 mm in size.[42] ACR LI-RADS guidelines recommend measuring the longest dimension of the entire lesion, from outer edge-to outer edge, including the capsule and excluding the surrounding perfusional abnormality, if any.[45] Ideally, measurement in the arterial phase should be avoided, because HCC can be associated with surrounding perfusional abnormalities (corona enhancement).

The fourth major criterion used for characterization and classification of hepatic lesions is the threshold growth. Both the current LI-RADS guidelines and Organ Procurement and Transplantation

Table 1
Summary of The American College of Radiology Liver Imaging Reporting And Data System guidelines (v2018) for untreated observation without pathologic proof in patients at high risk for HCC

LI-RADS Category	Definition	Probability of Malignancy	Recommendations and Implications
LR-NC	Cannot be categorized because of image degradation or omission	Not applicable	Repeat or alternative diagnostic imaging in ≤ 3 mo
LR-1	Definitely benign	0%	Return to surveillance in 6 mo
LR-2	Probably benign	18% (16% HCC)	Return to surveillance in 6 mo
LR-3	Intermediate probability of malignancy	39% (37% HCC)	Repeat or alternative diagnostic imaging in 3–6 mo
LR-4	Probably HCC	81% (74% HCC)	Multidisciplinary discussion for tailored workup, may include biopsy
LR-5	Definitely HCC	98% (95% HCC)	Multidisciplinary discussion for consensus management
LR-M	Probably or definitely malignant but not HCC specific	94% (37% HCC)	Multidisciplinary discussion for tailored workup, often includes biopsy
LR-TIV	Definite tumor in vein (TIV)		Multidisciplinary discussion for tailored workup, may include biopsy

Table 2
Summary of The American College of Radiology Liver Imaging Reporting And Data System computed tomography or MRI guidelines (v2018) for untreated observation without pathologic proof in patients at high risk for hepatocellular carcinoma

Arterial Phase Hyperenhancement (APHE)		No APHE		Nonrim APHE		
Size (mm)		<20	>20	<10	10–19	>20
Additional major features	None	LR-3	LR-3	LR-3	LR-3	LR-4
• Enhancing capsule	One	LR-3	LR-4	LR-4	LR-4[a]	LR-5
• Nonperipheral washout					LR-5[b]	
• Threshold growth	>Two	LR-4	LR-4	LR-4	LR-5	LR-5

[a] LR-4- if enhancing capsule.
[b] LR-5- if non-peripheral washout or threshold growth.

Network (OPTN)/UNOS criteria define threshold growth as an increase in diameter of the lesion by at least 50% within 6 months.[45,48] Doubling time for HCC (doubling of tumor volume) can range from 9 days to several years, with a median of 178 days for treatment naïve HCCs, and 82 days for recurrent HCCs after loco-regional treatment.[42]

LI-RADS guidelines also discusse 'ancillary' findings, which can be used to upgrade or downgrade an observation. The most common ancillary findings used to upgrade an observation include mild to moderate T2 hyperintensity, hepatobiliary phase hypointensity, and intralesional fat. The most frequent features used to downgrade an observation include marked T2 hyperintensity and stability (>2 years).

Clinical Implications of Liver Imaging Reporting and Data System

Various LI-RADS categories including the probability of malignancy in each category and clinical implications of each LI-RADS category are highlighted in **Table 1**. Lesions that demonstrate targetoid (peripheral rim) APHE and targetoid diffusion restriction are categorized as LI-RADS M observations (malignancy, not necessarily HCC). Observations categorized as LI-RADS M, therefore, require biopsy for definitive diagnosis. Observations categorized as LI-RADS 4 and LIRADS TIV may also require biopsy after multi-disciplinary discussion.

International Guidelines for Hepatocellular Carcinoma Diagnosis

Worldwide several guidelines are used for the diagnosis of HCC. The western guidelines (AASLD/LI-RADS, EASL, and CASL guidelines) aim at high specificity for diagnosis of HCC, with the primary intention being allocation of appropriate patients for liver transplant. On the contrary, the eastern guidelines (APASL 2017, KLCA-NCC 2018, JSH 2021, and CNLC 2019) aim at sensitivity with the primary aim of treating hypovascular pathologically early HCCs. Seo and colleagues found that the accuracy of CT for patient allocation based on the Milan criteria is comparable between AASLD/EASL, KLCSG-NCC, LI-RADS (v2014) and OPTN/UNOS guidelines, ranging from 81.5% to 83.3%.[49] However, a substantial proportion of HCCs in this study were under 2 cm in size and the AASLD/EASL-EORTC and KLCSG-NCC guidelines showed a significantly higher sensitivity (30.8%–41.0%) compared with the LI-RADS (v2014) and OPTN/UNOS guidelines (15.4%–18.0%), with no differences in the specificity.[49]

Imaging Modalities for Diagnosis of Hepatocellular Carcinoma: CT versus MRI

MRI is generally considered to be more sensitive and specific compared with CT for the diagnosis of HCC. The reported summarized sensitivity for detection of HCC varies from 48% to 95% for MRI and 31% to 92% for CT.[50] This is particularly true for lesions less than 2 cm in size (pooled sensitivity of 62% for MRI and 48% for CT).[50] Substantial discordance has been reported in LI-RADS categories assigned on CT and MRI with reported discordant rates of up to 77.2%.[51] A meta-analyses also revealed that on a per-lesion basis, MRI has been shown to be more sensitive than CT (sensitivity of 79% for MRI vs 72% for CT),[50] with head-to-head comparison studies revealing even greater discrepancy in sensitivity rates (80% for MRI vs 68% for CT).[50] Combination of CT and MRI has been reported to yield higher sensitivity, specificity, and accuracy compared with CT or MRI alone.[52] Specifically, in this study a combination of CT and MRI resulted in sensitivity 90.71%, statistically significantly higher than CT alone (54.1%), and marginally better than MRI alone (86.34%).

MRI Contrast Agents for Diagnosis of Hepatocellular Carcinoma: Extracellular versus Hepatobiliary Specific Contrast Agent

MRI with hepatobiliary specific contrast agent (Gadolinium ethoxybenzyl diethelenetriamine pentaacetic acid or gadoxetic acid or Gd-EOB-DTPA) has been found to be more sensitive than ECA-MRI. Approximately 50% of gadoxetic acid is taken up by the hepatocytes through organic anion transporting polypeptides (OATP1B1 and OATP1B3) located at the sinusoidal membranes and excreted into the bile via multidrug resistance protein 2 (MRP2) located at the bile-canalicular membranes. Hepatobiliary phase imaging is typically performed at 20 minutes after administration of the contrast, corresponding to the peak hepatic parenchymal enhancement. High grade dysplastic nodules and early HCC appear hypointense in HBP either because of lack of OATP uptake transporter or increased expression of excretion transporter (**Fig. 8**). A meta-analysis of 29 studies reported that addition of HBP in interpretation resulted in increased pooled sensitivity of EOB-MRI for detection of HCC from 49% to 76% (without HBP) to 75% to90% (with HBP).[53] Consequently, the current eastern guidelines for diagnosis of HCC consider hypointense signal on HBP after gadoxetic acid-enhanced MRI as a major feature for the diagnosis of HCC, thereby increasing the sensitivity of HCC diagnosis.[54] Although including the HBP hypointensity increases the sensitivity of HCC diagnosis (94%), it decreases the specificity (48%).[54] The western guidelines that aim at specificity for HCC diagnosis restrict the use of HBP hypointensity as

an ancillary finding.[55] The specificity of HCC diagnosis can be increased when using the portal venous phase washout alone as the major criteria (specificity: 98%), or by applying ancillary findings described by ACR LI-RADS (specificity: 87%).[56] Jeon and colleagues found that AASLD/LI-RADS and EASL guidelines yielded high specificity (97% and 92% respectively)[57] but the APASL guidelines yielded higher sensitivity (76%) compared with AASLD/LI-RADS (35%) and EASL guidelines (39%).[57] For lesions less than 2 cm, meta-analyses have shown that sensitivity of gadoxetic acid is statistically significantly higher (76%-83.6%), compared with CT (59.1%-68%) and extracellular contrast-enhanced MRI (63.8%-68%).[33,58] Another potential use of Gadoxetic acid enhanced MRI is differentiation of high-grade from low-grade dysplastic nodules. Over one-fourth of the hypovascular nodules with HBP hypointensity can progress to HCC, with cumulative incidence rates of 18%, 25%, and 30% at 1-, 2-, and 3-years respectively.[59]

Gadoxetic acid-enhanced MRI has, however, several limitations. Transient severe motion artifacts can occur in up to 22% of patients receiving gadoxetic acid, and usually affects the hepatic arterial-phase imaging, a vital component in assessing the major criterion for HCC diagnosis. Although up to 70% of lesions, which are hypointense on HBP, can be HCCs, 10% of lesions which are iso- or hyperintense on HBP can be HCCs.[60] Advanced cirrhosis or biliary obstruction can result in low quality HBP phase imaging, limiting the utility of gadoxetic acid (**Fig. 9**). Bilirubin competes with the gadoxetic acid for the uptake and excretion

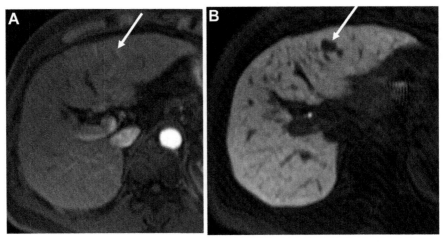

Fig. 8. MRI with gadoxetic acid in a 35 year with hepatitis B with persistently elevated alpha fetoprotein (AFP) and negative extracellular contrast agent enhanced MRI. A 1 cm hypointense lesion was seen on high blood pressure (HBP) (*B*) without Arterial phase hyperenhancement (APHE) (*A*). The lesion was not visible on other sequences. Biopsy confirmed the diagnosis of well-differentiated hepatocellular carcinoma (HCC).

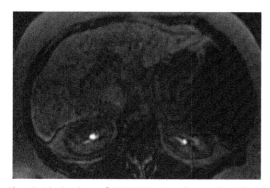

Fig. 9. Limitation of EOB-MRI in advanced cirrhosis with elevated total bilirubin. Numerous areas of heterogeneous hypointense signal on hepatobiliary phase because of reduced hepatocellular uptake and biliary excretion of the hepatobiliary contrast agent precludes accurate assessment for hepatocellular carcinoma (HCC).

transporter, resulting in both reduced hepatocellular uptake and biliary excretion of the contrast agent. Hwang and colleagues found that the optimal cut-off value of total bilirubin for predicting suboptimal HBP phase is 2.1 mg/dL.[61] Finally, unlike the commonly used macrocyclic extracellular contrast agents, gadoxetic acid is a linear agent with a theoretic increased risk of nephrogenic systemic fibrosis (NSF) and gadolinium deposition in brain. A systematic review and meta-analyses published in the year 2020 concludes that gadoxetic acid has similar safety profile to ACR group 2 gadolinium-based contrast agents for NSF, with a lower confidence for risk assessment because of fewer reported administrations in patients with severe renal impairment.[62] Similarly, this study concluded that there is incomplete information documenting the gadolinium retention in brain in patients who receive gadoxetic acid.[62] Clinical implications of gadolinium retention remain uncertain.

SUMMARY

Imaging diagnosis of cirrhosis and hepatocellular carcinoma has substantially evolved over the past decade. New serum tumor markers and advances in imaging have the potential to enable early detection of these tumors, thereby improving the overall survival. LI-RADS guidelines improve communication with referring physicians and patients, conveying an unambiguous estimate of HCC risk and enabling individualized management.

DISCLOSURE

The authors have nothing to disclose.

REFERENCES

1. Sung H, Ferlay J, Siegel RL, et al. Global Cancer Statistics 2020: GLOBOCAN Estimates of Incidence and Mortality Worldwide for 36 Cancers in 185 Countries. CA Cancer J Clin 2021;71(3): 209–49.
2. Rumgay H, Arnold M, Ferlay J, et al. Global burden of primary liver cancer in 2020 and predictions to 2040. J Hepatol 2022;77(6):1598–606.
3. McGlynn KA, Petrick JL, El-Serag HB. Epidemiology of Hepatocellular Carcinoma. Hepatology 2021; 73(Suppl 1):4–13.
4. European Association for the Study of the Liver. Electronic address eee, European Association for the Study of the L. EASL Clinical Practice Guidelines: Management of hepatocellular carcinoma. J Hepatol 2018;69(1):182–236.
5. Heidelbaugh JJ, Bruderly M. Cirrhosis and chronic liver failure: part I. Diagnosis and evaluation. Am Fam Physician 2006;74(5):756–62.
6. Bruden DJT, McMahon BJ, Townshend-Bulson L, et al. Risk of end-stage liver disease, hepatocellular carcinoma, and liver-related death by fibrosis stage in the hepatitis C Alaska Cohort. Hepatology 2017;66(1): 37–45.
7. Ludwig DR, Fraum TJ, Ballard DH, et al. Imaging biomarkers of hepatic fibrosis: reliability and accuracy of hepatic periportal space widening and other morphologic features on MRI. AJR Am J Roentgenol 2021;216(5):1229–39.
8. Loomba R, Sirlin CB, Ang B, et al. Ezetimibe for the treatment of nonalcoholic steatohepatitis: assessment by novel magnetic resonance imaging and magnetic resonance elastography in a randomized trial (MOZART trial). Hepatology 2015;61(4): 1239–50.
9. Chen J, Talwalkar JA, Yin M, et al. Early detection of nonalcoholic steatohepatitis in patients with nonalcoholic fatty liver disease by using MR elastography. Radiology 2011;259(3):749–56.
10. European Association for Study of L. Asociacion Latinoamericana para el Estudio del H. EASL-ALEH Clinical Practice Guidelines: Non-invasive tests for evaluation of liver disease severity and prognosis. J Hepatol 2015;63(1):237–64.
11. Kim BK, Tamaki N, Imajo K, et al. Head-to-head comparison between MEFIB, MAST, and FAST for detecting stage 2 fibrosis or higher among patients with NAFLD. J Hepatol 2022;77(6):1482–90.
12. Morisaka H, Motosugi U, Ichikawa S, et al. Magnetic resonance elastography is as accurate as liver biopsy for liver fibrosis staging. J Magn Reson Imaging 2018;47(5):1268–75.
13. Chowdhury AB, Mehta KJ. Liver biopsy for assessment of chronic liver diseases: a synopsis. Clin Exp Med 2023;23(2):273–85.

14. Zhang BH, Yang BH, Tang ZY. Randomized controlled trial of screening for hepatocellular carcinoma. J Cancer Res Clin Oncol 2004;130(7):417–22.

15. Singal AG, Pillai A, Tiro J. Early detection, curative treatment, and survival rates for hepatocellular carcinoma surveillance in patients with cirrhosis: a meta-analysis. PLoS Med 2014;11(4):e1001624.

16. Marrero JA, Kulik LM, Sirlin CB, et al. Diagnosis, staging, and management of hepatocellular carcinoma: 2018 practice guidance by the american association for the study of liver diseases. Hepatology 2018;68(2):723–50.

17. Kim DY, Kim JW, Kuromatsu R, et al. Controversies in surveillance and early diagnosis of hepatocellular carcinoma. Oncology 2011;81(Suppl 1):56–60.

18. Robinson A, Tavakoli H, Liu B, et al. Advanced hepatocellular carcinoma tumor stage at diagnosis in the 1945-1965 birth cohort reflects poor use of hepatocellular carcinoma screening. Hepatol Commun 2018;2(9):1147–55.

19. Liver cancer survival rates. Available at: https://www.cancer.org/cancer/types/liver-cancer/detection-diagnosis-staging/survival-rates.html. Accessed March 11, 2024.

20. Wolf E, Rich NE, Marrero JA, et al. Use of Hepatocellular carcinoma surveillance in patients with cirrhosis: a systematic review and meta-analysis. Hepatology 2021;73(2):713–25.

21. Tzartzeva K, Obi J, Rich NE, et al. Surveillance imaging and alpha fetoprotein for early detection of hepatocellular carcinoma in patients with cirrhosis: a meta-analysis. Gastroenterology 2018;154(6):1706–17018 e1.

22. Singal A, Volk ML, Waljee A, et al. Meta-analysis: surveillance with ultrasound for early-stage hepatocellular carcinoma in patients with cirrhosis. Aliment Pharmacol Ther 2009;30(1):37–47.

23. Colli A, Fraquelli M, Casazza G, et al. Accuracy of ultrasonography, spiral CT, magnetic resonance, and alpha-fetoprotein in diagnosing hepatocellular carcinoma: a systematic review. Am J Gastroenterol 2006;101(3):513–23.

24. Singal AG, Mittal S, Yerokun OA, et al. Hepatocellular carcinoma screening associated with early tumor detection and improved survival among patients with cirrhosis in the US. Am J Med 2017;130(9):1099–10106 e1.

25. Morgan TA, Maturen KE, Dahiya N, Sun MRM, Kamaya A, et al, American College of Radiology Ultrasound Liver I. US LI-RADS: ultrasound liver imaging reporting and data system for screening and surveillance of hepatocellular carcinoma. Abdom Radiol (NY) 2018;43(1):41–55.

26. Sevco TJ, Masch WR, Maturen KE, et al. Ultrasound (US) LI-RADS: Outcomes of Category US-3 Observations. AJR Am J Roentgenol 2021;217(3):644–50.

27. Tse JR, Shen L, Tiyarattanachai T, et al. Positive predictive value of LI-RADS US-3 observations:

28. Son JH, Choi SH, Kim SY, et al. Validation of US liver imaging reporting and data system version 2017 in patients at high risk for hepatocellular carcinoma. Radiology 2019;292(2):390–7.

29. Choi HH, Rodgers SK, Fetzer DT, et al. Ultrasound liver imaging reporting and data system (US LI-RADS): an overview with technical and practical applications. Acad Radiol 2021;28(10):1464–76.

30. Adeniji N, Dhanasekaran R. Current and emerging tools for hepatocellular carcinoma surveillance. Hepatol Commun 2021;5(12):1972–86.

31. Li H, Liu H, Yan LJ, et al. Performance of GALAD score and serum biomarkers for detecting NAFLD-related HCC: a systematic review and network meta-analysis. Expet Rev Gastroenterol Hepatol 2023;17(11):1159–67.

32. Yu NC, Chaudhari V, Raman SS, et al. CT and MRI improve detection of hepatocellular carcinoma, compared with ultrasound alone, in patients with cirrhosis. Clin Gastroenterol Hepatol 2011;9(2):161–7.

33. Roberts LR, Sirlin CB, Zaiem F, et al. Imaging for the diagnosis of hepatocellular carcinoma: A systematic review and meta-analysis. Hepatology 2018;67(1):401–21.

34. Lima PH, Fan B, Berube J, et al. Cost-Utility Analysis of Imaging for Surveillance and Diagnosis of Hepatocellular Carcinoma. AJR Am J Roentgenol 2019;213(1):17–25.

35. An JY, Pena MA, Cunha GM, et al. Abbreviated MRI for Hepatocellular Carcinoma Screening and Surveillance. Radiographics 2020;40(7):1916–31.

36. Vietti Violi N, Lewis S, Liao J, et al. Gadoxetate-enhanced abbreviated MRI is highly accurate for hepatocellular carcinoma screening. Eur Radiol 2020;30(11):6003–13.

37. Gupta P, Soundararajan R, Patel A, et al. Abbreviated MRI for hepatocellular carcinoma screening: A systematic review and meta-analysis. J Hepatol 2021;75(1):108–19.

38. Brunsing RL, Fowler KJ, Yokoo T, et al. Alternative approach of hepatocellular carcinoma surveillance: abbreviated MRI. Hepatoma Res 2020;6.

39. Goossens N, Singal AG, King LY, et al. Cost-effectiveness of risk score-stratified hepatocellular carcinoma screening in patients with cirrhosis. Clin Transl Gastroenterol 2017;8(6):e101.

40. Singal AG, Patibandla S, Obi J, et al. Benefits and harms of hepatocellular carcinoma surveillance in a prospective cohort of patients with cirrhosis. Clin Gastroenterol Hepatol 2021;19(9):1925–19232 e1.

41. Petrasek J, Singal AG, Rich NE. Harms of hepatocellular carcinoma surveillance. Curr Hepat Rep 2019;18(4):383–9.

42. Tang A, Bashir MR, Corwin MT, et al. Evidence Supporting LI-RADS Major Features for CT- and MR Imaging-

based Diagnosis of Hepatocellular Carcinoma: A Systematic Review. Radiology 2018;286(1):29–48.

43. Corwin MT, Lee AY, Fananapazir G, et al. Nonstandardized terminology to describe focal liver lesions in patients at risk for hepatocellular carcinoma: implications regarding clinical communication. AJR Am J Roentgenol 2018;210(1):85–90.

44. Park YN, Yang CP, Fernandez GJ, et al. Neoangiogenesis and sinusoidal "capillarization" in dysplastic nodules of the liver. Am J Surg Pathol 1998;22(6): 656–62.

45. American College of Radiology. Liver Imaging Reporting and Data System. Available at: https://www. acr.org/Clinical-Resources/Reporting-and-Data-Systems/LI-RADS. Accessed March 11, 2024.

46. Ishigami K, Yoshimitsu K, Nishihara Y, et al. Hepatocellular carcinoma with a pseudocapsule on gadolinium-enhanced MR images: correlation with histopathologic findings. Radiology 2009;250(2): 435–43.

47. Ishizaki M, Ashida K, Higashi T, et al. The formation of capsule and septum in human hepatocellular carcinoma. Virchows Arch 2001;438(6):574–80.

48. HRSA/OPTN Policy. Available at: https://optn.transplant. hrsa.gov/policies-bylaws/policies/. Accessed March 15, 2024.

49. Seo N, Kim MS, Park MS, et al. Optimal criteria for hepatocellular carcinoma diagnosis using CT in patients undergoing liver transplantation. Eur Radiol 2019;29(2):1022–31.

50. Lee YJ, Lee JM, Lee JS, et al. Hepatocellular carcinoma: diagnostic performance of multidetector CT and MR imaging-a systematic review and meta-analysis. Radiology 2015;275(1):97–109.

51. Corwin MT, Fananapazir G, Jin M, et al. Differences in liver imaging and reporting data system categorization between MRI and CT. AJR Am J Roentgenol 2016;206(2):307–12.

52. Basha MAA, AlAzzazy MZ, Ahmed AF, et al. Does a combined CT and MRI protocol enhance the diagnostic efficacy of LI-RADS in the categorization of hepatic observations? A prospective comparative study. Eur Radiol 2018;28(6):2592–603.

53. Pan J, Li W, Gu L, et al. Performance of adding hepatobiliary phase image in magnetic resonance imaging

for detection of hepatocellular carcinoma: a meta-analysis. Eur Radiol 2022;32(11):7883–95.

54. Joo I, Lee JM, Lee DH, et al. Noninvasive diagnosis of hepatocellular carcinoma on gadoxetic acid-enhanced MRI: can hypointensity on the hepatobiliary phase be used as an alternative to washout? Eur Radiol 2015;25(10):2859–68.

55. Zech CJ, Ba-Ssalamah A, Berg T, et al. Consensus report from the 8th International Forum for Liver Magnetic Resonance Imaging. Eur Radiol 2020; 30(1):370–82.

56. Joo I, Lee JM, Lee DH, et al. Retrospective validation of a new diagnostic criterion for hepatocellular carcinoma on gadoxetic acid-enhanced MRI: can hypointensity on the hepatobiliary phase be used as an alternative to washout with the aid of ancillary features? Eur Radiol 2019;29(4):1724–32.

57. Jeon SK, Lee JM, Joo I, et al. Comparison of guidelines for diagnosis of hepatocellular carcinoma using gadoxetic acid-enhanced MRI in transplantation candidates. Eur Radiol 2020;30(9):4762–71.

58. Hanna RF, Miloushev VZ, Tang A, et al. Comparative 13-year meta-analysis of the sensitivity and positive predictive value of ultrasound, CT, and MRI for detecting hepatocellular carcinoma. Abdom Radiol (NY) 2016;41(1):71–90.

59. Suh CH, Kim KW, Pyo J, et al. Hypervascular transformation of hypovascular hypointense nodules in the hepatobiliary phase of gadoxetic acid-enhanced MRI: a systematic review and meta-analysis. AJR Am J Roentgenol 2017;209(4):781–9.

60. Nakao S, Tanabe M, Okada M, et al. Liver imaging reporting and data system (LI-RADS) v2018: comparison between computed tomography and gadoxetic acid-enhanced magnetic resonance imaging. Jpn J Radiol 2019;37(9):651–9.

61. Hwang JA, Min JH, Kim SH, et al. Total bilirubin level as a predictor of suboptimal image quality of the hepatobiliary phase of gadoxetic acid-enhanced mri in patients with extrahepatic bile duct cancer. Korean J Radiol 2022;23(4):389–401.

62. Schieda N, van der Pol CB, Walker D, et al. Adverse events to the gadolinium-based contrast agent gadoxetic acid: systematic review and meta-analysis. Radiology 2020;297(3):565–72.

Evidence-Based Review of Current Cross-Sectional Imaging of Inflammatory Bowel Disease

Jesi Kim, MD[a,b,c], Bari Dane, MD[c],*

KEYWORDS

- Inflammatory bowel disease • Crohn's disease • Ulcerative colitis • Enterography

KEY POINTS

- Enterography allows for visualization of small bowel inflammation inaccessible to standard ileocolonoscopy, Crohn's disease complications, and quantification of disease activity.
- The Society of Abdominal Radiology Crohn's Disease-Focused Panel, the Society for Pediatric Radiology, and the American Gastroenterological Association have developed evidence-based consensus recommendations for interpreting and reporting enterography for small bowel Crohn's disease.
- Cross-sectional imaging is helpful for detecting complications in patients with ulcerative colitis who underwent total proctocolectomy with an ileal pouch–anal anastomosis.

INTRODUCTION

An estimated 1.2 million American were diagnosed with inflammatory bowel disease (IBD) in 2016.[1,2] Of those, approximately 490,000 were diagnosed with Crohn's disease (CD), 450,000 were diagnosed with ulcerative colitis (UC), and 250,000 were diagnosed with indeterminate colitis.[2] The prevalence of IBD has been rising. Patients with IBD often require biologic therapies that are costly and can have adverse side effects. Despite improvements in medical management, it is estimated that the 10 year cumulative risk for major abdominal surgery in CD is approximately 30%,[3,4] with some studies reporting up to 50%.[5,6]

Imaging is critical in the assessment of CD, as ileocolonoscopy can be falsely negative, and clinical parameters show poor correlation with disease activity. Approximately 50% of patients with CD may have false-negative ileoscopy due to the disease skipping the terminal ileum, disease only involving the intramural and mesenteric distal ileum, and disease only involving the upper gastrointestinal region.[7] There is also poor correlation of symptom-based clinical parameters such as the Crohn's disease activity index and Harvey–Bradshaw index with disease activity.[8,9] Therefore, accurate detection and characterization of disease with imaging can guide appropriate management. It has been established that computed tomography enterography (CTE) and MR enterography (MRE) are the most effective methods for imaging the small bowel in patients with CD according to an evidence-based consensus statement by the Society of Abdominal Radiology (SAR) Crohn's Disease-Focused Panel, the Society for Pediatric Radiology (SPR), and the American Gastroenterological Association (AGA).[10] This article reviews cross-sectional imaging of IBD including small bowel

[a] Department of Radiology, NYU Langone Health, New York, NY 10016, USA; [b] Diagnostic Radiology, NYU Grossman School of Medicine, 660 1st Avenue, New York, NY 10016, USA; [c] Department of Radiology, NYU Langone Health, 660 1st Avenue, New York, NY 10016, USA
* Corresponding author.
E-mail address: Bari.Dane@nyulangone.org

Radiol Clin N Am 62 (2024) 1025–1034
https://doi.org/10.1016/j.rcl.2024.05.003
0033-8389/24/© 2024 Elsevier Inc. All rights reserved, including those for text and data mining, AI training, and similar technologies.

CD and UC, with current evidence-based guidelines and information.

CT ENTEROGRAPHY AND MR ENTEROGRAPHY IMAGING TECHNIQUE

Patients fast for 4 to 6 hours prior to CTE or MRE to reduce filling defects within bowel and improve oral contrast consumption compliance.[11] CTE is a multi-detector CT examination that utilizes neutral oral and intravenous (IV) contrast.[12,13] CTE requires small bowel distention and the oral contrast agents utilized in CTE generally have lower attenuation (0–30 HU) to allow visualization of the interface between the bowel lumen and wall. A commercial 0.1% barium suspension (VoLumen or VoLumex, Bracco Diagnostics, Milan, Italy) and commercial sugar beverage (Breeza, Beekley Corp., Bristol, CT) are most commonly used, but water, milk, lactulose, polyethylene glycol, methylcellulose, sorbitol, and mannitol are all other possible alternative oral contrast agents.[12] A study of 4 commonly utilized contrast agents including water, methylcellulose, polyethylene glycol, and 0.1% barium suspension found that polyethylene glycol and 0.1% barium suspension provided more effective small bowel distention than water and methylcellulose.[14] Two studies showed similar bowel distention for a commercial sugar beverage (Breeza) and 0.1% barium suspension; however, patients were more likely to ingest the entire prescribed oral contrast volume when the commercial sugar beverage was utilized.[15,16] In patients with an intact gastrointestinal tract, 1.0 to 1.45 L is the target volume of oral contrast, and it should be administered 30 to 75 minutes prior to imaging.[13] The IV contrast is delivered by power injection at a rate greater than 3 mL/s and a scan delay 50 to 70 seconds. The enteric (late arterial) phase has the greatest level of bowel enhancement.[12,17] Table 1 shows details of our institutional CTE protocol.

MRE also utilizes oral as well as IV contrast and is specifically tailored toward assessing small bowel.[11] Commonly used oral contrast agents include 0.1% barium suspension, a commercial sugar beverage, polyethylene glycol, and methylcellulose. As water is normally absorbed, it may not provide adequate small bowel distention[18] but may be given immediately prior to the MRE to ensure stomach and duodenal distention.[18] Antiperistaltic medications, most commonly glucagon in the United States, are helpful for pharmacologic paralysis, particularly for post-contrast sequences.[11] T2-weighted fat-suppressed, diffusion-weighted, and post-contrast MR sequences with multiple time points may assist inflammation detection. Table 2 shows details of our institutional MRE protocol.

Table 1 Sample computed tomography enterography imaging technique	
Parameters	**Values**
kV	120 (single energy); 80 and 140 (dual-source dual-energy)
mAs	180–400 reference mAs
Detector collimation	0.6 mm
Field of view	Skin-to-skin
Gantry angle	None
Gantry rotation time	0.5 s
Pitch	0.6–0.9
Scan acquisition time	60 s (enterography phase)

CT ENTEROGRAPHY AND MR ENTEROGRAPHY UTILIZATION

Enterography allows for assessment of small bowel inflammation inaccessible to standard ileocolonoscopy, intramural, and penetrating disease.[10,19] Cross-sectional imaging is also highly sensitive for predicting postoperative recurrence, and patients with CD with imaging findings of inflammation are at increased risk for future recurrence.[20] Enterography can also be used for treatment response monitoring. In addition, imaging findings on enterography correlate with progression to surgery.[21,22]

There are different factors to consider when deciding among CT with positive oral contrast, CTE, and MRE (Table 2).[23] Positive oral contrast is useful for evaluating recent postoperative patients with concern for leak in the emergency department setting. Otherwise, in the outpatient setting, CTE and MRE are preferred in the imaging assessment of CD.[10] While the choice between CTE and MRE depends on a variety of factors including patient-related considerations, imaging access, and expertise, the following may be used to help guide imaging selection. CTE should be considered as the first cross-sectional enterography examination due to its superior spatial resolution or in an acutely symptomatic patient, whereas MRE may be performed for treatment response assessment or imaging of patients who are not acutely symptomatic. Additionally, patients with contraindications to MR imaging, claustrophobia, or allergy to gadolinium-based IV contrast should undergo CTE, whereas those with iodinated contrast allergy, younger patients, or perianal disease should undergo MRE. Finally, pregnant patients should undergo MRE, without IV

Table 2
Sample MR enterography imaging technique

Sequence	Coverage	TR/TE	Slice Thickness (mm)	FOV (mm)
Coronal HASTE	A, P	900/90	6	372 x 452
Axial HASTE	A, P	900/90	6	370 x 370
Axial T2 FS small FOV	Rectum	3280/105	4	200 x 200
Axial DWI (b = 0, 800)	A, P	7600/54	6	340 x 370
Axial T2 rectum	Rectum	3280/105	4	200 x 200
GRASP pre- and post DCE	A, P	4.08/1.65	3	325 x 325
Coronal VIBE post-contrast (Cartesian)	A, P	4.56/2.38	3	256 x 179
Radial VIBE high spatial resolution post-contrast	P, TI	4/1.76	2.5–3	350 x 350
Axial VIBE small field-of-view post-contrast	Rectum	4.9/2.21	2	280 x 280
Axial VIBE post-contrast (Cartesian)	Liver	3.07/1.47	2.5–3	325 x 325

contrast.[10,24] Table 3 summarizes indications for CTE and MRE in CD.

CROHN'S DISEASE IMAGING FINDINGS

Standardized nomenclature ensures clear, consistent reporting for gastroenterologists and surgeons. Additionally, it ensures consistency that referring providers can rely upon to determine future management. The consensus recommendations by SAR, SPR, and AGA for interpreting and reporting CTE and MRE for small bowel CD showed strong inter-radiologist agreement for key CD phenotypes.[25] These are reviewed here.

Active Inflammation

Imaging findings of inflammation in CD are strongly correlated with histologic inflammation (Table 4).[26–28] Segmental mural hyperenhancement is defined as increased attenuation or signal intensity on an IV contrast-enhanced CT or MR examination in a non-contracted small bowel segment in comparison with nearby normal small bowel. Mural enhancement is often asymmetric and stratified. Asymmetric inflammation in CD is often more severe along the mesenteric border, which is a specific feature of CD.[19,29] Stratified mural hyperenhancement is defined as either hyperenhancement of the inner (bilaminar), or both the inner and outer (trilaminar) aspects of the bowel wall.[27,28,30,31] While bowel wall hyperenhancement is a sign of active inflammation, it is not used to describe severity of disease due to physiologic and technical factors affecting acquisition and the degree of bowel wall enhancement.[10] Fig. 1 shows active terminal ileitis with luminal narrowing.

Mural edema, evident as high signal intensity on T2-weighted fat-suppressed images on MRE, is a finding of active inflammation.[32] Restricted diffusion can also be used to detect the presence of inflammation but is a nonspecific sign. Therefore, diffusion-weighted imaging should be used in conjunction with contrast-enhanced T1-weighted and/or fat-suppressed T2-weighted MR images to confidently report active inflammation. False positive high signal intensity on diffusion-weighted images may occur in inadequately distended bowel.

Table 3
When to consider computed tomography enterography or MR enterography

CT Enterography	MR Enterography
First cross-sectional enterography	Disease surveillance
Older patient (over 35 years old)	Younger patient (under 35 years old)
Known Crohn's disease with acute exacerbation, suspect complex penetrating disease with possible future surgical intervention	Evaluate not acutely ill patients or assess response to therapy
Low-dose computed tomography techniques	Pregnancy (without IV contrast)
Imaging access and expertise	Imaging access and expertise

Table 4
Imaging findings of small bowel inflammation in Crohn's disease

Imaging Findings	Description/Definition
Segmental mural hyperenhancement	Increased attenuation or signal intensity in contrast-enhanced scan in non-contracted segment compared to normal nearby small bowel segments
Asymmetric	Mesenteric border is often more affected than the antimesenteric border
Stratified (bilaminar or trilaminar)	Inner-wall hyperenhancement
Homogeneous, symmetric	Transmural hyperenhancement
Wall thickening	
Mild	3–5 mm
Moderate	5–9 mm
Severe	10 mm or greater
Intramural edema	Can only be seen on MR and is defined as hyperintense signal on fat-saturated T2-weighted images
Ulcerations	Small focal breaks in the intraluminal surface of the bowel wall with focal extension of air or oral contrast into the inflamed bowel wall

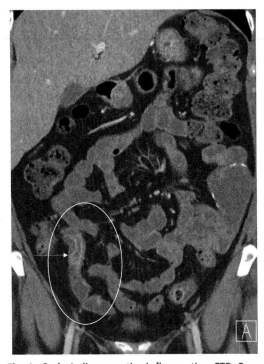

Fig. 1. Crohn's disease active inflammation CTE. Coronal image from CTE in 56 year old woman with Crohn's disease shows active terminal ileal inflammation with luminal narrowing (*oval*), but no upstream dilation to suggest stricture. Note the asymmetric wall thickening, with greater involvement along the mesenteric border than antimesenteric border, and the mural stratification with a bilaminar appearance. An area of ulceration is also shown (*arrow*).

Ulcerations appear as small breaks in the luminal surface with extension of air or oral contrast into the inflamed bowel wall. Ulcerations on imaging correlate with endoscopically severe disease.[33,34] The degree of wall thickening may also be used in the assessment of disease severity, with mild wall thickening between 3 and 5 mm, moderate from 5 to 9 mm, and severe 10 mm or greater. Mild inflammation rarely causes luminal narrowing.[10]

When active inflammation is present, the presence or absence of luminal narrowing, length of intestinal inflammatory involvement, and location relative to the ileocecal valve or the ligament of Treitz should be reported. Additionally, if prior imaging is available, the report should comment on whether the extent and severity of disease is improved, stable, or worse from the prior examination.

Strictures

Strictures form due to complex interactions of inflammatory cells, cytokines, mesenchymal cells, and enteric flora.[10,35] Additionally, there has been increased recognition of the role of abnormal smooth muscle proliferation in strictures.[36–38] CD strictures often have a combination of inflammation, fibrosis, and smooth muscle hypertrophy.[38] While predominantly inflammatory strictures may be treated with medical therapy, strictures predominantly containing fibrosis or smooth muscle hypertrophy may require endoscopic or surgical management.

Strictures are defined as a bowel segment with wall thickening, luminal narrowing, and upstream dilation of 3 cm or greater (Fig. 2). A "probable" stricture can be diagnosed when the upstream lumen is less than 3 cm, and multiple pulse sequences on MR or serial imaging examinations demonstrate fixed luminal narrowing. However, upstream dilation may not always be present if there are multiple strictures or penetrating disease.[39] These strictures would unfortunately not be diagnosed based on the current cross-sectional imaging stricture definitions. When a stricture is present, the presence or absence of active inflammation should be reported.

Currently, the diagnostic criteria for CD-associated strictures on cross-sectional imaging differ from that of the endoscopic definition. In addition, differentiation between predominantly inflammatory strictures and predominantly fibrotic strictures remains challenging.[40] As mentioned earlier, this differentiation is helpful in determining the treatment course. Additionally, there has been an increased interest in developing a robust system for evaluation of fibrotic strictures as imaging will likely play a crucial role in defining efficacy of antifibrotic therapies.[40]

Penetrating Disease

Penetrating disease occurs due to transmural inflammation in CD and includes sinus tracts, fistulas, inflammatory masses, abscesses, and perforation (Table 5). A sinus tract is a blind-ending tract that extends beyond the bowel serosa but does not reach an adjacent organ or skin. A fistula is an extraenteric tract extending from the bowel lumen to another epithelialized surface. Fistulas should be described by the 2 epithelized

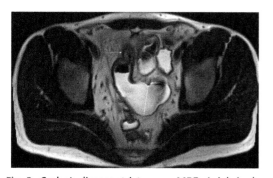

Fig. 2. Crohn's disease stricture on MRE. Axial single-shot fast-spin echo image through the pelvis in an MRE in a 19 year old man with Crohn's disease shows a segment of distal ileum (*arrow*) demonstrating luminal narrowing, wall thickening, and upstream dilation greater than 3 cm (*white line*), which is highly compatible with a stricture.

structures they connect (eg, enterocutaneous, enterovesical, and enteroenteric). Fistulas may be described as simple or complex. A simple fistula is defined as a single extraenteric tract (Fig. 3), whereas a complex fistula has more than one fistulous tract and often has an asterisk or star-shaped appearance. An inflammatory mass is defined as dense mesenteric inflammation without a well-defined fluid component or discrete wall adjacent to a bowel segment with mural inflammation. These are often seen in the presence of complex fistulas. In the past, the term *phlegmon* was used; however, the use of this term is discouraged due to its ambiguous definition. An abscess is a fluid collection with rim enhancement and well-defined wall on IV contrast-enhanced CTE or MRE. Free perforation is a very rare complication of CD. The presence of complex fistulas, inflammatory masses, and abscesses are associated with greater surgical complexity with greater estimated blood loss, conversion to open surgery, and need for fecal diversion, even in patients undergoing a primary ileocolic resection.[41] There is a strong correlation between stricture formation and penetrating disease.[42,43]

Perianal Disease

Perianal disease is also a common manifestation of CD. Approximately 25% of patients with CD present with perianal fistulas.[10] Consequently, dedicated imaging of the anal sphincters and perineum is often performed, with MR imaging being the best imaging modality for perianal assessment.[10] However, patients presenting to the emergency department with perianal abscess often first undergo CT to identify or exclude abscess. The presence or absence of perianal disease should be evaluated for and reported, because it often requires clinical management. If an abscess is present, patients will require antibiotics with possible drainage to treat the abscess prior to initiating therapy with immunosuppressive or biologic medication.[44] The Parks classification may be used for reporting perianal fistulas.[45] Perianal fistulas should be described as intersphincteric (Fig. 4), transphincteric, suprasphincteric, or extrasphincteric.

Perienteric and Extraintestinal Findings

Perienteric findings associated with small bowel CD include perienteric edema or fat stranding, which are present in more severe disease. Engorged vasa recta, also known as the "comb sign," results from current or previous bowel inflammation. Findings of chronicity include sacculations and fibrofatty proliferation.[46] Sacculations

Table 5
Imaging findings of penetrating disease in Crohn's disease

Imaging Findings	Description/Definition
Sinus tract	Blind-ending tract that extends beyond the bowel serosa but does not reach and adjacent organ or skin
Fistula	Extraenteric tract between bowel lumen to another epithelialized surface
Simple fistula	Single extraenteric tract
Complex fistula	More than one extraenteric tract
Inflammatory mass	Dense mesenteric inflammation without a well-defined fluid component or discrete wall
Abscess	Fluid collection with rim enhancement

result from shortening along the mesenteric border with ballooning along the antimesenteric border. Fibrofatty proliferation is hypertrophy of the mesenteric fat adjacent to diseased bowel segments due to repeated inflammation. Mesenteric venous thrombosis or occlusion has been described in CD. It is important to distinguish between acute mesenteric thrombosis and chronic mesenteric vein thrombosis. Chronic peripheral mesenteric vein occlusion has been shown to anatomically correspond with small bowel segments with active or prior CD inflammation. In addition, acute and chronic mesenteric vein thrombosis/occlusion has been correlated with increased risk for stricture and surgery in a retrospective study.[47] Lymphadenopathy up to 1.5 cm in short axis is considered reactive in IBD.

Extraintestinal findings include sacroiliitis, primary sclerosing cholangitis (PSC), avascular necrosis of the hips, nephrolithiasis, cholelithiasis, and pancreatitis (type 2 autoimmune pancreatitis and due to cholelithiasis).[10] Many patients with CD present with back pain, and the detection of sacroiliitis allows for identification of the cause and therapy facilitation. PSC can be seen in both CD and UC; however, it is more common in UC. On MR cholangiopancreatography (MRCP), PSC bile ducts may have a beaded appearance, whereas on CT isolated intrahepatic biliary dilation may be evident.

QUANTITATIVE CROHN'S DISEASE ACTIVITY ASSESSMENT

Recently, there have been efforts to quantify disease activity using CTE and MRE. Dual-energy CT allows for the determination of iodine density, which reflects only the iodine content within a voxel. Iodine density has been shown to be a surrogate marker of perfusion. Prior studies have shown that dual-energy CTE-obtained iodine density correlates with active inflammation in CD.[9,48–51] In

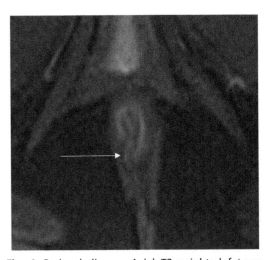

Fig. 3. Simple enteroenteric fistula in CD. Axial T2-weighted fat-suppressed MR image through the pelvis from an MRE shows a simple fluid-filled enteroenteric fistula (*arrow*) connecting 2 adjacent ileal segments.

Fig. 4. Perianal disease. Axial T2-weighted fat-suppressed image through the anus from an MRE in a 23 year old man with Crohn's disease shows a right posterior 7:00 lithotomy position intersphincteric perianal fistula (*arrow*).

addition, photon-counting CT enterography iodine density can be used to distinguish mild from moderate-to-severe active inflammation.[52]

MRE has also been used for disease quantification. There are several MR-based scoring systems that can be used to quantify disease activity, including the MR index of activity (MaRIA) and simplified MaRIA scores.[53] The MaRIA uses wall thickening, mural contrast enhancement, presence of mural edema, and ulcerations as independent predictors for presence and severity of inflammation.[54,55] The simplified MaRIA may be performed for inflammation assessment without IV contrast and is easier to use, without compromising accuracy.[55]

ULCERATIVE COLITIS IMAGING FINDINGS

Patients with UC are at increased risk for colorectal cancer (4.5% over 20 years), so total proctocolectomy is indicated.[56] Many patients currently opt for total proctocolectomy with ileal pouch-anal anastomosis (IPAA), as this allows avoidance of a lifelong ostomy and ensures maintenance of anal sphincter integrity. Patients with UC are also at risk for megacolon. Consequently, in patients with UC and acute abdominal pain, the first examination performed is often radiography to exclude pneumoperitoneum.[57] CT is often the primary imaging examination performed in the emergency department or inpatient setting. Imaging findings on CT and MR include contiguous colitis extending from the rectum to the more proximal colon (Table 6). A backwash ileitis may also be evident in patients with pancolitis.

Ileal Pouch-Anal Anastomosis Imaging

There are a variety of pouch configurations, but the J-pouch is the most common. In this configuration, the distal 15 to 20 cm of ileum is folded onto itself to create a reservoir, and the apex is anastomosed with the anal transition zone to create the IPAA.

Common complications of IPAA surgery include leak, stricture, inflammation, and twist or volvulus.[58,59] Leaks occur in the immediate postoperative period, and most commonly occur at the IPAA, but may also occur at the pouch body staple lines or stapled tip of the J pouch.[58] Tip of the J leaks is sometimes overlooked, and it is important to maintain a high index of suspicion. If a tract arises more than 6 months after surgery, it may indicate a Crohn's phenotype. In female patients, pouch–vaginal fistulas can occur due to inadvertent stapling of the posterior vaginal wall to the IPAA. These also often occur in the immediate postoperative period, and a delayed presentation could indicate a Crohn's phenotype.

Strictures

Strictures most commonly occur at the pouch outlet, such as the IPAA. These may also occur in the pre-pouch ileum/inlet or pouch body. IPAA strictures may be related to ischemia or anastomotic dehiscence. A pre-pouch ileum stricture with associated penetrating complications is strongly suggestive of the Crohn's phenotype.

Inflammation

Inflammation can present as cuffitis, pouchitis, or pre-pouch ileum inflammation. Cuffitis is defined as inflammation of retained rectal mucosa distal to the IPAA in patients who did not undergo complete mucosectomy. Cuffitis is thought to be a recurrence of UC, so the initial treatment is mesalamine.[59] Pouchitis often coexists with cuffitis (Fig. 5).[59] Pouchitis is multifactorial and may be from colonic metaplasia inciting a recurrence of UC or from stasis of fecal material. It is the most common late complication of IPAA surgery, and unlike cuffitis, the initial treatment is antibiotics.[59] Pre-pouch ileum inflammation can occur from pouchitis with associated backwash ileitis or Crohn's phenotype. While pouch surgery is often performed for UC, some patients may ultimately

Table 6		
Imaging modalities and common indications for ulcerative colitis		
CT with Positive Oral Contrast	Water-Soluble Contrast Enema	MR Imaging
Acute presentation or recent postoperative patient	Assess for pouch and anastomotic integrity	Assess for subacute or chronic postoperative complications
May evaluate chronic missed pouch leak	Evaluate for stricture and pouch emptying	Evaluate for perianal fistula and pre-pouch ileum
Evaluate for perforation, abscess, leak, bowel obstruction, and mesenteric or portal thrombus	Evaluate for leak, sinus tract, fistula, and abscess in acute or chronic setting	Evaluate for pouchitis, cuffitis, and rectal cuff or anal transitional zone length

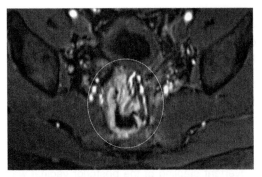

Fig. 5. Pouchitis. Axial T1-weighted fat-suppressed contrast-enhanced MR image through the pelvis in a 30 year old man with UC following proctocolectomy with a J-pouch shows pouch wall thickening and avid enhancement (*white oval*) in the setting of pouchitis.

be diagnosed with CD after their proctocolectomy. Lastly, twisting at the IPAA results from a surgical error during IPAA stapling. On the other hand, volvulus is a torque at the pouch inlet and may be due to adhesions near the presacral region.

Extraintestinal Findings

Extraintestinal manifestations of UC are also important to report. In particular, patients with UC are at increased risk for PSC. In addition to the risk of cholangiocarcinoma in patients with PSC, UC patients with PSC are at greater risk for colon cancer, particularly in the ascending colon. Patients with concomitant PSC benefit from dedicated MRCP imaging.

SUMMARY

CTE and MRE play an important role in the detection of intramural, proximal small bowel inflammation, and extraintestinal manifestations in patients with IBD. In addition, enterography can assist with quantification of disease activity, distribution of disease, and detection of complications including penetrating disease. Consistent, accurate reporting ensures clear communication with referrers and allows for improved patient care.[59]

CLINICS CARE POINTS

- CTE and MRE allow for assessment of the small bowel, which is largely inaccessible to standard ileocolonoscopy.
- CTE and MRE enable identification of Crohn's disease complication and detection of extraintestinal manifestations.

- Pelvic MR is a valuable imaging tool in the assessment of patients who underwent ileal pouch-anal anstomosis surgery.

DISCLOSURES

B. Dane receives speaker honorarium and research support from Siemens Healthineers, Germany. J. Kim has no conflict of interest to report.

REFERENCES

1. Lewis JD, Parlett LE, Jonsson Funk ML, et al. Incidence, prevalence, and racial and ethnic distribution of inflammatory bowel disease in the United States. Gastroenterology 2023;165(5):1197–1205 e1192.
2. Ye Y, Manne S, Treem WR, et al. Prevalence of inflammatory bowel disease in pediatric and adult populations: recent estimates from large National Databases in the United States, 2007-2016. Inflamm Bowel Dis 2020;26(4):619–25.
3. Lichtenstein GR, Loftus EV, Isaacs KL, et al. ACG clinical guideline: management of Crohn's Disease in adults. Am J Gastroenterol 2018;113(4):481–517.
4. Torres J, Mehandru S, Colombel JF, et al. Crohn's disease. Lancet 2017;389(10080):1741–55.
5. Inoue A, Bartlett DJ, Shahraki N, et al. Predicting risk of surgery in patients with small bowel crohn's disease strictures using computed tomography and magnetic resonance enterography. Inflamm Bowel Dis 2022;28(11):1677–86.
6. Peyrin-Biroulet L, Loftus EV Jr, Colombel JF, et al. The natural history of adult Crohn's disease in population-based cohorts. Am J Gastroenterol 2010;105(2):289–97.
7. Samuel S, Bruining DH, Loftus EV Jr, et al. Endoscopic skipping of the distal terminal ileum in Crohn's disease can lead to negative results from ileocolonoscopy. Clin Gastroenterol Hepatol 2012; 10(11):1253–9.
8. Deepak P, Fletcher JG, Fidler JL, et al. Predictors of durability of radiological response in patients with small bowel Crohn's disease. Inflamm Bowel Dis 2018;24(8):1815–25.
9. Dane B, Sarkar S, Nazarian M, et al. Crohn Disease active inflammation assessment with iodine density from dual-energy CT enterography: comparison with histopathologic analysis. Radiology 2021; 301(1):144–51.
10. Bruining DH, Zimmermann EM, Loftus EV Jr, et al, Society of Abdominal Radiology Crohn's Disease-Focused P. Consensus recommendations for evaluation, interpretation, and utilization of computed tomography and magnetic resonance enterography in patients with small bowel Crohn's Disease. Gastroenterology 2018;154(4):1172–94.

11. American College of Radiology. ACR-SAR-SPR Practice Parameter for the Performance of Magnetic Resonance (MR) Enterography. 2020; Available at: MR-Enterog.pdf (acr.org). Accessed June 24, 2024.

12. American College of Radiology. ACR-SAR-SPR Practice Parameter for the Performance of Computed Tomography (CT) Enterography. 2020; Available at: CT-Entero.pdf (acr.org). Accessed June 24, 2024.

13. Gandhi NS, Dillman JR, Grand DJ, et al. Computed tomography and magnetic resonance enterography protocols and techniques: survey of the Society of Abdominal Radiology Crohn's Disease Disease-Focused Panel. Abdom Radiol (NY) 2020;45(4): 1011–7.

14. Young BM, Fletcher JG, Booya F, et al. Head-to-head comparison of oral contrast agents for cross-sectional enterography: small bowel distention, timing, and side effects. J Comput Assist Tomogr 2008;32(1):32–8.

15. Dillman JR, Towbin AJ, Imbus R, et al. Comparison of two neutral oral contrast agents in pediatric patients: a prospective randomized study. Radiology 2018;288(1):245–51.

16. Kolbe AB, Fletcher JG, Froemming AT, et al. Evaluation of Patient Tolerance and Small-Bowel Distention With a New Small-Bowel Distending Agent for Enterography. AJR Am J Roentgenol 2016;206(5): 994–1002.

17. Schindera ST, Nelson RC, DeLong DM, et al. Multidetector row CT of the small bowel: peak enhancement temporal window–initial experience. Radiology 2007;243(2):438–44.

18. Grand DJ, Guglielmo FF, Al-Hawary MM. MR enterography in Crohn's disease: current consensus on optimal imaging technique and future advances from the SAR Crohn's disease-focused panel. Abdom Imag 2015;40(5):953–64.

19. Guglielmo FF, Anupindi SA, Fletcher JG, et al. Small Bowel Crohn Disease at CT and MR Enterography: Imaging Atlas and Glossary of Terms. Radiographics 2020;40(2):354–75.

20. Bachour SP, Shah RS, Lyu R, et al. Test Characteristics of Cross-sectional Imaging and Concordance With Endoscopy in Postoperative Crohn's Disease. Clin Gastroenterol Hepatol 2022;20(10):2327–2336 e2324.

21. Dane B, Qian K, Krieger R, et al. Correlation between imaging findings on outpatient MR enterography (MRE) in adult patients with Crohn disease and progression to surgery within 5 years. Abdom Radiol (NY) 2022;47(10):3424–35.

22. Grass F, Fletcher JG, Alsughayer A, et al. Development of an Objective Model to Define Near-Term Risk of Ileocecal Resection in Patients with Terminal Ileal Crohn Disease. Inflamm Bowel Dis 2019;25(11): 1845–53.

23. Expert Panel on Gastrointestinal I, Kim DH, Chang KJ, et al. ACR Appropriateness Criteria(R) Crohn Disease. J Am Coll Radiol 2020;17(5S):S81–99.

24. Guimaraes LS, Fidler JL, Fletcher JG, et al. Assessment of appropriateness of indications for CT enterography in younger patients. Inflamm Bowel Dis 2010;16(2):226–32.

25. Dane B, Qian K, Gauvin S, et al. Inter-reader agreement of the Society of Abdominal Radiology-American Gastroenterological Association (SAR-AGA) consensus reporting for key phenotypes at MR enterography in adults with Crohn disease: impact of radiologist experience. Abdom Radiol (NY) 2021;46(11):5095–104.

26. Bodily KD, Fletcher JG, Solem CA, et al. Crohn Disease: mural attenuation and thickness at contrast-enhanced CT Enterography–correlation with endoscopic and histologic findings of inflammation. Radiology 2006; 238(2):505–16.

27. Church PC, Turner D, Feldman BM, et al. Systematic review with meta-analysis: magnetic resonance enterography signs for the detection of inflammation and intestinal damage in Crohn's disease. Aliment Pharmacol Ther 2015;41(2):153–66.

28. Qiu Y, Mao R, Chen BL, et al. Systematic review with meta-analysis: magnetic resonance enterography vs. computed tomography enterography for evaluating disease activity in small bowel Crohn's disease. Aliment Pharmacol Ther 2014;40(2):134–46.

29. Tolan DJ, Greenhalgh R, Zealley IA, et al. MR enterographic manifestations of small bowel Crohn disease. Radiographics 2010;30(2):367–84.

30. Horsthuis K, Bipat S, Bennink RJ, et al. Inflammatory bowel disease diagnosed with US, MR, scintigraphy, and CT: meta-analysis of prospective studies. Radiology 2008;247(1):64–79.

31. Siddiki H, Fletcher JG, Hara AK, et al. Validation of a lower radiation computed tomography enterography imaging protocol to detect Crohn's disease in the small bowel. Inflamm Bowel Dis 2011;17(3): 778–86.

32. Steward MJ, Punwani S, Proctor I, et al. Non-perforating small bowel Crohn's disease assessed by MRI enterography: derivation and histopathological validation of an MR-based activity index. Eur J Radiol 2012;81(9):2080–8.

33. Rimola J, Ordas I, Rodriguez S, et al. Magnetic resonance imaging for evaluation of Crohn's disease: validation of parameters of severity and quantitative index of activity. Inflamm Bowel Dis 2011;17(8):1759–68.

34. Rimola J, Rodriguez S, Garcia-Bosch O, et al. Magnetic resonance for assessment of disease activity and severity in ileocolonic Crohn's disease. Gut 2009;58(8):1113–20.

35. Rieder F, Zimmermann EM, Remzi FH, et al. Crohn's disease complicated by strictures: a systematic review. Gut 2013;62(7):1072–84.

36. Abu-Ata N, Dillman JR, Rubin JM, et al. Ultrasound shear wave elastography in pediatric stricturing small bowel Crohn disease: correlation with histology and second harmonic imaging microscopy. Pediatr Radiol 2023;53(1):34–45.

37. Lu C, Gui X, Chen W, et al. Ultrasound Shear Wave Elastography and Contrast Enhancement: Effective Biomarkers in Crohn's Disease Strictures. Inflamm Bowel Dis 2017;23(3):421–30.

38. Chen W, Lu C, Hirota C, et al. Smooth Muscle Hyperplasia/Hypertrophy is the Most Prominent Histological Change in Crohn's Fibrostenosing Bowel Strictures: A Semiquantitative Analysis by Using a Novel Histological Grading Scheme. J Crohns Colitis 2017;11(1):92–104.

39. Stocker D, King MJ, El Homsi M, et al. Luminal Narrowing Alone Allows an Accurate Diagnosis of Crohn's Disease Small Bowel Strictures at Cross-Sectional Imaging. J Crohns Colitis 2021;15(6):1009–18.

40. Bettenworth D, Bokemeyer A, Baker M, et al. Assessment of Crohn's disease-associated small bowel strictures and fibrosis on cross-sectional imaging: a systematic review. Gut 2019;68(6):1115–26.

41. Dane B, Remzi FH, Grieco M, et al. Preoperative cross-sectional imaging findings in patients with surgically complex ileocolic Crohn's disease. Abdom Radiol (NY) 2023;48(2):486–93.

42. Oberhuber G, Stangl PC, Vogelsang H, et al. Significant association of strictures and internal fistula formation in Crohn's disease. Virchows Arch 2000;437(3):293–7.

43. Kelly JK, Preshaw RM. Origin of fistulas in Crohn's disease. J Clin Gastroenterol 1989;11(2):193–6.

44. Gecse KB, Bemelman W, Kamm MA, et al, World Gastroenterology Organization, International Organisation for Inflammatory Bowel Diseases IOIBD, European Society of Coloproctology and Robarts Clinical Trials. A global consensus on the classification, diagnosis and multidisciplinary treatment of perianal fistulising Crohn's disease. Gut 2014;63(9):1381–92.

45. Parks AG, Gordon PH, Hardcastle JD. A classification of fistula-in-ano. Br J Surg 1976;63(1):1–12.

46. Li XH, Feng ST, Cao QH, et al. Degree of Creeping Fat Assessed by Computed Tomography Enterography is Associated with Intestinal Fibrotic Stricture in Patients with Crohn's Disease: A Potentially Novel Mesenteric Creeping Fat Index. J Crohns Colitis 2021;15(7):1161–73.

47. Naik Vietti N, Vietti Violi N, Schoepfer AM, et al, Swiss Inflammatory Bowel Disease Cohort Study G. Prevalence and clinical importance of mesenteric venous thrombosis in the Swiss Inflammatory Bowel Disease Cohort. AJR Am J Roentgenol 2014;203(1):62–9.

48. Dane B, Duenas S, Han J, et al. Crohn's Disease Activity Quantified by Iodine Density Obtained From Dual-Energy Computed Tomography Enterography. J Comput Assist Tomogr 2020;44(2):242–7.

49. Dane B, Kernizan A, O'Donnell T, et al. Crohn's disease active inflammation assessment with iodine density from dual-energy CT enterography: comparison with endoscopy and conventional interpretation. Abdom Radiol (NY) 2022;47(10):3406–13.

50. Dane B, Garada A, O'Donnell T, et al. Crohn Disease Prognostication With Semiautomatic Dual-Energy Computed Tomography Enterography-Derived Iodine Density. J Comput Assist Tomogr 2021;45(2):171–6.

51. Dane BDS, Han J, O'Donnell T, et al. Crohn's disease activity quantified by iodine density obtained from dual-energy CT enterography. JCAT 2020.

52. Dane B, Qian K, Soni R, et al. Crohn's disease inflammation severity assessment with iodine density from photon counting CT enterography: comparison with endoscopic histopathology. Abdom Radiol (NY) 2024;49(1):271–8.

53. Minordi LM, Larosa L, Belmonte G, et al. Crohn's disease activity before and after medical therapy evaluated by MaRIA score and others parameters in MR Enterography. Clin Imag 2020;62:1–9.

54. Rimola J, Alvarez-Cofino A, Perez-Jeldres T, et al. Comparison of three magnetic resonance enterography indices for grading activity in Crohn's disease. J Gastroenterol 2017;52(5):585–93.

55. Ordas I, Rimola J, Alfaro I, et al. Development and Validation of a Simplified Magnetic Resonance Index of Activity for Crohn's Disease. Gastroenterology 2019;157(2):432–439 e431.

56. Gros B, Kaplan GG. Ulcerative Colitis in Adults: A Review. JAMA 2023;330(10):951–65.

57. Eghbali E, Akhavi Milani A, Shirmohamadi M, et al. CT features of toxic megacolon: A systematic review. Radiography 2021;27(2):716–20.

58. Dane B, Huang C, Luk L, et al. Contrast enema, CT, and small bowel series of the ileal pouch. Abdom Radiol (NY) 2023;48(9):2935–43.

59. Huang C, Remzi FH, Dane B, et al. Reporting Templates for MRI and Water-Soluble Contrast Enema in Patients With Ileal Pouch-Anal Anastomosis: Experience From a Large Referral Center. AJR Am J Roentgenol 2021;217(2):347–58.

Ultrasound Contrast Agents
Current Role in Adults and Children for Various Indications

Krishna Mundada, MD[a], John S. Pellerito, MD, FSRU, FAIUM[b],
Benjamin Srivastava[c], Margarita V. Revzin, MD, MS, FAIUM, FSRU, FSAR[d],*

KEYWORDS

- CEUS in abdomen and pelvis • CEUS of the liver and renal masses
- CEUS in trauma and pediatric population and interventions

KEY POINTS

- CEUS is a technique that uses contrast agents for real-time recording and evaluation of tissue perfusion, microvasculature, and architecture.
- In the United States, UCAs are currently only approved for 2D-echocardiography, focal hepatic abnormalities, and urologic conditions in children such as vesiculoureteral reflux (contrast-enhanced VUR, in Europe).
- CEUS has the potential to address many limitations of conventional ultrasound and other cross-sectional imaging modalities beyond the currently approved uses.

INTRODUCTION/BACKGROUND

Contrast-enhanced ultrasound (US) (CEUS) is a technique that uses contrast agents for real-time recording and evaluation of tissue perfusion, microvasculature, and architecture. There are 3 generations of ultrasound contrast agents (UCAs) that have been developed and marketed. UCAs are currently only approved for 2D-echocardiography, focal hepatic abnormalities, and urologic conditions in children such as vesiculoureteral reflux (VUR) (contrast-enhanced VUR, in Europe). Other uses of UCAs are considered off-label indications of CEUS. However, CEUS has the potential to address many limitations of conventional US and other cross-sectional imaging modalities beyond the currently approved uses.

The first-generation UCA has been off market since 2014, whereas the newer second- and third-generation UCAs are now widely available. First-generation contrast agents were composed of air-filled microbubbles and albumin microbubbles, which made them highly soluble in blood and - tissues, leading to rapid distribution and shorter circulation time, a drawback that was addressed by the newer agents. An example of a first-generation UCA is the Schering-manufactured Levovist, which had a resonance range (RR) of 2 to 3 MHz.

Second-generation gas microbubbles were created to increase the stability of the contrast agents in the circulation and enhance their resonance response. These microbubbles (2–6 μm in size) are dense and filled with hydrophobic gases

[a] Department of Nuclear Medicine, Seth G.S. Medical College and K.E.M Hospital, Mumbai; [b] Department of Radiology, Division of US, CT and MRI, Peripheral Vascular Laboratory, North Shore - Long Island Jewish Health System; [c] Wilton Public High School, Wilton, CT 06897, USA; [d] Department of Radiology and Biomedical Imaging, Yale School of Medicine, New Haven, CT, USA
* Corresponding author.
E-mail address: margarita.revzin@yale.edu

0033-8389/24/© 2024 Elsevier Inc. All rights reserved, including those for text and data mining, AI training, and similar technologies.

radiologic.theclinics.com

encapsulated by a shell composed of various chemicals, including but not limited to galactose, albumin, lipid, and polymers.[1] The substantial difference in acoustic impedance at gas fluid/tissue interfaces provides strong acoustic backscatter, and gas microbubbles resonate in the acoustic beam at frequencies used in diagnostic US, thus enhancing the blood pool detected on US. The capsule or shell of the microbubbles contributes to its stability and resonant properties. The higher densities of gases such as perfluorocarbons (used in the perflutren contrast agent, called DEFINITY), with an RR of 1.5 to 4 MHz, and sulfur hexafluoride (used in LUMASON in the United States and outside of the United States as SonoVue), with an RR of 1.8 to 3.2 MHz, make them last longer in the vascular circulation because of their slow diffusion across the capsule membrane and less solubility in the blood, thus increasing microbubble stability over a longer period.[2] Sonazoid is another contrast agent (not approved by the Food and Drug Administration [FDA]). Compared with other second-generation agents, Sonazoid has the ability to be taken up by the hepatic Kupffer cells in the late postvascular phase thus allowing differentiation of masses lacking *Kupffer* cells from the background liver parenchyma (eg, metastases to the liver), increasing diagnostic capability and accuracy.[3] In general, microbubbles are smaller than red blood cells and flow throughout the human microcirculation at physiologic transit times, effectively functioning as surrogate markers of perfusion.

CONTRAST-ENHANCED ULTRASOUND TECHNIQUE

Dynamic intravenous (IV) CEUS is a technique that uses time-intensity curve (TIC) analysis to evaluate tissue perfusion via a bolus or infusion of a contrast agent. This method not only helps in defining vascular architecture of an organ but also, if present, compares vascularity and perfusion of a mass to the normal tissue parenchyma of an organ of interest. Thus, TICs are a graphic display of contrast perfusion, allowing representation of the time of arrival of contrast to the region of interest (ROI) and peak time of contrast within the ROI. TIC curves are analyzed using TIC software. The data from an ROI are added over a normal curve for comparative analysis, and several parameters are evaluated. These parameters include time parameters such as *time zero* offset, which is time of injection to first appearance of microbubbles on the ROI and *time to peak*, which is autocalculated based on the corresponding time marker of the nadir, that is, between injection and contrast

arrival to the time to peak enhancement. The time from 5% to 95% intensity is called the *wash in time*, whereas the time from peak to zero value is called *washout time*. The difference between the maximum and minimum intensities is called the *peak intensity (Tp)*. The mean time taken for the bubbles from arrival to the end of ROI is called the *mean transit time*. The area under the curve represents the total blood volume and is useful in therapy monitoring trials and follow-up examinations[4] (**Fig. 1**).

3D CEUS is a promising more advanced version of CEUS, which is based on acquisition of data to create tissue volumes. This technique reconstructs stereoscopic images of tissue essentially defining tumor characteristics, vascularity, and rim enhancement patterns in a three-dimensional construct. This feature has proven particularly valuable for chemoembolization or postprocedural response assessment. Various softwares are available on the market to enhance and optimize the results from CEUS real-time imaging by removing artifacts, detecting information even from low concentration of contrast, and so on. Contrast US dispersion imaging and contrast-tuned imaging (by Esaote) are a few examples of such software. These advancements have elevated CEUS as a modality, making it a competitive alternative application compared with other diagnostic techniques such as magnetic resonance (MR) imaging.

CONTRAST-ENHANCED ULTRASOUND ADVANTAGES AND DISADVANTAGES

CEUS possesses several inherent advantages over other cross-sectional modalities using contrast agents, that is, computed tomography (CT) and MR imaging. These advantages include

1. A real-time approach without the need for a predefined scan time.
2. Portability and intraoperative use, facilitating bedside examination in critically ill patients; this also reduces examination related time and risks.
3. Cost-effectiveness.
4. No renal toxicity or clearance (can be used at any level of renal function).
5. No ionizing radiation.
6. Strong safety profile, with low adverse events and side effects reported from approved contrast-enhanced agents.
7. Repeat bolus in a single session is possible due to a safe renal and adverse reaction profile.
8. No claustrophobia, unlike MR imaging, and occasionally CT.

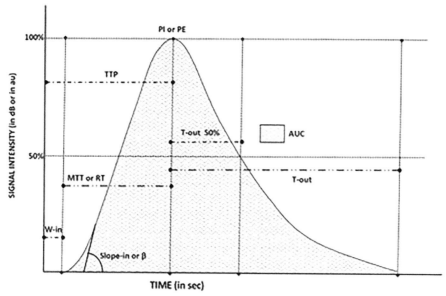

Fig. 1. Graphic representation of the time-intensity curve and the calculated perfusion parameters. Wash-in time (W-in): the time when organ/vascular enhancement first occurs, measured in seconds; time to peak (TTP): the time needed to reach the peak intensity (PI), measured in seconds; mean transit time (MTT) or rise time (RT): the time difference between the time needed to reach the PI and the time since the beginning of region of interest (ROI) enhancement, measured in seconds; PI or peak enhancement (PE): the maximum ROI enhancement, measured in decibel (dB) or acoustic units (au); washout time (T-out): the time difference between the 50% PI values in the washout and peak intensity value, measured in seconds (several studies also consider T-out as the time needed for the descending slope to reach a contrast signal intensity of 0); area under the curve (AUC): intensities of the entire enhancement period, measured in dB or au (several studies also differentiate wash-in AUC [before PI] and washout AUC [after PI]); slope in or β: the coefficient of the wash in slope, it reflects the mean blood flow velocity in the region of interest, measured in dB or au. (*From* Tenuta M, Sesti F, Bonaventura I, et al. Use of contrast enhanced ultrasound in testicular diseases: A comprehensive review. Andrology. 2021;9(5):1369–82.)

9. CEUS can be used when both CT and MR imaging are contraindicated due to allergies to iodinated or gadolinium-based contrast material.

However, there are some *disadvantages* of CEUS worth mentioning:

1. CEUS shares most disadvantages with conventional US such as operator dependency and is affected by bowel gas and patient body habitus, scars, wounds, overlying devices, limited trained personnel available especially after hours, and so on.
2. Variations in reproducibility of results and findings due to operator bias may hinder further research and categorization of pathologic findings.
3. Often only one mass/focal abnormality can be visualized at a time (limited field of view).
4. Difficulties in assessment of patients with altered surgical anatomy.
5. Rare but severe adverse reactions to UCAs:
   a. In patients with no known allergy to polyethylene glycol (PEG) the chance of life-threatening anaphylactoid reaction has been reported to be 0.001% without any fatalities.
   b. Clinical signs of contrast reaction include but are not limited to hypotension, palpitations, erythema, and warmth sensation on the face, dizziness, malaise, headache, nausea, and vomiting.[5]
   d. UCAs are contraindicated in patients with adverse reaction to PEG, a molecule commonly found in vaccines, specifically in coronavirus disease 2019 vaccines. Many UCAs are formulated with PEG to stabilize their phospholipid shell. The PEGylated molecules incorporate into the microbubble monolayer shell and stabilize the particles against coalescence with other microbubbles and interaction with blood plasma proteins.[6]

DEFINITY and LUMASON also share the PEG molecule in their preparation and should not be administered in patients who have reported previous reactions. Immediate hypersensitivity reactions with resulting fatalities have been reported in this patient population.[7]

In April 2021, the American College of Radiology issued a warning against the use of DEFINITY and LUMASON in patients with PEG allergy.

USES OF CONTRAST-ENHANCED ULTRASOUND
Contrast-Enhanced Ultrasound in the Abdomen and Pelvis

Given CEUS' strong advantages with a relatively high safety profile, it has several potential applications, including detecting and distinguishing benign from malignant masses and pathologic conditions, as well as vascular complications in the abdomen and pelvis.

Contrast-enhanced ultrasound in characterization of benign and malignant hepatic tumors

CEUS has been widely used in evaluation of focal liver abnormalities. Hepatocellular tumors and focal hepatic abnormalities are by far the most well-characterized masses using CEUS.[8]

In the noncirrhotic adult and pediatric liver CEUS can aid in further characterization of hepatic masses initially incidentally discovered on US. CEUS is also helpful in the evaluation of incompletely characterized masses detected on noncontrast or on IV contrast-enhanced CT and MR imaging.[9] Specific contrast enhancement patterns in the arterial phase (10–40 seconds after contrast injection), portal venous phase (45 seconds 2 minutes), the late phase (after 2 minutes to clearance of contrast from the blood pool, after 5 minutes), and postvascular phase (uptake by Kupffer cells) allow detailed mass characterization and diagnosis.[10]

Benign masses and hepatic conditions including *hemangiomas, focal nodular hyperplasia (FNH), hepatic adenoma, and focal fat* demonstrate characteristic presentations on CEUS, allowing accurate diagnosis and obviating additional imaging with other cross-sectional modalities. For example, early arterial centripetal filling and hyperenhancement on portal and delayed imaging is a pattern characteristic of hemangiomas, whereas a centrifugal pattern of enhancement is seen with FNH (**Table 1**).

Characteristic contrast-enhanced ultrasound imaging appearance of benign liver masses

On CEUS, small hemangiomas (less than 2 cm) demonstrate a prominent progressive centripetal filling pattern of enhancement and larger hemangiomas show discontinuous peripheral nodular enhancement during the early arterial phase, with progression of more central enhancement in the later arterial phase of imaging (**Fig. 2A–D**). Hemangiomas remain either isoechoic or hyperechoic in the late and portal phases of imaging and are almost never hypoechoic.[11,12] Internal nonenhancement within a hemangioma signifies thrombosis.

In the pediatric population, two types of hemangiomas are described: infantile and congenital. Although congenital hemangiomas usually show a similar pattern of enhancement to adult hemangiomas, an infantile hemangioma may show washout in the late phase, making their diagnosis more challenging.[13]

Focal fat on CEUS demonstrates an enhancement pattern similar to the rest of the liver parenchyma on all phases of imaging.[14]

FNH, a benign process mostly found in females, can be easily differentiated from other hepatic masses using CEUS.[15] FNH is characterized by arterial phase hyperenhancement (APHE) with sustained enhancement during later phases of imaging, often with a central nonenhanced stellate scar.[16] Arterial phase enhancement with centrifugal filling and enhancement of the vessels from the center of the mass to the periphery results in a spoke-wheel appearance and is a hallmark that differentiates FNH from other liver masses.

Hepatic adenomas may have various patterns of enhancement due to their different histologic types, the presence of fat, and hemorrhagic components, making their CEUS enhancement features inconsistent.[10] These adenomas may show either arterial enhancement characteristic of benign masses with sustained enhancement in the portal phase or weak washout in the later phase, making their differentiation from hepatocellular carcinoma (HCC) challenging, putting emphasis on patient history and demographics (eg, a young woman on oral contraceptives is more likely to have a hepatic adenoma, versus a patient with underlying liver cirrhosis who will likely have HCC).[10]

CEUS may be challenging in the differentiation of regenerative nodules from dysplastic nodules. When regenerative nodules are larger than 5 mm (macronodules), they may be differentiated on CEUS from dysplastic nodules by demonstration of a hypo- to isoechoic pattern of enhancement on the arterial phase and are isoechoic to the remaining liver on the late phase. In contrast, dysplastic nodules usually show diffuse contrast enhancement in the arterial phase and a late phase isoechoic appearance.[17]

Contrast-enhanced ultrasound in evaluation and characterization of malignant hepatic tumors

CEUS has been recognized as a first- or second-line modality for characterization and diagnosis

Table 1
Characteristic CEUS features of benign and malignant liver tumors

Tumor	Phase: Arterial	Phase: Portal	Phase: Late	Other Characteristics
Hemangioma	Centripetal	Hyper/iso	Hyper/iso	Rarely: nonenhancing areas corresponding to central thrombus
FNH	Centrifugal	Iso	Iso	Central stellate scar is hypoechoic "spoke-wheel" appearance of the vessels distributed from the center to the periphery
Focal fatty infiltration	Iso: most common. Hyper also being reported	Iso	Iso	Will never show washout in portal and late phases
Adenoma	Centripetal	Iso	Hypo/iso/ hyper	Nonenhancing areas: intratumoral hemorrhage, fat components, or necrosis. The diagnosis and pattern remain subtype dependent[33]
HCC	Hyperenhancement (APHE) with late arterial iso	Iso	Hypo	Late/slow washout. Areas of nonenhancement confirm necrosis. May demonstrate hypo- or isoarterial enhancement (no APHE). Rapid washout or no washout may also be rarely observed
Cholangiocarcinoma	Hyperenhancement	Hypo	Hypo	Peripheral arterial rim enhancement. Early washout
Metastatic	Transient arterial enhancement with rapid marked washout. Note that the pattern of arterial enhancement may depend on tumor vascularity and type			Punched-out holes, or black tumors on the background of liver enhancement on the portal venous phase. Peripheral arterial rim enhancement may be seen

Abbreviation: APHE, arterial phase hyperenhancement.

of observations found on surveillance US for HCC. CEUS is also a useful problem-solving technique in liver imaging, demonstrating the ability to resolve indeterminate observations seen on MR imaging examinations.[18]

Unlike benign hepatic masses, malignant tumors are characterized not by their arterial enhancement but by their washout pattern. Arterial enhancement in malignant tumors is highly variable and cannot be used for differentiation of tumors. Washout patterns help to make an accurate diagnosis of malignant neoplasms. The time of washout and the intensity are both helpful features. When washout is seen early, before 1 minute, it is referred to as *early (or rapid) washout*. Washout occurring after 1 minute is referred to as *late washout*. Intensity of the tumor at washout can be *mild*, where some contrast is remaining within the tumor, or it may be *marked*, with the

tumor appearing completely black relative to the remaining liver parenchyma, also known as a punched-out hole within the enhanced liver (this is before 2 minutes following contrast injection). In general, hepatocellular malignancies such as HCC typically demonstrate late and weak washout and nonhepatocellular malignancies, such as cholangiocarcinoma, usually show rapid and marked washout.[19–21]

As mentioned earlier, Sonazoid microbubbles can be used during the hepatobiliary phase of imaging to detect and characterize tumors containing Kupffer cells.[20]

Contrast-enhanced ultrasound in the diagnosis of metastases

Metastases, independent of their primary origin (lung, breast, colon, and so on), usually demonstrate transient arterial hypervascularity with rapid

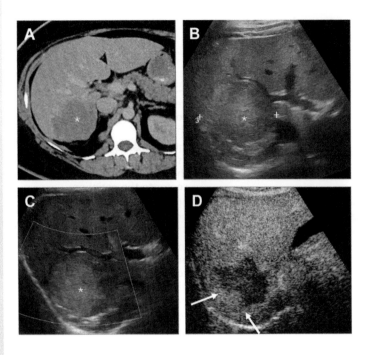

Fig. 2. Hepatic hemangioma in a 49-year-old man with an incidentally discovered hepatic mass on CT. (*A*) Axial contrast-enhanced CT of the abdomen and pelvis shows a lobular hypodense nonspecific mass in the right hepatic lobe (*asterisk* in *A*). (*B, C*) Gray-scale (*B*) and color Doppler (*C*) images of the liver in the transverse plane demonstrate a hyperechoic slightly heterogeneous mass (*asterisks* in *B, C*) with no substantial flow on color Doppler (*asterisk* in *C*). (*D*) CEUS image shows the right hepatic mass with peripheral nodular discontinuous enhancement indicating a hemangioma (*arrows*).

marked washout, appearing as black holes on the background of enhancing liver parenchyma during the washout stage (portal venous phase) (**Fig.** 3A, B).

Contrast-enhanced ultrasound in the diagnosis of hepatocellular carcinoma

HCCs arise from hepatocytes in pre-existing benign hepatic nodules, most commonly in the setting of liver disease/cirrhosis, by the process called *hepatocarcinogenesis*. The initial step in hepatocarcinogenesis is formation of a regenerative nodule, which undergoes progressive atypia, resulting in the development of a dysplastic nodule, which eventually becomes replaced with cancerous tissue. Variations in angiogenesis are responsible for differences in HCC vascularity and patterns of enhancement and washout on CEUS. Therefore, differentiation between dysplastic nodules and well-differentiated HCC on imaging can be challenging.[22,23] The classic HCC pattern of enhancement on CEUS includes APHE with late and weak washout (**Fig.** 4A, B). It should be noted that HCC may demonstrate hypo- or isoarterial enhancement (no APHE), and either rapid or no washout, thus overlapping with nonhepatocellular malignancies.[24]

Contrast-enhanced ultrasound in the diagnosis of intrahepatic cholangiocarcinoma

Intrahepatic cholangiocarcinoma (ICC) is a relatively rare malignancy, with incidence of 10% to 20% of all types of cholangiocarcinomas, representing only 3% of all gastrointestinal malignancies. ICC usually occurs in normal liver in older patients, especially those with risk factors such as choledocholithiasis, primary sclerosing cholangitis, hepatitis B and C, among other etiologies.[25,26] ICC has been detected more frequently in patients with chronic liver disease, and therefore, should be distinguished from HCC in this patient population.[27] On CEUS ICC shows variable arterial enhancement ranging from hypo- to hyperenhancement. Rim enhancement may also be seen. Similar to other nonhepatocellular cancers, ICC demonstrates rapid and marked washout.[27]

One area of research is the use of ultrasonics (an imaging software based on the radiomics model of CT and MR imaging), which has shown promising results, with high sensitivity and specificity for diagnosing and differentiating combined hepatocellular cholangiocarcinoma versus HCC.[28] Features of ICCs on CEUS are further specified by their subtypes. ICCs are divided into 3 different types depending on the location. A mass-forming ICC shows 4 types of enhancement pattern: irregular rimlike enhancement, heterogeneous or homogeneous hyperenhancement, and heterogeneous hypoenhancement. Hyperenhancement in the tumor signifies increased tumor burden, whereas late enhancement and hypoenhancement indicate more fibrous stroma. Mass-forming ICCs will usually show hypoenhancement in both portal and late phases. Smaller ICCs may show more diffuse

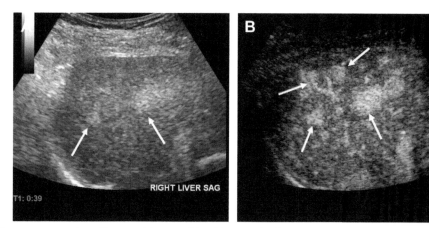

Fig. 3. Liver metastases in a 59-year-old man with a history of colon cancer. Fusion gray-scale (A) and CEUS (B) images of the liver obtained in the sagittal plane demonstrate slightly heterogeneous liver parenchyma with a few geographic, poorly-defined areas of hyperechogenicity without discrete masses seen (arrows in A). Note multiple arterially hyperenhancing masses seen on CEUS (arrows in B), which are compatible with liver metastases.

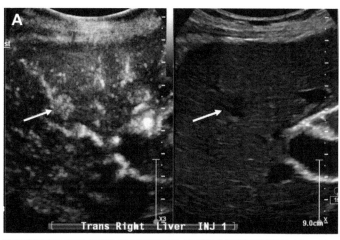

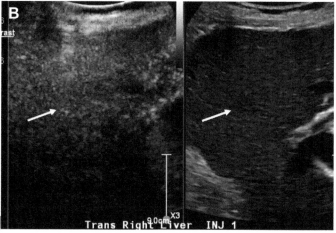

Fig. 4. LI-RADS 5 hepatic observation in an 83-year-old woman status postliver transplant 15 years ago. (A) Fusion CEUS and gray-scale images obtained in the arterial phase at 30 seconds demonstrate a hypoechoic observation with woman following liver transplant APHE (arrows in A). (B) Fusion gray-scale CEUS image through the observation obtained at 4-minute post–contrast injection shows late weak washout (arrows in B). LI-RADS 5, highly suspicious for HCC. Pathology confirmed HCC.

hyperenhancement, whereas larger ones can show peripheral rim hyperenhancement due to more fibrous content in the larger ICCs.[29,30]

Periductal infiltrating ICC tends to spread via bile ducts toward the porta hepatis and shows heterogeneous enhancement with hypoenhancement during the portal and late phases.[31] Intraductal growing ICC typically shows homogeneous hyperenhancement, with a few reported heterogeneous patterns of hyperenhancement and late and portal phase hypoenhancement.[32,33]

Contrast-Enhanced Ultrasound Liver Reporting and Data System

CEUS is a major component of the Liver Reporting and Data System (LI-RADS). Similar to MR imaging LI-RADS, CEUS LI-RADS is a standardized system for description of technique, interpretation, reporting, and assessment of risk management of patients at high risk for the development of HCC. Observations that are stratified as LI-RADS 1 or 2 correspond to a very low risk of malignancy, and LI-RADS 5 observations are most likely HCC. LI-RADS 5 nodules require the presence of at least 3 features in an at-risk patient: size greater than 1 cm, nonrim APHE, and late and mild washout at greater than 1 minute following US contrast administration (see Fig. 4A-D). This category is highly specific for characterization of nodules (with specificity of 100%), thus nodules can be treated without the need for a biopsy.[34]

Contrast-Enhanced Ultrasound and Tumor Treatment Outcome Monitoring

CEUS and dynamic CEUS applications are safe and cost-effective alternatives to IV contrast-enhanced computed tomography (CECT) and contrast-enhanced magnetic resonance imaging (CEMRI) for treatment outcome monitoring and assessment of microvessel perfusion during all vascular phases. CEUS provides high spatial resolution and can be used repeatedly as a serial follow-up of the tumor after various therapeutic applications (chemoembolization, immunotherapy, or radiofrequency ablation) (Fig. 5A, B). The European Federation of Societies for Ultrasound in Medicine and Biology highlights the role of CEUS not only in the characterization and detection of focal liver nodules but also in monitoring tumor response after locoregional and systemic HCC treatments.[4,35,36] Drawbacks such as operator dependance as well as limited acoustic windowing and tumor location and multiplicity may reduce CEUS reproducibility. Additionally, multinodularity, hypoenhancement in pretreatment CEUS, and

infiltrative diffuse growth pattern are conditions that affect CEUS efficacy. When performed four weeks after the therapeutic procedure, CEUS demonstrates high sensitivity and specificity of 88% and 99% for the identification of residual unablated tumors when compared with CECT (92% and 99%, respectively).[12,13] Similar to other cross-sectional modalities, one of the limitations of CEUS is the presence of reactive inflammation to thermal injury around a treated nodule, resulting in persistence of hyperemic halos around ablated tissue, potentially mimicking residual disease. CEUS can also be used to assess the perfusion pattern of recurrent HCC after radiofrequency ablation (RFA). It has been shown that after ablation, recurrent HCC demonstrates more homogeneous enhancement in the arterial phase, with a poorly defined border at the peak, and more inner necrotic areas when compared with initial HCC. Similarly posttherapeutic CEUS monitoring of patients after transcatheter chemoebmbolization (TACE)-treated tumors demonstrates positive results, with the reported detection rate of residual HCC masses being statistically significantly higher with CEUS performed after 1 day than with CECT performed after 1 month (95.7% vs 78.7%, $P<.05$).[37,38] Other studies showed that CEUS at 3 days after drug-eluting beads (DEB-TACE) allowed the early assessment of therapeutic efficacy with no enhancement and peripheral ring enhancement suggestive of a positive outcome.

Dynamic CEUS (D-CEUS) applications are promising because they enable a quantitative assessment of tumor perfusion earlier when compared with the current reference standard.[36]

Contrast-Enhanced Ultrasound and Renal Masses

CEUS is an excellent application for the evaluation of the global perfusion of the kidneys, permitting better delineation of the renal hila and assessment of potential renal infarcts (Fig. 6A, B). In addition to assessment of renal perfusion, CEUS is also used for the evaluation of renal masses. CECT and CEMRI are considered the standard techniques at present for diagnosing and characterizing renal masses.[39] However, both these techniques have a few negative aspects, including cost-effectiveness, radiation exposure, longer examination time, and the potential for contrast nephrotoxicity/contrast reactions. CEUS has shown equivalent if not higher accuracy for the diagnosis of renal tumors than CECT and CEMRI.[40] A recent study by Herms and colleagues[41] underscores the importance of CEUS in diagnosing and following up cystic renal

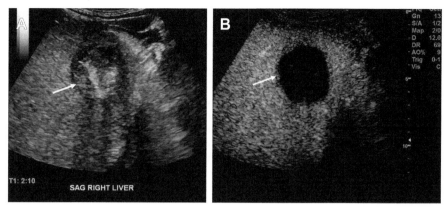

Fig. 5. Postablation of liver HCC in a 67-year-old man with liver cirrhosis. Fusion gray-scale (A) and CEUS (B) images of the liver obtained in the sagittal plane demonstrate a nonspecific heterogeneous area in the region of prior HCC ablation (arrow, B). On CEUS the focus demonstrates no enhancement compatible with necrosis and absence of tumor recurrence or residual disease (arrow, B).

masses. The study showed that CEUS-based Bosniak classification accurately identified and assigned a higher grade to histopathologically proven carcinomas when compared with the classic Bosniak classification based on CT and MR imaging characteristics of renal cysts.[41] CEUS Bosniak classification describes Bosniak 1 to 3 as benign cysts, which show lack of enhancement within the cyst and cyst wall. Bosniak 2F masses are best described as "presumably benign, however, containing mildly complex features," and therefore, management with surveillance imaging is advised. Bosniak 3 masses are indeterminate and can be either benign or malignant. Some of the benign Bosniak 3 masses include abscess or changes in the previously identified prior cyst in the setting of a trauma. Therefore, knowledge of prior history

and clinical correlation can help in accurate assessment. Bosniak 3 cystic masses may demonstrate smooth thickened (≥4 mm) walls or irregular thickened (>3 mm) walls and need surveillance or surgical management depending on septation enhancement pattern and patient clinical history and past medical history.[41,42] If no prior history is helpful in determining benignity of the cystic mass, they are usually resected due to the high risk of malignancy (49%–78%).[43] Bosniak 4 cystic masses are likely (85%–100%) malignant cystic tumors, that is, they contain solid components and thickened walls. Bosniak 4 cystic masses that are not malignant (up to 15%), such as cystic masses with nodular but nonenhancing components, can be differentiated from malignant tumors on CEUS. Further characteristics of solid renal tumors such as renal cell

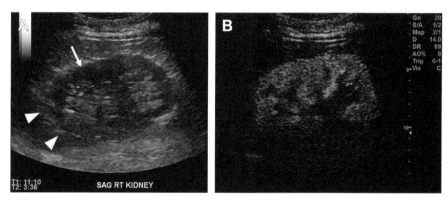

Fig. 6. Normal perfusion of the renal parenchyma on CEUS in a 36-year-old man with suggestion of renal cortical thinning on gray scale and possible infarct. Fusion gray-scale (A) and arterial phase CEcUS (B) images obtained in the sagittal projection demonstrate increased echogenicity of the upper pole of the right kidney (arrow) and thinning of the renal cortex (arrowheads). CEUS image shows normal cortical thickness (arrow) and no areas of lack of perfusion to suggest an infarct. Note that intrarenal collecting system visualization is substantially improved on CEUS.

carcinomas (RCCs) and their subtypes have also been studied.

Clear cell RCCs (cRCCs) are the most common of all RCCs. cRCCs are highly vascularized, thus demonstrating early arterial hyperenhancement with washout in the venous and late phases.[44] Papillary-type RCC (pRCC) are typically hypoenhancing tumors on arterial phase imaging (Fig. 7A, B). CEUS has an advantage over CT in the diagnosis of papillary cancer, which may appear as complicated cysts in the latter due to the contrast time lag.[45,46] A study by Xue and colleagues[47] described the pRCC pattern as slow enhancement, early washout, and hypoenhancement that helps differentiate them from cRCCs. Chromophobe RCC has the most favorable prognosis and shows intermediate intensity curves on CEUS.

Benign renal masses such as angiomyolipomas (AMLs) can mimic RCCs on CEUS and may be difficult to differentiate especially if they are smaller than 4 cm, and in the case of AMLs, are lipid poor. Recent advancements in CEUS technique with the utilization of both qualitative and quantitative characteristics improved accuracy and specificity in the diagnosis and differentiation of the RCC from benign renal masses.[48,49] Evidence has also favored tumor size as one of the most important parameters when evaluating renal masses.[50] Recently, a prospective study demonstrated 100% specificity of CEUS in differentiation of benign from malignant small tumors (<4 cm), as hypovascularity in the arterial phase was seen in only malignant and not benign masses.[51]

Apart from differentiating renal masses, CEUS can also play a major role in diagnosing complicated

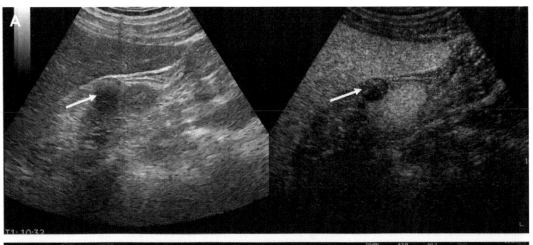

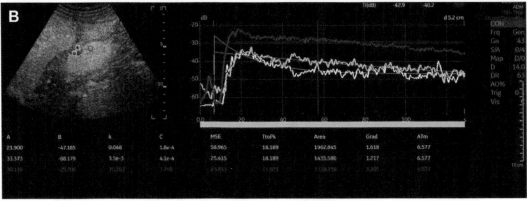

Fig. 7. Right renal cell carcinoma in an 84-year-old man with hematuria. (A) Fusion gray-scale (left) and CEUS (right) images of the right kidney obtained in the transverse view demonstrate a heterogeneously enhancing mass in the upper pole of the right kidney (arrows in A, B). Based on relatively slow pattern of enhancement the mass likely is papillary-type RCC, with the tumor being hypoechoic relative to the remaining normal renal parenchyma as seen on the arterial phase of imaging. (B) Time-intensity curve demonstrates enhancement of the mass to be slower than normal parenchyma (turquoise and yellow curves). The red curve represents normal renal parenchymal enhancement adjacent to the mass. The findings increase confidence that the RCC type is most likely papillary.

renal infections, especially in patients with increased creatinine levels. Kidneys generally appear hypoenhancing in pyelonephritis due to loss of renal architecture and vascular congestion. Renal abscess may remain nonenhancing or can show a central focal defect with rim enhancement (**Table 2**).[52]

Contrast-Enhanced Ultrasound in Gastrointestinal Disorders

Active inflammatory bowel disease (IBD) is often associated with increased vascularity in the mesentery and neoangiogenesis of the bowel wall. Thus, increased mural blood flow on Doppler has been considered a sign of active IBD, whereas inactive IBD or IBD in remission shows absent hyperemia.[53–55] However, Doppler fails to depict microvasculature at the capillary level, which plays a role in the determination of disease acuity and activity.

CEUS provides subjective and objective parameters defining microvasculature and reflecting inflammation in the bowel wall and mesentery, which is useful in diagnosing flare-ups in inflammatory bowel disorders. These parameters help aid diagnosis along with nonspecific and often disputed active inflammatory markers.[56] A systematic review with a meta-analysis performed by Searfin and colleagues[57] that included 332 cases showed a high sensitivity of 94% and a moderately high specificity of 79% in the diagnosis of Crohn disease. These statistics are comparable with that of CT and MR. Pairing B-mode US, which has been shown to be more specific in visualization of structural changes related to IBD, along with CEUS, may improve the overall diagnostic specificity and overall accuracy.[58] Focal enhancement of the entire thickness of the intestinal wall or enhancement of only submucosa and mucosa layers indicate acute Crohn disease.

These results combined with increased bowel wall thickness have previously shown to be promising in diagnosing and differentiating active versus quiescent Crohn disease.[59] Additional usage of TICs allows quantification of bowel fractional blood volume, blood flow, and transit time, all of which are helpful in the assessment of the degree of bowel wall inflammation. CEUS is also beneficial in resolving challenging cases where colonic content may obstruct the view or in the presence of other gastrointestinal pathologies, such as inflammatory polyps or neoplasms.[60]

Contrast-Enhanced Ultrasound in Gallbladder Disease

CEUS shows utility in the evaluation of gallbladder pathologies, including but not limited to gallbladder neoplasms, and differentiation of gallbladder sludge from gallbladder neoplasms.[61] However, data are still inconclusive for the use of CEUS in the differentiation of gallbladder polyps from malignancy (**Fig. 8**).[62]

Contrast-Enhanced Ultrasound in the Evaluation of Pancreatic Masses

Currently UCAs are not approved for direct use in the detection and characterization of pancreatic masses. However, CEUS has the potential to rival CT evaluation in offering high sensitivity and specificity for the diagnosis of pancreatic adenocarcinoma, and hence it is often used off label in the assessment of pancreatic masses. On CEUS, ductal adenocarcinomas appear as hypoenhancing masses on all phases of imaging due to the typically intense desmoplastic reaction and hypovascular profile of the tumor. The microbubble contrast agents help delineate the boundaries

Table 2
Characteristic CEUS features of benign and malignant renal tumors

	Arterial Contrast Medium Behavior	Venous Contrast Medium Behavior	Late Phase
Clear cell renal cell carcinoma	Hyperenhancement	Washout	Persistent washout
Papillary renal cell carcinoma	Hypoenhancement	Hypoenhancement	Hypoenhancement
Chromophobe renal cell carcinoma	Hypoenhancement	Hypoenhancement	Hypoenhancement
Oncocytoma	Indifferent	Indifferent	Indifferent
Angiomyolipoma	Indifferent	Indifferent	Indifferent
Metastasis/lymphoma	Hypoenhancement	Hypoenhancement	Hypoenhancement
Pseudotumor	Isoenhancement	Isoenhancement	Isoenhancement
Pyelonephritis	Hypoenhancement	Hypoenhancement	Hypoenhancement
Renal abscess	Nonenhancing	Nonenhancing	Nonenhancing

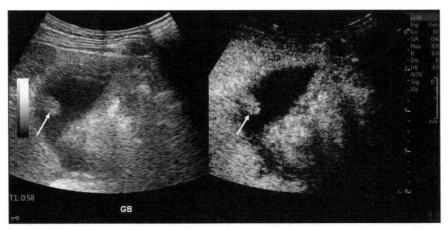

Fig. 8. Gallbladder carcinoma in a 68-year-old woman with right upper quadrant pain. Fusion gray-scale (*left*) and CEUS (*right*) images of a mildly distended gallbladder show a polypoid echogenic mass projecting into the gallbladder lumen (*arrow*). CEUS image shows enhancement of the polypoid mass that was confirmed on pathology to be gallbladder adenocarcinoma (*arrow*).

and extent of disease for surgical planning and for improving biopsy yields.[63] Assessment of patency and involvement of the adjacent related vasculature adds additional benefits in preoperative evaluation.

In contrast to pancreatic adenocarcinomas, pancreatic neuroendocrine tumors appear hypervascular and show rapid and intense enhancement in the early arterial phase, making the differentiation from adenocarcinoma possible with CEUS.[64,65] Exocrine tumors often do not infiltrate pancreatic ducts, unlike adenocarcinomas.[66] Various benign pancreatic tumors and cystic masses including serous cystadenomas and mucinous cystadenomas (MCAs) as well as intraductal papillary mucinous neoplasms can demonstrate characteristic features on CEUS. For example, serous cystadenomas typically contain multiple small (less than 2 cm) cysts resulting in a honeycomb appearance, with enhancing septations seen on CEUS.[67] MCAs usually demonstrate solitary cysts or cysts larger than 2 cm and are known for their potential for malignant transformation. MCAs can be monitored using CEUS. Pseudocysts, a complication after pancreatitis, may resemble MCAs, but unlike MCAs, they are homogeneously anechoic and avascular on CEUS.[67,68] Intraductal papillary mucinous neoplasms are located either in the main duct or in tributary ducts/ductules. Diagnosis of intraductal papillary mucinous neoplasm involves identification of an accompanying dilated duct communicating with the cyst along with presence of unilocular or multilocular cystic masses, with or without vascularized papillary projections inside the cysts. Autoimmune pancreatitis can have features similar to those of

pancreatic carcinoma due to lack of enhancement. CEUS has found a role in accurately differentiating inflammatory conditions such as pancreatitis and pancreatic adenocarcinoma based on differences in TICs.[69]

Contrast-Enhanced Ultrasound in the Assessment of Splenic Findings

Similar to pancreatic abnormalities, UCAs have not been approved for use in evaluating splenic masses, therefore their use is an off-label indication. However, contrast offers a natural advantage over conventional US while examining splenic masses. In contrast to pancreatic tail masses or lymph nodes, which typically demonstrate early washout, normal spleen parenchyma shows a late phase of microbubble trapping resulting in persistent enhancement. When compared with conventional US, CEUS improves differentiation of splenic masses such as lymphoma and metastases from benign entities.[70] A few common benign splenic masses include hemangioma, hamartoma, lymphangioma, splenic infarction, and complex cysts (**Fig. 9**A, B).

The behavior of splenic metastases is similar to that of hepatic metastases, including early washout and disorganized vessels.[71] Lymphomas typically show early arterial enhancement and rapid washout in the venous phase. Delayed enhancement in malignant tumors is due to the absence of sinusoidal spaces and reticuloendothelial system cells that are seen in normal parenchyma and benign masses. Early-phase isoenhancement with persistent enhancement in the late phase is suggestive of a benign process, including vascular

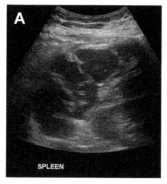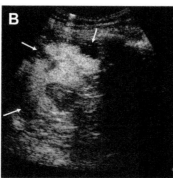

Fig. 9. (*A*, *B*) Splenic infarcts in a 64-year-old man with history of atrial fibrillation and back pain. Gray-scale image of the spleen in the sagittal plane shows heterogeneous splenic parenchyma. CEUS image obtained in similar projection demonstrates focal wedge-shape defects (*arrows*) in the subcapsular location of the spleen, indicating multiple infarcts.

malformations or hamartomas.[72,73] Benign masses also show slow or incomplete washout.[74] It is more challenging to accurately diagnose atypical splenic hemangiomas that contain necrosis or calcification, making CEUS pertinent. The typical centripetal pattern seen in liver hemangiomas is not common in splenic hemangiomas.[75]

Contrast-Enhanced Ultrasound in the Diagnosis of Adrenal Pathology

The use of CEUS has not been well studied in adrenal nodules and masses when compared with the relatively extensive data on renal tumors; this is likely because only around 10% of fewer of adrenal nodules and masses are functional and produce symptoms. Malignancy is seen in only 5% of cases.[76] Triphasic CECT remains the modality of choice in differentiating and diagnosing adrenal findings; however, characteristics of malignant and benign adrenal nodules and masses on CEUS have been reported in various studies with suggestions to use it as a screening tool given its high sensitivity.[77] Adrenal nodules and masses show 4 different types of enhancement patterns (1) early arterial enhancement (<20 seconds) with an early peak and washout, (2) arterial enhancement with peak enhancement after 30 seconds, (3) minimal/late enhancement that occurs after 40 seconds, and (4) no substantial enhancement. Malignant tumors often show the first 2 patterns, whereas the other 2 are seen in benign processes.[78] Similarly, parametric mapping of adrenal nodules and masses was studied by Stapa and colleagues,[79] who did not show any significant replicable pattern to differentiate between hyperplasia and adenomas.

Vascular Applications of Contrast-Enhanced Ultrasound and Monitoring Stent Graft Status

CEUS is an optimal modality for evaluation of vascular patency, either arterial or venous, including

but not limited to near occlusion, arterial dissection, plaque characterization/ulceration, and thrombus in vein assessment (**Figs. 10**A, B and **11**A, B).[80]

CEUS has been proved to add value in the evaluation of patients who underwent endovascular abdominal aortic aneurysm repair (EVAR), where a bifurcated abdominal stent graft is placed across the lumen of the aorta and iliac arteries to exclude the aneurysm from arterial circulation. The procedure has a high success rate but needs long-term monitoring for complications including endoleaks, fractures, graft migration, increase in aneurysm size, and so on. CEUS is effective in the diagnosis of endoleaks. Endoleak types include lack of a tight seal between the stent graft edge and the wall of the aorta (type 1a, 1b); the presence of a feeding vessel (type 2), either via the inferior mesenteric or lumbar arteries (**Fig. 12**); and loss of stent graft integrity due to compromise by stent-graft fracture (type 3). CT angiography with 3D reconstruction is at present the reference standard in the assessment of endoleaks, whereas color Doppler has shown to have a high specificity and variable sensitivity.[81,82] Mirza and colleagues[83] in their meta-analysis in 2010 found that CEUS can provide a sensitivity of 98% in diagnosing any type of endoleak in post-EVAR patients. SonoVue is currently approved for vascular imaging including imaging of the stent grafts. Presence of UCA within the aneurysm sac is diagnostic of endoleak. Immediate extravasation is seen in type 1 and type 3 endoleaks, whereas a delay of more than 5 seconds is seen in a type 2 endoleak.[83] Endoleak evaluation with CEUS also allows measurement of the aneurysm sac diameter. 3D CEUS for endoleak detection is another promising technique that combines 3D duplex US images with US contrast, enhancing blood flow leaks.[84,85]

A few CEUS disadvantages in the evaluation of the post-EVAR complications are worth mentioning, including restricted examination windows, interference due to bowel gas, and limitations

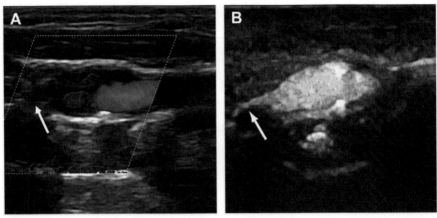

Fig. 10. Internal carotid artery near-complete occlusion in a 76 year-old woman presenting with multiple transient ischemic attacks. (A) Color Doppler image obtained in the sagittal plane over the right carotid system demonstrates flow at the bifurcation; however, no flow is seen at the origin and in the proximal internal carotid artery (ICA) (arrow in A), raising concern for complete ICA occlusion. (B) CEUS image in the arterial phase of imaging obtained in the sagittal plane demonstrates small amount of flow, also known as the "string sign" at the origin of the ICA (arrow in B) with adjacent soft plaque indicating incomplete occlusion, allowing for a change in patient management with plaque removal as a part of carotid endarterectomy.

due to patient body habitus and overlying ascites, if present. Reflection of sound by the stent, inability to recognize stent graft migration, and limited assessment for stent fracture/kinking are additional potential limitations. Complementary use of radiographs with CEUS can help to avoid some of these limitations.[86] The high sensitivity of CEUS for the detection of very small and clinically insignificant endoleaks decreases the efficacy of this application—often, patients with such small type 1 and type 2 endoleaks are managed conservatively without additional interventions. Therefore, CEUS

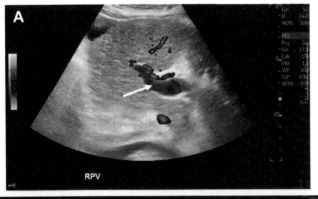

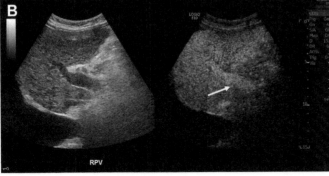

Fig. 11. Patency assessment of the main portal vein in a 69-year-old man with cirrhosis and elevated liver function test results. (A) Color Doppler image of the liver obtained in sagittal plane through the porta hepatis demonstrates nonfilling of the portal vein with color (arrow in A). This finding could be related to poor optimization of Doppler parameters, slow flow, absence of flow due to portal vein thrombosis, or artifact. (B) Fusion CEUS with gray-scale images through porta hepatis demonstrate clear enhancement of the portal vein on the CEUS confirming patency of the portal vein and absence of thrombosis (arrow in B).

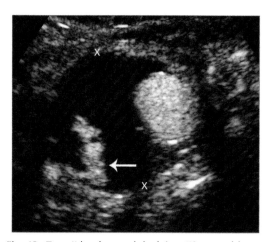

Fig. 12. Type II lumbar endoleak in a 72-year-old man with history of endovascular stent graft repair with increasing size of the infrarenal abdominal aneurysm. CEUS image obtained in the transverse view through the level of the aneurysm sac shows flow in the lumen of the sac extending from the posterior wall into the sac lumen (*arrow*), indicating a type II endoleak from the lumbar artery. Note white calipers identifying the aneurysm sac. Calipers show the sizde of the abdominal aortic aneurysm.

should be reserved for the evaluation of those post-EVAR patients whose aneurysm sac has increased in size or if there is a high clinical concern for other post-EVAR complications, including limb occlusion or development of an aortoenteric fistula.[86]

Therapeutic and Guidance Use of Contrast-Enhanced Ultrasound in the Abdomen and Pelvis

CEUS has also gained traction in US-guided procedures: biopsy, abscess drainage, percutaneous nephrostomy placement, various biliary interventions, thermal tumor ablations, and diagnosis of vascular complications.

Recently, CEUS gained acceptance as a guidance tool for thermal ablation of hepatic tumors not seen on conventional US. A study conducted in 2011 showed that CEUS-guided microwave ablation had a treatment efficacy of 99.05%, with fewer than 2% ablated tumors reporting progression.[87,88]

CEUS also plays a role in the detailed assessment of abscesses, especially if the abscess is multiloculated. In contrast to conventional US, CEUS provides better assessment of avascular portions of an abscess, delineating areas of septations and loculations within the affected parenchyma. CEUS aids in detection of communications between multiloculated abscess compartments, as the microbubbles move between the loculations.[89]

CEUS helps assess positioning of percutaneous drainage catheters, as well as detect catheter occlusion and malfunction. The ability of the technique to confer spatial information on necrotic areas and delineate vascular regions finds use in both drainage and biopsy, improving biopsy positive yields. This becomes clinically relevant, as poor differentiation of a target abnormality remains a common reason for a failed biopsy.[90]

In the setting of percutaneous nephrostomy, the nonenhancing pelvicalyceal system is imaged against a background of vascular renal cortex, which helps direct the nephrostomy tube toward the targeted calyx, avoiding cortical vascular injury. Postinsertion evaluation of functional drainage of urine can be simultaneously performed by injecting the UCA into the tube and observing the contrast bubbles' movement into the bladder—a technique called CEUS nephrostography. This method increases the success rate of accurate and optimal tube placement. Repeated attempts can be made by destroying the microbubbles and injecting new microbubbles on the second attempt. This method is different from a fluoroscopic-guided catheterization in which the injected CT contrast may interfere with repeated attempts of the procedure.[91]

Research around the therapeutic role of CEUS is also taking large strides. CEUS can serve as a vehicle of therapeutic drug delivery to an area of interest. A drug can be incorporated within the microbubble covered with the lipid-soluble shell and delivered by the bloodstream to the target area where it is then released from the lipid shell with the use of the US beam bursting the protective shell. A large concentration of a drug can be achieved locoregionally with a decreased risk of systemic side effects. In the recent past, one of the main limitations of this potential drug delivery application was the inability of microbubbles to cross blood-barrier and become incorporated into the targeted organ or structure's interstitium.[92,93] However, the introduction of focused US with microbubbles promises unprecedented advantages for blood-brain barrier disruption over existing intracranial drug delivery methods, as well as a substantial number of tunable parameters that affect its safety and efficacy.[94]

Contrast-Enhanced Ultrasound in Pelvic Diseases

The FDA has not yet approved CEUS for the evaluation of gynecologic or obstetric disorders. The safety of UCAs in pregnant women is not known; therefore, before CEUS, it is required to obtain a urine pregnancy test. Despite the aforementioned limitations, studies have shown that CEUS can help differentiate between various intrauterine pathologies based on patterns of enhancement.[95] The normal enhancement of the uterus begins with enhancement of the uterine artery followed by myometrium, myometrial-endometrial junction, and finally, endometrium.

The appearance of fibroids has been studied according to their size, with larger fibroids showing peripheral rim hyperenhancement (pseudocapsule) and centralized homogeneous and heterogeneous enhancement more prominent than the myometrium, whereas smaller fibroids (<2 cm) showing isoenhancement with no peripheral rim enhancement (pseudocapsule not enhanced). The washout in fibroids is faster when compared with the surrounding myometrium.[96] A few studies have also attempted to differentiate leiomyosarcomas, which show poorly defined borders when compared with the smooth borders seen in fibroids; the study reported earlier enhancement of feeding vessels than the surrounding myometrium.[97,98] Endometrial cancers show twisted and irregular blood vessels on 3D CEUS. Another clue is significantly lower perfusion time parameters and higher intensity parameters compared with other endometrial processes.[99,100] CEUS is also used for the differentiation of benign ovarian entities such as hemorrhagic cysts from neoplasms (**Fig. 13**A, B).

Ovarian tumors: A large meta-analysis by Qiao and colleagues[101] has shown CEUS to have high sensitivity and specificity for the differentiation of benign and malignant ovarian tumors. Malignant tumors tend to show early peak enhancement time and peak enhancement intensity when compared with benign tumors. This finding may be secondary to the presence of atrioventricular

(AV) shunts and neovascularization associated with malignancy. Another study showed that increased (time to peak intensity − arrival time) of the mass/(time to peak intensity −arrival time) of the uterus and ascending slope time are highly specific and sensitive markers for malignant tumors.[102,103] Further studies are needed to analyze if additional findings by CEUS are clinically relevant and affect treatment management and patient outcome.[104] Nevertheless, the diagnostic reliability of the technique remains high.[105]

Therapeutic and Interventional Use of Contrast-Enhanced Ultrasound in Gynecology

CEUS used for assessing postuterine artery embolization and post–microwave ablation and evaluating post-high intensity fociused ultrasound (HIFU) outcomes demonstrating fibroid perfusion has comparable efficacy to MR imaging.[106–108]

Contrast-Enhanced Ultrasound in Urology

Prostatic carcinomas (Pca) are often evaluated with multiparametric MRI (mpMRI). Although not in use in routine practice, ongoing efforts to detect and improve the role of CEUS have been under investigation in the past decade. A few studies on the use of CEUS in prostate cancer before and after treatment have shown a high biopsy yield, increased specificity and sensitivity, as well as easier and cost-effective posttreatment analysis.[109]

Pretreatment
When compared with conventional US guidance and 10-core systematic repeat biopsy strategy, CEUS has been shown to be an effective technique in performance of transrectal ultrasound

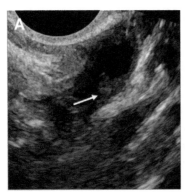 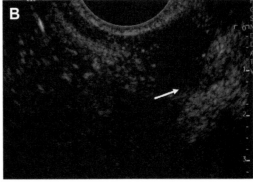

Fig. 13. Left ovarian cystic mass in a 72-year-old asymptomatic woman. (*A*) Gray-scale image of the left adnexa obtained via transvaginal (TV) approach demonstrates a cystic mass with suggestion of solid intramural components (*arrow*). (*B*) CEUS image of the same area shows no enhancement of the solid component (*arrow*) to suggest tumor vascularity indicating a benign entity, likely a blood clot.

prostate biopsy with improved detection rate and use of fewer biopsy passes.[110,111] Whether targeted biopsies are actually effective over systematic biopsies has not been established to our knowledge. The meta-analysis carried out by van Hove and colleagues[112] analyzing 6 CEUS targeted biopsies showed no added advantage of the technique. However, none of these studies included quantification parameters of CEUS, which have shown a reduction in biopsy core procedures (63.1%) with a 5.6% miss of clinically important Pca.[112,113] Similarly, a D-CEUS comparison with patients undergoing radical prostatectomy in 19 samples also reported an accuracy of 81% in detecting malignant regions and improving prostatic biopsy yield.[114] Thus, further studies on dynamic contrast enhancement with parametric mapping may be useful in the overall assessment of targeted biopsies.

The study by Lu and colleagues[115] on the use of contrast US in patients with various prostate-specific antigen (PSA) levels showed a high detection rate, even in patients with a relatively low concentration of PSA. The rise time and time to peak are two parameters that have shown the best results for quantitative detection of cancerous regions in tissue.[116] Features of prostatic malignancy on CEUS include focal hyperenhancement, rapid hyperenhancement, rapid washout (10–20 seconds), and asymmetrical distribution of blood vessels in the prostate. CEUS helps detect microcirculation in the tumor bed that is not revealed by Doppler US.[117]

Posttreatment

Unlike pretreatment analysis of prostatic tumors using mpMRI, analysis of treated tumoral foci with focal therapy is not well established. Assessment of tumor microcirculation with CEUS and mpMRI image fusions post-HIFU treatment has shown changes as early as 24 hours after treatment.[118,119] CEUS along with or without concomitant mpMRI for detecting missed clinically significant cancer post-HIFU may have utility as well.[120]

Contrast-Enhanced Ultrasound in Thyroid and Parathyroid Abnormalities

A recent 2022 article by Ruan and colleagues proposed a CEUS TIRADS scoring system. The scoring system considers 9 different parameters: 4 contrast-dependent parameters and 5 conventional US parameters. When performed together, TIRADS with CEUS has shown to improve diagnostic efficiency in studies comparing TIRADS and CEUS stand-alone with their combined diagnostic outcomes.[121]

The parameters of the scoring system include *echogenicity* (hyper/isoechoic [0 points], hypoechoic [1 point], and very hypoechoic [1 point]), *shape* (wider than tall [0 points] and taller than wide [1 point]), *margin* (smooth [0 point] or irregular/lobulated [1 point]), *extrathyroidal extension* (absent [0 points] or present [1 point]), *echogenic foci* (no calcification [0 points], rim calcification [1 point], macrocalcification [1 point], punctate echogenic foci [2 points]), *enhancement direction* (scattered [0 points], centripetal/centrifugal [1 point]), *peak intensity* (none/iso [0 points], hyper or hypo [1 point]), and *ring enhancement characteristic* (nonsolid [0 points], and solid [1 point]).[122]

Thyroid scoring system (TR1): 0 points TR 2: 1 point TR 3: 2 points TR 4 (A, B, and C with 3, 4, and 5 points respectively).[122] This study needs further validation and trials to discern clinical relevance and additional practical value over conventional US. Besides the scoring system, specific patterns can also be used to identify benign and malignant nodules.

Thyroid adenomas show *fast in-slow out* pattern. Specifically, the washout is either very slow with prominent edge postwashout or it does not occur by the late phase. Complete washout in the late phase is the most consistent finding of thyroid carcinomas. Other features including irregular ring enhancement, microcalcifications, and inhomogeneous hypoenhancement are also seen.[123] Lymph nodal metastases are identified by the absence of echogenic hila, the presence of microcalcification or cystic changes, and intensity to peak time.[124] However, the contradictory findings on peripheral ring enhancement patterns in studies by different authors prompt further trials and systematic reviews. An irregular pattern of rim enhancement is often noted in malignancy against a regular pattern seen in benign nodules.[125] A large meta-analysis and systematic review showed CEUS sensitivity and specificity of 85% and 82% for the diagnosis of malignant thyroid nodules.[126] Other nodular foci such as multinodular goiter show homogeneous isoenhancement with no specific differentiation pattern in thyroid parenchymal vascularization and that of the nodule. Inhomogeneous hyperenhancement is seen in liquefaction necrosis and hemorrhage[127]; however, inhomogeneous hypoenhancement patterns have also been reported.[128] In the setting of thyroiditis, heterogeneous enhancement is highly suggestive of malignancy. Thus, contrast may help to detect secondary malignancies in autoimmune thyroiditis. The combination of imaging features of CEUS along with time to peak, peak intensity, and quantitative parameters may show higher accuracy in diagnosing malignancy and differentiating it from nodular Hashimoto thyroiditis.[129]

Parathyroid

Preoperative localization of parathyroid adenomas (PAs) in primary hyperparathyroidism has been under research due to increasing use of minimally invasive parathyroidectomy replacing neck dissection. In patients with no visualization of PAs on conventional US, further imaging with a nuclear medicine scan (multiplexed ion beam imaging [MIBI] scans) is typically performed, followed by "4D" CT. Recent studies have compared the CEUS with 4D CT and have found similar sensitivity and specificity of these 2 examinations.[130] CEUS (with Sonozoid contrast agent) has also been used to analyze outcomes post–microwave ablation of PAs and has shown promising results. The potential clinical role of CEUS in differentiating PA from parathyroid hyperplasia (PH) has not yet been established.

On CEUS PA demonstrates early hyperenhancement with more distinct rim enhancement and late phase central washout. Centripetal enhancement is usually observed, which helps to differentiate PA from a lymph node that demonstrates centrifugal enhancement.

PH commonly shows early homogeneous enhancement with early washout; however, these findings are inconsistent. Quantitatively the wash in and washout rates and contrast signal intensity were significantly higher in PH than PA, providing an important groundwork for differentiating focal abnormalities with qualitative similarities.[131]

Contrast-Enhanced Ultrasound in Emergency Imaging

Contrast-enhanced ultrasound in trauma

Several studies have shown focused assessment with sonography for trauma to be excellent for revealing intraperitoneal free fluid, making it a routine practice for patients with blunt abdominal trauma. However, detection of solid organ injury in the absence of free fluid remains low.[132]

Solid organ injury shows nonenhancing defects against a well-enhanced background. Hematomas appear as heterogeneously enhancing areas with ill-defined borders, whereas subcapsular hematomas appear as nonenhancing lentiform areas. Absence of organ perfusion indicates complete avulsion of the vascular pedicle. Active extravasation appears as round or oval hyperechoic bands or serpentinelike hyperechoic jets, which is a shared feature with traumatic AV fistulas. Similarly, CEUS can play an important role in the follow-up of minor hepatic and splenic injuries.[133]

Contrast-enhanced ultrasound in ovarian and testicular pathologies

Acute ovarian pathologies Ovarian torsion is a gynecologic emergency seen in women of all ages, often affecting the right ovary more than the left due to the presence of the sigmoid colon that anchors the left ovary. Other predilections include the presence of a benign ovarian mass such as a teratoma that acts as a leading point.[134] The first-line modality for diagnosis is pelvic US with Doppler, but a continued strong clinical suspicion with a negative Doppler can be followed by CT or MR imaging. This approach is especially important as presence of blood flow in Doppler cannot be used to exclude intermittent torsion. CEUS in chronic torsion has shown reduction in vascularity when compared with the contralateral ovary. However, further studies are required for establishment of diagnostic findings and criteria.[135]

SonoVue contrast has been used off label in pediatric patients with ovarian torsion, with a reported high sensitivity of 94.1% and a specificity of 100%.[95,136] Findings include increased ovarian volume, inhomogeneous adnexal parenchymal echogenicity, and lack of contrast enhancement.

Acute testicular pathologies

The role of CEUS has not been found to be superior to Doppler and conventional US in cases of acute scrotum to exclude or diagnose torsion.[137] CEUS can aid in differentiation of the testicular masses from infarcts (**Fig. 14**A, B). Additionally, its potential use for diagnosing and differentiating benign and malignant testicular tumors, especially when they are small, vascular, and demonstrate well-defined margins, is promising. On CEUS, characteristic hyperenhancement is noted with almost all malignant testicular masses. **Table 3** summarizes different hyperenhancement patterns in testicular malignancies.

Contrast-Enhanced Ultrasound in Transplant Imaging

CEUS is a safe modality for initial imaging in patients with acute rejection of a renal allograft and vascular complications. CEUS is superior to Doppler for visualization of tissue perfusion (**Fig. 15**). Estimation of renal blood flow from CEUS has been shown to closely correlate with corresponding creatinine values, thus improving the diagnostic capability of US in the assessment of transplant organ rejection.[138,139] CEUS demonstrated equivalent sensitivity and specificity in the evaluation of patients who underwent renal transplant when compared with CECT. Thus, CEUS showed a sensitivity of 100%, a specificity of 66.7%, a positive predictive value of 71.4%, and a negative predictive value of 100% for the detection of vascular complications, which is similar to other cross-sectional imaging modalities.[140]

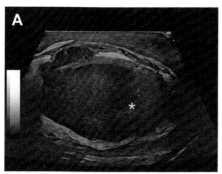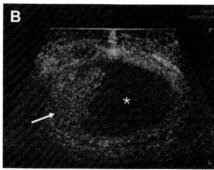

Fig. 14. Partial right testicular infarct in a 58-year-old man following inguinal hernia repair with right scrotal pain and swelling. Fusion gray-scale (*A*) and CEUS (*B*) images of the right testicle obtained in the sagittal plane demonstrate a hypoechoic heterogeneous area with irregular borders, which shows no enhancement on CEUS, indicating an infarct (*asterisks* in *A*, *B*). Note that the normally perfused remaining parenchyma of the upper pole of the testis is much better appreciated on CEUS (*arrow* in *B*).

Both Doppler and CEUS can be used to accurately diagnose renal artery stenosis. Complete absence of contrast enhancement with absence of flow on Doppler is seen in transplant renal artery thrombosis. It should be noted that absence of blood flow on Doppler in the renal artery may also be a sign of acute rejection. Therefore, CEUS increases confidence in the diagnosis of this severe complication.[141] Transplant renal vein thrombosis usually seen a week after surgery is a major cause of graft loss requiring prompt treatment. When the renal vein is occluded, the kidney enlarges due to congestion, the renal cortex appears hypoechoic and slightly heterogeneous, and there is absence of flow in the main renal vein on color and spectral Doppler. Arterial flow may demonstrate a characteristic reversal of flow in diastole. However, in some situations, visualization of the renal vein may be challenging due to edema, deep positioning of the transplant, and poor Doppler parameter optimization. This challenge can be compensated with the use of CEUS, where the absence of venous flow and the presence of pulsatile and high-resistance flow in renal parenchyma during the early corticomedullary phase attributable to organ congestion have been reported.[142] Quantitative analysis using TIC-derived analysis and abnormal quantitative indices has shown good potential in rejection detection. Acute rejection shows an increase in time to peak, whereas non-rejection-related acute tubular necrosis in grafts will show an increased mean transit time and regional blood volume.[143]

Contrast-Enhanced Ultrasound in the Pediatric Population

UCAs are considered safe in both adults and children.[144] Children have shown lower rates of contrast reactions when compared with adults.[145] The technique is used to evaluate liver abnormalities, pneumonia, congenital abnormalities in renal outflow, renal tumors, and pancreatic and bowel abnormalities, along with splenic malformations and hypoxic brain injury.

Renal and Adrenal Abnormalities

CEUS is frequently used for the evaluation of VUR and urethral obstruction (contrast-enhanced voiding urosonography). SonoVue is approved by the European Union (but not in the United States) for VUR assessment in children.[146] Other indications include recurrent infection, renal scarring secondary to reflux nephropathy, altered tract anatomy (ie, ureteroceles, ectopic ureter, and duplications), prenatal

Table 3
Different hyperenhancement patterns in testicular malignancies

Tumor	CEUS Finding
Non–germ cell tumors: a. Leydig cell tumor b. Sertoli cell tumor c. Lymphomas and leukemias	a. Homogenously hyperenhancing b. Hyperenhancing
Seminoma	Homogeneous hyperenhancing
Teratomas	Heterogeneously hyperenhancing
Yolk sac and choriocarcinomas	Hyperenhancing
Mixed germ cell tumor	Homogenously or inhomogeneously hyperenhancing

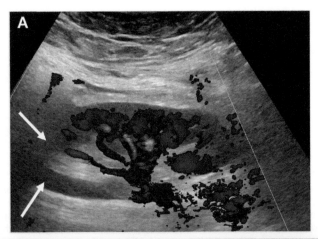

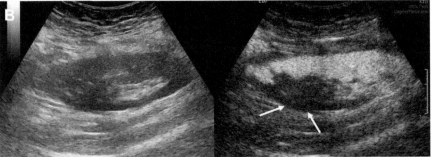

Fig. 15. Renal transplant infarct in a 56-year-old woman with increased serum creatinine. (*A*) Color Doppler image in the sagittal plane demonstrates a lack of color perfusion of the upper pole of the right lower quadrant renal transplant, concerning for an infarct (*arrows*). (*B*) Fusion gray-scale (*left*) and CEUS (*right*) images of the renal transplant show area of nonenhancement in the upper pole confirming renal transplant partial infarct (*arrows*).

ureterohydronephrosis, and urethral abnormalities. Vesicular conditions including diverticulum, urogenital sinus, anterior and posterior urethral valves, strictures, and ectasia can also be diagnosed using the technique.[147,148] Besides these, it can also be used to diagnose and differentiate between uncomplicated focal pyelonephritis and abscess (as discussed previously) in children with complicated infections and poor disease improvement on treatment.

Renal pseudotumors are embryonic remnants of renal masses that form part of the normal kidney and can even be functional as in the case of a hypertrophied column of Bertin. CEUS is a reliable technique to distinguish normal perfusion patterns and medullary pyramids to identify pseudotumors. Metanephric adenomas are benign tumors seen in children; they have been reported to be hyperenhancing in the arterial phase with subsequent hypoenhancement in late phases; however, these findings were not replicated in other studies.[149,150] The potential role of contrast US in the diagnosis of Wilms tumor and tumor characterization during

various phases remains to be investigated to our knowledge.

Brain

The open anterior fontanelle in children improves US visualization of brain parenchyma and intracranial contents. Conventional US is often the first-line and preferred diagnostic modality in the evaluation of various intracranial pathologies such as intraventricular hemorrhage, infections, and congenital anomalies. The off-label use of CEUS shows promise in diagnosis of hypoxic-ischemic injury changes. Hypoxic injury will present with nonenhancement and loss of gray-white matter differentiation. Congenital anomalies such as vein of Galen malformations can be easily diagnosed using contrast agents and has advantage over conventional US as it can help assess flow after embolization.[151]

Another potential use is for pediatric strokes; although strokes occur rarely in children, studies have shown successful assessment of stroke using quantitative parameters and delayed time to peak. Similarly thrombolytic treatment and reperfusion follow-up becomes convenient. Robust research in the field can potentially revolutionize and bring stroke treatment to peripheral and underserved areas.[152] A prospective indication for CEUS is for diagnosing infectious conditions including meningitis, cerebritis, and ventriculitis. An abscess can be easily differentiated from other focal abnormalities due to characteristic nonenhancement with a hyperenhancing rim appearance on CEUS.[153] CEUS fusion imaging with MR imaging also aids in intraoperative real-time imaging of tumor extent and vascularity for appraisal of tissue perfusion.[154]

Contrast-enhanced ultrasound in pneumonia
SonoVue marketed as LUMASON is the only UCA that has been used for pulmonary US imaging so far; however, it has not yet been approved by the FDA. Determining the presence of enhancement is important to identify avascular/hypoperfused regions, especially in conditions such as necrotizing pneumonia. As a rule of thumb contrast enhancement that occurs within 8 to 10 seconds after injection is due to supply via the pulmonary arterial circulation, whereas that coming from the bronchial arteries is delayed (due to time lag for contrast reaching left ventricle); similarly, an early washout is present when the contrast circulates out before the adjacent normal lung parenchyma.[155] It helps in delineating necrotizing nonenhancing areas or abscess cavities, which is often difficult to do with Doppler and conventional B-mode US.

CEUS can also depict complex parapneumonic effusions and expedites therapeutic decisions. Similarly in complex abscess cavities with thickened septations, drainage catheter patency and incomplete drainage can be assessed by injecting microbubble contrast via a catheter; this helps guide intrapleural fibrinolysis.[156,157]

CEUS can be used to biopsy pleural metastases from pediatric malignancies including Ewing sarcoma, Wilms tumor, hepatoblastoma, and osteosarcoma and to monitor treatment progression after chemotherapy. However, further large-scale research is needed to better define any conclusive role in this area.[158,159]

Contrast-Enhanced Ultrasound and Ultrasound Contrast Agents in Drug Delivery

Microbubbles have the potential to advance medical science far beyond diagnostic imaging. Currently, extensive research is underway to identify and explore the uses of microbubble contrast agents in drug delivery and targeted therapies. The use of microbubbles ensures targeted drug or gene delivery, enhanced delivery by overcoming the blood-brain barrier, and controlled release using an US probe.[160] Research and application for inner ear drug delivery, Alzheimer disease, Parkinson disease, intranasal drug delivery, and many other potential applications is presently advancing.[161,162] Microbubble contrast agents have been used for the identification of atherosclerotic plaque nature and plaque characterization with neovascularization for fragility assessment and risk assessment of thromboembolic events.[163] When oscillated at a given frequency, microbubbles have shown to create disruption-mediated cavitation foci, effectively enhancing thrombolysis and efficacy of thrombolytic drugs.[164]

Another potential area is the use of the technique to direct ligand-bound microbubbles toward diseased tissue. Animal-based experimentation has shown success in VCAM1 and P-selectin receptor-specific ligand-bound microbubble aggregation in inflamed vascular tissue.[163] The use of this delivery method in cancer diagnosis is a potential area for future studies. Similarly, use of microbubbles insonated with focused US and microbubble-enhanced unfocused US has shown to increase the permeability of the blood-brain barrier, thus allowing diagnostic as well as therapeutic agents to permeate brain parenchyma.

SUMMARY

IV CEUS is an advanced US imaging technique with the potential to diversify and enhance diagnostic applications, therapeutic use, and effectiveness of interventional procedures in both the adult and pediatric population. The technique has a high potential in the field of interventional oncology and could potentially even outperform other crosssectional modalities for real-time tissue analysis. This technique shows great promise for the identification of various systemic pathologies without the need of protracted or radiation-intensive scans, an added advantage in emergency cases and in the pediatric population. Contrast agents for drug deliveries and targeted therapy have the potential to revolutionize the future of oncology. However, there are well-recognized limitations and barriers to the use of CEUS including operator dependance, difficulty in evaluation of patients with large body habitus or those with substantial bowel gas, and limited field of view in CEUS when compared with CT and MR imaging. Additionally, high workload of radiologists, lack of trained personnel to perform and assist in performance of this procedure, and limited hospital and private practice facility resources make utilization and widespread use of the CEUS application much more challenging.

CLINICS CARE POINTS

- CEUS can be used to accurately characterise solid organ masses.
- CEUS is an excellent modality for evaluation of vascular patency, active extravasation, and neovascularty in a neoplasm.

REFERENCES

1. Ajmal S. Contrast-enhanced ultrasonography: review and applications. Cureus 2021;13(9):e18243.
2. Malone CD, Fetzer DT, Monsky WL, et al. Contrast-enhanced US for the Interventional Radiologist: Current and Emerging Applications. Radiographics 2020;40(2):562–88.
3. Lee JY, Minami Y, Choi BI, et al. The AFSUMB consensus statements and recommendations for the clinical practice of contrast-enhanced ultrasound using sonazoid. J Med Ultrasound 2020; 28(2):59–82.
4. Dietrich CF, Averkiou MA, Correas JM, et al. An EFSUMB introduction into Dynamic Contrast-Enhanced Ultrasound (DCE-US) for quantification of tumour perfusion. Ultraschall der Med 2012; 33(4):344–51.
5. Piscaglia F, Bolondi L, Italian Society for Ultrasound in M, Biology Study Group on Ultrasound Contrast A. The safety of Sonovue in abdominal applications: retrospective analysis of 23188 investigations. Ultrasound Med Biol 2006;32(9): 1369–75.
6. Abou-Saleh RH, Swain M, Evans SD, et al. Poly(ethylene glycol) lipid-shelled microbubbles: abundance, stability, and mechanical properties. Langmuir 2014;30(19):5557–63.
7. Soni M, McGovern M, Jacob R, et al. Ultrasound-enhancing agents and associated adverse reactions: a potential connection to the COVID-19 vaccines? J Am Soc Echocardiogr 2022;35(2):241–2.
8. D'Onofrio M, Crosara S, De Robertis R, et al. Contrast-enhanced ultrasound of focal liver lesions. AJR Am J Roentgenol 2015;205(1):W56–66.
9. AIUM practice parameter for the performance of contrast-enhanced ultrasound. J Ultrasound Med 2024;43(3):E8–19.
10. Barr RG, Wilson SR, Lyshchik A, et al. Contrast-enhanced ultrasound: state of the art in North America. Ultrasound Q 2020;36(3):206–17.
11. Quaia E, Calliada F, Bertolotto M, et al. Characterization of focal liver lesions with contrast-specific US modes and a sulfur hexafluoride-filled microbubble contrast agent: diagnostic performance and confidence. Radiology 2004;232(2):420–30.
12. Quaia E, Bertolotto M, Dalla Palma L. Characterization of liver hemangiomas with pulse inversion harmonic imaging. Eur Radiol 2002;12(3):537–44.
13. El-Ali AM, McCormick A, Thakrar D, et al. Contrast-enhanced ultrasound of congenital and infantile hemangiomas: preliminary results from a case series. AJR Am J Roentgenol 2020;214(3):658–64.
14. Shiozawa K, Watanabe M, Ikehara T, et al. Evaluation of hemodynamics in focal steatosis and focal spared lesion of the liver using contrast-enhanced ultrasonography with sonazoid. Radiol Res Pract 2014; 2014:604594.
15. Nguyen BN, Flejou JF, Terris B, et al. Focal nodular hyperplasia of the liver: a comprehensive pathologic study of 305 lesions and recognition of new histologic forms. Am J Surg Pathol 1999;23(12): 1441–54.
16. Piscaglia F, Lencioni R, Sagrini E, et al. Characterization of focal liver lesions with contrast-enhanced ultrasound. Ultrasound Med Biol 2010;36(4): 531–50.
17. Kim TK, Jang HJ. Contrast-enhanced ultrasound in the diagnosis of nodules in liver cirrhosis. World J Gastroenterol 2014;20(13):3590–6.
18. Hu J, Bhayana D, Burak KW, et al. Resolution of indeterminate MRI with CEUS in patients at high risk for hepatocellular carcinoma. Abdom Radiol (NY) 2020;45(1):123–33.
19. Burrowes DP, Kono Y, Medellin A, et al. Radio-Graphics update: contrast-enhanced US approach to the diagnosis of focal liver masses. Radiographics 2020;40(4):E16–20.
20. Wu Q, Liu Y, Sun D, et al. Protocol of Kupffer phase whole liver scan for metastases: a single-center prospective study. Front Med 2022;9:911807.
21. Yang HK, Burns PN, Jang HJ, et al. Contrast-enhanced ultrasound approach to the diagnosis of focal liver lesions: the importance of washout. Ultrasonography 2019;38(4):289–301.
22. Rawla P, Sunkara T, Muralidharan P, et al. Update in global trends and aetiology of hepatocellular carcinoma. Contemp Oncol 2018;22(3):141–50.
23. Younossi ZM. Non-alcoholic fatty liver disease - A global public health perspective. J Hepatol 2019; 70(3):531–44.
24. Jang HJ, Kim TK, Burns PN, et al. Enhancement patterns of hepatocellular carcinoma at contrast-enhanced US: comparison with histologic differentiation. Radiology 2007;244(3):898–906.
25. Banales JM, Marin JJG, Lamarca A, et al. Cholangiocarcinoma 2020: the next horizon in mechanisms and management. Nat Rev Gastroenterol Hepatol 2020;17:557–88.
26. Banales JM, Cardinale V, Carpino G, et al. Expert consensus document: cholangiocarcinoma: current knowledge and future perspectives consensus statement from the European Network for the Study of

Cholangiocarcinoma (ENS-CCA). Nat Rev Gastroenterol Hepatol 2016;13:261–80. Available at: https://www.cancer.org/cancer/types/bile-duct-cancer/about/key-statistics.html#:~:text=bileductcancer?-,Howcommonisbileductcancer?,ismuchmorecommon there.

27. Wilson SR, Burns PN, Kono Y. Contrast-enhanced ultrasound of focal liver masses: a success story. Ultrasound Med Biol 2020;46(5):1059–70.

28. Li CQ, Zheng X, Guo HL, et al. Differentiation between combined hepatocellular carcinoma and hepatocellular carcinoma: comparison of diagnostic performance between ultrasomics-based model and CEUS LI-RADS v2017. BMC Med Imag 2022; 22(1):36.

29. Yoshida Y, Imai Y, Murakami T, et al. Intrahepatic cholangiocarcinoma with marked hypervascularity. Abdom Imag 1999;24(1):66–8.

30. Valls C, Guma A, Puig I, et al. Intrahepatic peripheral cholangiocarcinoma: CT evaluation. Abdom Imag 2000;25(5):490–6.

31. Guo LH, Xu HX. Contrast-enhanced ultrasound in the diagnosis of hepatocellular carcinoma and intrahepatic cholangiocarcinoma: controversy over the ASSLD guideline. BioMed Res Int 2015;2015: 349172.

32. Xu HX, Chen LD, Liu LN, et al. Contrast-enhanced ultrasound of intrahepatic cholangiocarcinoma: correlation with pathological examination. Br J Radiol 2012;85(1016):1029–37.

33. Manichon AF, Bancel B, Durieux-Millon M, et al. Hepatocellular adenoma: evaluation with contrast-enhanced ultrasound and MRI and correlation with pathologic and phenotypic classification in 26 lesions. HPB Surg 2012;2012:418745.

34. Wilson SR, Lyshchik A, Piscaglia F, et al. CEUS LI-RADS: algorithm, implementation, and key differences from CT/MRI. Abdom Radiol (NY) 2018; 43(1):127–42.

35. Dietrich CF, Nolsoe CP, Barr RG, et al. Guidelines and Good Clinical Practice Recommendations for Contrast-Enhanced Ultrasound (CEUS) in the liver-update 2020 WFUMB in cooperation with EFSUMB, AFSUMB, AIUM, and FLAUS. Ultrasound Med Biol 2020;46(10):2579–604.

36. Faccia M, Garcovich M, Ainora ME, et al. Contrast-enhanced ultrasound for monitoring treatment response in different stages of hepatocellular carcinoma. Cancers 2022;14(3).

37. Takizawa K, Numata K, Morimoto M, et al. Use of contrast-enhanced ultrasonography with a perflubutane-based contrast agent performed one day after transarterial chemoembolization for the early assessment of residual viable hepatocellular carcinoma. Eur J Radiol 2013;82(9):1471–80.

38. Watanabe Y, Ogawa M, Kumagawa M, et al. Utility of contrast-enhanced ultrasound for early therapeutic evaluation of hepatocellular carcinoma after transcatheter arterial chemoembolization. J Ultrasound Med 2020;39(3):431–40.

39. Ljungberg B, Albiges L, Abu-Ghanem Y, et al. European association of urology guidelines on renal cell carcinoma: the 2022 update. Eur Urol 2022; 82(4):399–410.

40. Furrer MA, Spycher SCJ, Buttiker SM, et al. Comparison of the diagnostic performance of contrast-enhanced ultrasound with that of contrast-enhanced computed tomography and contrast-enhanced magnetic resonance imaging in the evaluation of renal masses: a systematic review and meta-analysis. Eur Urol Oncol 2020;3(4):464–73.

41. Herms E, Weirich G, Maurer T, et al. Ultrasound-based "CEUS-Bosniak" classification for cystic renal lesions: an 8-year clinical experience. World J Urol 2023;41(3):679–85.

42. Cantisani V, Bertolotto M, Clevert DA, et al. EFSUMB 2020 proposal for a contrast-enhanced ultrasound-adapted bosniak cyst categorization - position statement. Ultraschall der Med 2021; 42(2):154–66.

43. Smith AD, Remer EM, Cox KL, et al. Bosniak category IIF and III cystic renal lesions: outcomes and associations. Radiology 2012;262(1):152–60.

44. Cairns P. Renal cell carcinoma. Cancer Biomarkers 2010;9(1–6):461–73.

45. Graumann O, Osther SS, Karstoft J, et al. Bosniak classification system: a prospective comparison of CT, contrast-enhanced US, and MR for categorizing complex renal cystic masses. Acta Radiol 2016;57(11):1409–17.

46. Chen Y, Wu N, Xue T, et al. Comparison of contrast-enhanced sonography with MRI in the diagnosis of complex cystic renal masses. J Clin Ultrasound 2015;43(4):203–9.

47. Xue LY, Lu Q, Huang BJ, et al. Papillary renal cell carcinoma and clear cell renal cell carcinoma: Differentiation of distinct histological types with contrast - enhanced ultrasonography. Eur J Radiol 2015;84(10):1849–56.

48. Dipinto P, Canale V, Minelli R, et al. Qualitative and quantitative characteristics of CEUS for renal cell carcinoma and angiomyolipoma: a narrative review. J Ultrasound 2024;27(1):13–20.

49. Geyer T, Schwarze V, Marschner C, et al. Diagnostic Performance of Contrast-Enhanced Ultrasound (CEUS) in the evaluation of solid renal masses. Medicina (Kaunas) 2020;56(11).

50. Zhu J, Li N, Zhao P, et al. Contrast-enhanced ultrasound (CEUS) of benign and malignant renal tumors: distinguishing CEUS features differ with tumor size. Cancer Med 2023;12(3):2551–9.

51. Tufano A, Drudi FM, Angelini F, et al. Contrast-Enhanced Ultrasound (CEUS) in the evaluation of renal masses with histopathological validation-results from a

prospective single-center study. Diagnostics 2022; 12(5).

52. Rinaldo C, Grimaldi D, Di Serafino M, et al. An update on pyelonephritis: role of contrast enhancement ultrasound (CEUS). J Ultrasound 2023;26(2): 333–42.

53. Mitchell DG. Color Doppler imaging: principles, limitations, and artifacts. Radiology 1990;177(1): 1–10.

54. Castellano MA, Scheeffer V, Petersen V, et al. Evaluation of bowel wall flow by color Doppler ultrasound in the assessment of inflammatory bowel disease activity in pediatric patients. Radiol Bras 2023;56(5):242–7.

55. Ahmed R, Debian H, Fawzi M, et al. Diagnosis of inflammatory bowel disease by abdominal ultrasound and color Doppler techniques. Curr Med Imaging 2021;17(9):1085–93.

56. Lahiff C, Safaie P, Awais A, et al. The Crohn's disease activity index (CDAI) is similarly elevated in patients with Crohn's disease and in patients with irritable bowel syndrome. Aliment Pharmacol Ther 2013;37(8):786–94.

57. Serafin Z, Bialecki M, Bialecka A, et al. Contrast-enhanced ultrasound for detection of Crohn's disease activity: systematic review and meta-analysis. J Crohns Colitis 2016;10(3):354–62.

58. Ripolles T, Martinez-Perez MJ, Blanc E, et al. Contrast-enhanced ultrasound (CEUS) in Crohn's disease: technique, image interpretation and clinical applications. Insights Imaging 2011;2(6):639–52.

59. Paredes JM, Ripolles T, Cortes X, et al. Contrast-enhanced ultrasonography: usefulness in the assessment of postoperative recurrence of Crohn's disease. J Crohns Colitis 2013;7(3):192–201.

60. Medellin A, Merrill C, Wilson SR. Role of contrast-enhanced ultrasound in evaluation of the bowel. Abdom Radiol (NY) 2018;43(4):918–33.

61. Liu LN, Xu HX, Lu MD, et al. Contrast-enhanced ultrasound in the diagnosis of gallbladder diseases: a multi-center experience. PLoS One 2012;7(10): e48371.

62. Piscaglia F, Nolsoe C, Dietrich CF, et al. The EFSUMB Guidelines and Recommendations on the Clinical Practice of Contrast Enhanced Ultrasound (CEUS): update 2011 on non-hepatic applications. Ultraschall der Med 2012;33(1):33–59.

63. Sidhu PS, Cantisani V, Dietrich CF, et al. The EFSUMB Guidelines and Recommendations for the Clinical Practice of Contrast-Enhanced Ultrasound (CEUS) in non-hepatic applications: update 2017 (Long Version). Ultraschall der Med 2018;39(2): e2–44.

64. D'Onofrio M, Crosara S, Signorini M, et al. Comparison between CT and CEUS in the diagnosis of pancreatic adenocarcinoma. Ultraschall der Med 2013;34(4):377–81.

65. Jia WY, Gui Y, Chen XQ, et al. Evaluation of the diagnostic performance of the EFSUMB CEUS Pancreatic Applications guidelines (2017 version): a retrospective single-center analysis of 455 solid pancreatic masses. Eur Radiol 2022;32(12):8485–96.

66. D'Onofrio M, Mansueto G, Falconi M, et al. Neuroendocrine pancreatic tumor: value of contrast enhanced ultrasonography. Abdom Imag 2004; 29(2):246–58.

67. D'Onofrio M, Zamboni G, Faccioli N, et al. Ultrasonography of the pancreas. 4. Contrast-enhanced imaging. Abdom Imag 2007;32(2):171–81.

68. D'Onofrio M, Caffarri S, Zamboni G, et al. Contrast-enhanced ultrasonography in the characterization of pancreatic mucinous cystadenoma. J Ultrasound Med 2004;23(8):1125–9.

69. Vitali F, Pfeifer L, Janson C, et al. Quantitative perfusion analysis in pancreatic contrast enhanced ultrasound (DCE-US): a promising tool for the differentiation between autoimmune pancreatitis and pancreatic cancer. Z Gastroenterol 2015;53(10): 1175–81.

70. Yang R, Lu Q, Xu J, et al. Value of contrast-enhanced ultrasound in the differential diagnosis of focal splenic lesions. Cancer Manag Res 2021;13:2947–58.

71. von Herbay A, Barreiros AP, Ignee A, et al. Contrast-enhanced ultrasonography with SonoVue: differentiation between benign and malignant lesions of the spleen. J Ultrasound Med 2009;28(4):421–34.

72. Gorg C, Graef C, Bert T. Contrast-enhanced sonography for differential diagnosis of an inhomogeneous spleen of unknown cause in patients with pain in the left upper quadrant. J Ultrasound Med 2006;25(6):729–34.

73. Stang A, Keles H, Hentschke S, et al. Incidentally detected splenic lesions in ultrasound: does contrast-enhanced ultrasonography improve the differentiation of benign hemangioma/hamartoma from malignant lesions? Ultraschall der Med 2011;32(6):582–92.

74. Stang A, Keles H, Hentschke S, et al. Differentiation of benign from malignant focal splenic lesions using sulfur hexafluoride-filled microbubble contrast-enhanced pulse-inversion sonography. AJR Am J Roentgenol 2009;193(3):709–21.

75. Catalano O, Lobianco R, Sandomenico F, et al. Real-time contrast-enhanced ultrasound of the spleen: examination technique and preliminary clinical experience. Radiol Med 2003;106(4):338–56.

76. Dietrich CF, Correas JM, Dong Y, et al. WFUMB position paper on the management incidental findings: adrenal incidentaloma. Ultrasonography 2020;39(1):11–21.

77. Aggarwal A, Das CJ. Contrast-enhanced ultrasound in evaluation of adrenal lesions with CT/MRI correlation. Br J Radiol 2021;94(1120): 20201170.

78. Friedrich-Rust M, Glasemann T, Polta A, et al. Differentiation between benign and malignant adrenal mass using contrast-enhanced ultrasound. Ultraschall der Med 2011;32(5):460–71.

79. Slapa RZ, Kasperlik-Zaluska AA, Migda B, et al. Application of parametric ultrasound contrast agent perfusion studies for differentiation of hyperplastic adrenal nodules from adenomas-Initial study. Eur J Radiol 2015;84(8):1432–5.

80. Mehta KS, Lee JJ, Taha AG, et al. Vascular applications of contrast-enhanced ultrasound imaging. J Vasc Surg 2017;66(1):266–74.

81. Karthikesalingam A, Al-Jundi W, Jackson D, et al. Systematic review and meta-analysis of duplex ultrasonography, contrast-enhanced ultrasonography or computed tomography for surveillance after endovascular aneurysm repair. Br J Surg 2012;99(11):1514–23.

82. Smith T, Quencer KB. Best practice guidelines: imaging surveillance after endovascular aneurysm repair. AJR Am J Roentgenol 2020;214(5):1165–74.

83. Mirza TA, Karthikesalingam A, Jackson D, et al. Duplex ultrasound and contrast-enhanced ultrasound versus computed tomography for the detection of endoleak after EVAR: systematic review and bivariate meta-analysis. Eur J Vasc Endovasc Surg 2010;39(4):418–28.

84. Abbas A, Hansrani V, Sedgwick N, et al. 3D contrast enhanced ultrasound for detecting endoleak following endovascular aneurysm repair (EVAR). Eur J Vasc Endovasc Surg 2014;47(5):487–92.

85. Lowe C, Abbas A, Rogers S, et al. Three-dimensional contrast-enhanced ultrasound improves endoleak detection and classification after endovascular aneurysm repair. J Vasc Surg 2017; 65(5):1453–9.

86. Cantisani V, Grazhdani H, Clevert DA, et al. EVAR: Benefits of CEUS for monitoring stent-graft status. Eur J Radiol 2015;84(9):1658–65.

87. Kim TK, Khalili K, Jang HJ. Local ablation therapy with contrast-enhanced ultrasonography for hepatocellular carcinoma: a practical review. Ultrasonography 2015;34(4):235–45.

88. Liu F, Yu X, Liang P, et al. Contrast-enhanced ultrasound-guided microwave ablation for hepatocellular carcinoma inconspicuous on conventional ultrasound. Int J Hyperther 2011;27(6):555–62.

89. Kishina M, Koda M, Tokunaga S, et al. Usefulness of contrast-enhanced ultrasound with Sonazoid for evaluating liver abscess in comparison with conventional B-mode ultrasound. Hepatol Res 2015;45(3):337–42.

90. Sainani NI, Arellano RS, Shyn PB, et al. The challenging image-guided abdominal mass biopsy: established and emerging techniques 'if you can see it, you can biopsy it'. Abdom Imag 2013;38(4):672–96.

91. Guo X, Zhang Z, Liu Z, et al. Assessment of the contrast-enhanced ultrasound in percutaneous nephrolithotomy for the treatment of patients with nondilated collecting system. J Endourol 2021; 35(4):436–43.

92. Mitchell MJ, Billingsley MM, Haley RM, et al. Engineering precision nanoparticles for drug delivery. Nat Rev Drug Discov 2021;20(2):101–24.

93. Shakya G, Cattaneo M, Guerriero G, et al. Ultrasound-responsive microbubbles and nanodroplets: A pathway to targeted drug delivery. Adv Drug Deliv Rev 2024;206:115178.

94. Song KH, Harvey BK, Borden MA. State-of-the-art of microbubble-assisted blood-brain barrier disruption. Theranostics 2018;8(16):4393–408.

95. Olinger K, Liu X, Khoshpouri P, et al. Added value of contrast-enhanced US for evaluation of female pelvic disease. Radiographics 2024;44(2):e230092.

96. Wang W, Wang Y, Tang J. Safety and efficacy of high intensity focused ultrasound ablation therapy for adenomyosis. Acad Radiol 2009;16(11): 1416–23.

97. Li Z, Zhang P, Shen H, et al. Clinical value of contrast-enhanced ultrasound for the differential diagnosis of specific subtypes of uterine leiomyomas. J Obstet Gynaecol Res 2021;47(1):311–9.

98. Zhang XL, Zheng RQ, Yang YB, et al. The use of contrast-enhanced ultrasound in uterine leiomyomas. Chin Med J (Engl). 2010;123(21):3095–9.

99. Zhou HL, Xiang H, Duan L, et al. Application of combined two-dimensional and three-dimensional transvaginal contrast enhanced ultrasound in the diagnosis of endometrial carcinoma. BioMed Res Int 2015;2015:292743.

100. Liu Y, Xu Y, Cheng W, et al. Quantitative contrast-enhanced ultrasonography for the differential diagnosis of endometrial hyperplasia and endometrial neoplasms. Oncol Lett 2016;12(5):3763–70.

101. Qiao JJ, Yu J, Yu Z, et al. Contrast-enhanced ultrasonography in differential diagnosis of benign and malignant ovarian tumors. PLoS One 2015;10(3): e0118872.

102. Shentu W, Zhang Y, Gu J, et al. Contrast-enhanced ultrasonography for differential diagnosis of adnexal masses. Front Oncol 2022;12:968759.

103. Orden MR, Jurvelin JS, Kirkinen PP. Kinetics of a US contrast agent in benign and malignant adnexal tumors. Radiology 2003;226(2):405–10.

104. Sconfienza LM, Perrone N, Delnevo A, et al. Diagnostic value of contrast-enhanced ultrasonography in the characterization of ovarian tumors. J Ultrasound 2010;13(1):9–15.

105. Xu A, Nie F, Liu T, et al. Adnexal masses: diagnostic performance of contrast-enhanced ultrasound using the simple rules from the international ovarian tumor analysis group. Int J Gynaecol Obstet 2022;157(3):568–73.

106. Henri M, Florence E, Aurore B, et al. Contribution of contrast-enhanced ultrasound with Sonovue to describe the microvascularization of uterine fibroid tumors before and after uterine artery embolization. Eur J Obstet Gynecol Reprod Biol 2014;181: 104–10.

107. Peng S, Hu L, Chen W, et al. Intraprocedure contrast enhanced ultrasound: the value in assessing the effect of ultrasound-guided high intensity focused ultrasound ablation for uterine fibroids. Ultrasonics 2015;58:123–8.

108. Jiang N, Xie B, Zhang X, et al. Enhancing ablation effects of a microbubble-enhancing contrast agent ("SonoVue") in the treatment of uterine fibroids with high-intensity focused ultrasound: a randomized controlled trial. Cardiovasc Intervent Radiol 2014; 37(5):1321–8.

109. Dias AB, O'Brien C, Correas JM, et al. Multiparametric ultrasound and micro-ultrasound in prostate cancer: a comprehensive review. Br J Radiol 2022; 95(1131):20210633.

110. Xie SW, Li HL, Du J, et al. Contrast-enhanced ultrasonography with contrast-tuned imaging technology for the detection of prostate cancer: comparison with conventional ultrasonography. BJU Int 2012; 109(11):1620–6.

111. Mitterberger M, Horninger W, Aigner F, et al. Contrast-enhanced colour Doppler-targeted vs a 10-core systematic repeat biopsy strategy in patients with previous high-grade prostatic intraepithelial neoplasia. BJU Int 2010;105(12):1660–2.

112. van Hove A, Savoie PH, Maurin C, et al. Comparison of image-guided targeted biopsies versus systematic randomized biopsies in the detection of prostate cancer: a systematic literature review of well-designed studies. World J Urol 2014;32(4): 847–58.

113. Postema AW, Frinking PJ, Smeenge M, et al. Dynamic contrast-enhanced ultrasound parametric imaging for the detection of prostate cancer. BJU Int 2016;117(4):598–603.

114. Wildeboer RR, Postema AW, Demi L, et al. Multiparametric dynamic contrast-enhanced ultrasound imaging of prostate cancer. Eur Radiol 2017;27(8): 3226–34.

115. Lu DY, Shen L, Cai JR, et al. [Clinical value of contrast-enhanced ultrasonography in the diagnosis of prostate cancer in patients with different PSA concentrations]. Zhonghua Nan ke Xue 2018; 24(1):50–4.

116. Maxeiner A, Fischer T, Schwabe J, et al. Contrast-Enhanced Ultrasound (CEUS) and quantitative perfusion analysis in patients with suspicion for prostate cancer. Ultraschall der Med 2019;40(3):340–8.

117. Postema AW, Scheltema MJ, Mannaerts CK, et al. The prostate cancer detection rates of CEUS-targeted versus MRI-targeted versus systematic TRUS-guided biopsies in biopsy-naive men: a prospective, comparative clinical trial using the same patients. BMC Urol 2017;17(1):27.

118. Apfelbeck M, Clevert DA, Ricke J, et al. Contrast enhanced ultrasound (CEUS) with MRI image fusion for monitoring focal therapy of prostate cancer with high intensity focused ultrasound (HIFU)1. Clin Hemorheol Microcirc 2018;69(1–2): 93–100.

119. Apfelbeck M, Chaloupka M, Schlenker B, et al. Follow-up after focal therapy of the prostate with high intensity focused ultrasound (HIFU) using contrast enhanced ultrasound (CEUS) in combination with MRI image fusion. Clin Hemorheol Microcirc 2019;73(1):135–43.

120. Bacchetta F, Martins M, Regusci S, et al. The utility of intraoperative contrast-enhanced ultrasound in detecting residual disease after focal HIFU for localized prostate cancer. Urol Oncol 2020;38(11): 846 e1–e7.

121. Zhao H, Liu X, Lei B, et al. Diagnostic performance of thyroid imaging reporting and data system (TI-RADS) alone and in combination with contrast-enhanced ultrasonography for the characterization of thyroid nodules. Clin Hemorheol Microcirc 2019; 72(1):95–106.

122. Ruan J, Xu X, Cai Y, et al. A practical CEUS thyroid reporting system for thyroid nodules. Radiology 2022;305(1):149–59.

123. Zhang Y, Luo YK, Zhang MB, et al. Diagnostic accuracy of contrast-enhanced ultrasound enhancement patterns for thyroid nodules. Med Sci Monit 2016;22:4755–64.

124. Zhan J, Diao XH, Chen Y, et al. Homogeneity parameter in contrast-enhanced ultrasound imaging improves the classification of abnormal cervical lymph node after thyroidectomy in patients with papillary thyroid carcinoma. BioMed Res Int 2019; 2019:9296010.

125. Radzina M, Ratniece M, Putrins DS, et al. Performance of contrast-enhanced ultrasound in thyroid nodules: review of current state and future perspectives. Cancers 2021;13(21).

126. Trimboli P, Castellana M, Virili C, et al. Performance of contrast-enhanced ultrasound (CEUS) in assessing thyroid nodules: a systematic review and meta-analysis using histological standard of reference. Radiol Med 2020;125(4):406–15.

127. Jiang J, Shang X, Wang H, et al. Diagnostic value of contrast-enhanced ultrasound in thyroid nodules with calcification. Kaohsiung J Med Sci 2015;31(3): 138–44.

128. He Y, Wang XY, Hu Q, et al. Value of contrast-enhanced ultrasound and acoustic radiation force impulse imaging for the differential diagnosis of benign and malignant thyroid nodules. Front Pharmacol 2018;9:1363.

129. Yang L, Zhao H, He Y, et al. Contrast-enhanced ultrasound in the differential diagnosis of primary thyroid lymphoma and nodular hashimoto's thyroiditis in a background of heterogeneous parenchyma. Front Oncol 2020;10:597975.

130. Lerner A, Grant EG, Acharya J, et al. Utility of contrast-enhanced ultrasound and 4-dimensional computed tomography for preoperative detection and localization of parathyroid adenomas compared with surgical results. J Ultrasound Med 2022;41(9): 2295–306.

131. Pavlovics S, Radzina M, Niciporuka R, et al. Contrast-enhanced ultrasound qualitative and quantitative characteristics of parathyroid gland lesions. Medicina (Kaunas) 2021;58(1).

132. Valentino M, Serra C, Zironi G, et al. Blunt abdominal trauma: emergency contrast-enhanced sonography for detection of solid organ injuries. AJR Am J Roentgenol 2006;186(5):1361–7.

133. Manetta R, Pistoia ML, Bultrini C, et al. Ultrasound enhanced with sulphur-hexafluoride-filled microbubbles agent (SonoVue) in the follow-up of mild liver and spleen trauma. Radiol Med 2009;114(5):771–9.

134. Guile SL, Mathai JK. Ovarian Torsion. StatPearls. Treasure Island (FL) ineligible companies. Disclosure: Josephin Mathai declares no relevant financial relationships with ineligible companies.2024.

135. Bardin R, Perl N, Mashiach R, et al. Prediction of adnexal torsion by ultrasound in women with acute abdominal pain. Ultraschall der Med 2020;41(6): 688–94.

136. Trinci M, Danti G, Di Maurizio M, et al. Can contrast enhanced ultrasound (CEUS) be useful in the diagnosis of ovarian torsion in pediatric females? A preliminary monocentric experience. J Ultrasound 2021;24(4):505–14.

137. Moschouris H, Stamatiou K, Lampropoulou E, et al. Imaging of the acute scrotum: is there a place for contrast-enhanced ultrasonography? Int Braz J Urol 2009;35(6):692–702 [discussion -5].

138. Wang X, Yu Z, Guo R, et al. Assessment of postoperative perfusion with contrast-enhanced ultrasonography in kidney transplantation. Int J Clin Exp Med 2015;8(10):18399–405.

139. Miller A 3rd, Scanlan RA, Lee JS, et al. Volatile compounds produced in sterile fish muscle (Sebastes melanops) by Pseudomonas perolens. Appl Microbiol 1973;25(2):257–61.

140. David E, Del Gaudio G, Drudi FM, et al. Contrast enhanced ultrasound compared with MRI and CT in the evaluation of post-renal transplant complications. Tomography 2022;8(4):1704–15.

141. Akbar SA, Jafri SZ, Amendola MA, et al. Complications of renal transplantation. Radiographics 2005; 25(5):1335–56.

142. Alvarez Rodriguez S, Hevia Palacios V, Sanz Mayayo E, et al. The usefulness of contrast-enhanced ultrasound in the assessment of early kidney transplant function and complications. Diagnostics 2017;7(3).

143. Como G, Da Re J, Adani GL, et al. Role for contrast-enhanced ultrasound in assessing complications after kidney transplant. World J Radiol 2020;12(8):156–71.

144. Ntoulia A, Anupindi SA, Back SJ, et al. Contrast-enhanced ultrasound: a comprehensive review of safety in children. Pediatr Radiol 2021;51(12): 2161–80.

145. Dillman JR, Trout AT, Davenport MS. Allergic-like contrast media reaction management in children. Pediatr Radiol 2018;48(12):1688–94.

146. Marschner CA, Ruebenthaler J, Schwarze V, et al. Comparison of computed tomography (CT), magnetic resonance imaging (MRI) and contrast-enhanced ultrasound (CEUS) in the evaluation of unclear renal lesions. Röfo 2020;192(11):1053–9.

147. Duran C, Beltran VP, Gonzalez A, et al. Contrast-enhanced voiding urosonography for vesicoureteral reflux diagnosis in children. Radiographics 2017;37(6):1854–69.

148. Hains DS, Cohen HL, McCarville MB, et al. Elucidation of renal scars in children with vesicoureteral reflux using contrast-enhanced ultrasound: a pilot study. Kidney Int Rep 2017;2(3):420–4.

149. Ignee A, Straub B, Schuessler G, et al. Contrast enhanced ultrasound of renal masses. World J Radiol 2010;2(1):15–31.

150. Quaia E, Siracusano S, Bertolotto M, et al. Characterization of renal tumours with pulse inversion harmonic imaging by intermittent high mechanical index technique: initial results. Eur Radiol 2003; 13(6):1402–12.

151. Hwang M, Barnewolt CE, Jungert J, et al. Contrast-enhanced ultrasound of the pediatric brain. Pediatr Radiol 2021;51(12):2270–83.

152. Wiesmann M, Meyer K, Albers T, et al. Parametric perfusion imaging with contrast-enhanced ultrasound in acute ischemic stroke. Stroke 2004; 35(2):508–13.

153. Plut D, Prutki M, Slak P. The use of Contrast-Enhanced Ultrasound (CEUS) in the evaluation of the neonatal brain. Children 2023;10(8).

154. Mattei L, Prada F, Legnani FG, et al. Neurosurgical tools to extend tumor resection in hemispheric low-grade gliomas: conventional and contrast enhanced ultrasonography. Childs Nerv Syst 2016;32(10): 1907–14.

155. Caremani M, Benci A, Lapini L, et al. Contrast enhanced ultrasonography (CEUS) in peripheral lung lesions: A study of 60 cases. J Ultrasound 2008;11(3):89–96.

156. Deganello A, Rafailidis V, Sellars ME, et al. Intravenous and intracavitary use of contrast-enhanced ultrasound in the evaluation and management of

complicated pediatric pneumonia. J Ultrasound Med 2017;36(9):1943–54.

157. Wrightson JM, Davies RJ. The approach to the patient with a parapneumonic effusion. Semin Respir Crit Care Med 2010;31(6):706–15.

158. Yusuf GT, Rafailidis V, Moore S, et al. The role of contrast-enhanced ultrasound (CEUS) in the evaluation of scrotal trauma: a review. Insights Imaging 2020;11(1):68.

159. Lassau N, Chami L, Benatsou B, et al. Dynamic contrast-enhanced ultrasonography (DCE-US) with quantification of tumor perfusion: a new diagnostic tool to evaluate the early effects of antiangiogenic treatment. Eur Radiol 2007;17(Suppl 6):F89–98.

160. Hernot S, Klibanov AL. Microbubbles in ultrasound-triggered drug and gene delivery. Adv Drug Deliv Rev 2008;60(10):1153–66.

161. Liao AH, Wang CH, Weng PY, et al. Ultrasound-induced microbubble cavitation via a transcanal or transcranial approach facilitates inner ear drug delivery. JCI Insight 2020;5(3).

162. Lin CY, Hsieh HY, Chen CM, et al. Non-invasive, neuron-specific gene therapy by focused ultrasound-induced blood-brain barrier opening in Parkinson's disease mouse model. J Control Release 2016;235: 72–81.

163. Steinl DC, Kaufmann BA. Ultrasound imaging for risk assessment in atherosclerosis. Int J Mol Sci 2015;16(5):9749–69.

164. Hua X, Liu P, Gao YH, et al. Construction of thrombus-targeted microbubbles carrying tissue plasminogen activator and their in vitro thrombolysis efficacy: a primary research. J Thromb Thrombolysis 2010;30(1):29–35.

Trauma and 'Whole' Body Computed Tomography
Role, Protocols, Appropriateness, and Evidence to Support its Use and When

Daniela Galan, MD[a],*, Kim M. Caban, MD[a], Leandro Singerman, MD[a],
Thiago A. Braga, MD[a], Fabio M. Paes, MD, MBA[a],
Douglas S. Katz, MD, FACR, FSAR, FASER[b], Felipe Munera, MD[a]

KEYWORDS

- Whole body CT in trauma • Dual-energy CT in trauma • Vascular injury • Diaphragmatic injury
- Bowel injury • Structured reporting • Artificial intelligence

KEY POINTS

- Non-invasive imaging with whole-body computed tomography (WBCT) is an excellent tool for the prompt screening, diagnosis, management, and surveillance of potentially life-threatening trauma-related injuries in the significantly or severely injured patient; however, its role in those without obvious injury is debatable.
- WBCT may be used to identify unexpected critical injuries and incidental findings that may affect mortality and morbidity, thereby making it appropriate despite associated costs and radiation exposure.
- The decision to utilize WBCT in trauma is ultimately that of the managing medical/surgical team.

INTRODUCTION

The criteria for patient selection and the possible techniques and protocols for whole-body computed tomography (WB-CT) for blunt polytrauma have evolved and have changed over the past number of years since the first articles on the topic of severely injured trauma patients with WB-CT appeared in the imaging literature.1 Imaging plays a crucial role in the immediate evaluation of the trauma patient, particularly using multi-detector CT, and especially in moderately to severely injured trauma patients. There are specific areas of relative consensus, while other aspects of WB-CT use remain controversial and are subject to opinion/debate based on the current literature.

The initial assessment of trauma patients relies on a combination of physical examination, laboratory investigations, chest and pelvis radiography, and focused sonography to triage whether patients need emergent surgery or not. Hemodynamically stable patients typically undergo further imaging evaluation with CT based on the results of those investigations and the mechanism of injury. In many patients, CT is the initial imaging examination performed on 1 or more body parts. Facilitated by advances in CT technology, WB-CT has emerged as the preferred method to diagnose injuries quickly and accurately in these patients. It has become routine practice in most trauma centers, replacing assessment with standard radiography and selective use of CT.[1]

[a] Department of Radiology, Jackson Memorial Hospital, University of Miami-Miller School of Medicine, 1611 Northwest 12th Avenue, West Wing 279, Miami, FL 33136, USA; [b] Department of Radiology, NYU Grossman Long Island School of Medicine, NYU Langone Hospital - Long Island, 259 First Street, Mineola, NY 11501, USA
* Corresponding author.
E-mail address: dcg112@med.miami.edu

Radiol Clin N Am 62 (2024) 1063–1076
https://doi.org/10.1016/j.rcl.2024.06.001
0033-8389/24/© 2024 Elsevier Inc. All rights are reserved, including those for text and data mining, AI training, and similar technologies.

The article focuses on the appropriate patient selection for WB-CT in blunt trauma patients and discusses current evidence and controversies. The authors explore indications and contraindications for scanning, framed within the context of existing evidence-based trauma surgery algorithms and published clinical trials. The article discusses existing imaging protocols and highlights the pros and cons of various CT imaging approaches. It also includes a practical discussion of key injuries which require surgical or endovascular intervention, and specific findings that radiologists should be aware of that may determine or influence the approach and technique. The review emphasizes evidence-based practical tips for maximizing the efficiency of imaging interpretation based on known injury associations. The authors review the utility of dual-energy applications, radiation considerations, incidental findings, structured reporting advances in artificial intelligence, and post-processing techniques, as well as potential diagnostic pitfalls.

INDICATIONS AND RATIONALE FOR WHOLE-BODY COMPUTED TOMOGRAPHY IN POLYTRAUMA

The use of WB-CT in polytrauma patients has become a crucial component of modern trauma care. It undoubtedly helps guide the trauma team in identifying potentially life-threatening injuries, allowing for timely and effective treatment to patients.[2,3] However, the appropriate selection of patients for which WB-CT provides evidence-based benefits remains a complex issue with varying perspectives.[4–11] In a prospective study,[12] 1403 severely injured trauma patients were randomly assigned to WB-CT scanning or standard workup, concluding that immediate WB-CT scans does not reduce in-hospital mortality compared to standard radiological work-up, supporting the decision to perform WB-CT based on the identification of risk factors for severe trauma, which ultimately relies on the trauma surgical team. The American College of Radiology Appropriateness Criteria recommends using clinical judgment to determine which patients should receive WBCT versus selective CT for major trauma.[13] The radiologist is often unaware of the factors that influence the decision to proceed with a WB-CT, which include the mechanism of trauma, the severity and multiplicity of external injuries, conditions at the trauma site, and the patient's mental status/ Glasgow Coma Scale score.[2]

More WB-CT is being performed routinely in hemodynamically stable polytrauma patients with negative clinical examinations and questionable risk factors for severe trauma. The capability of detecting any clinically significant trauma not apparent on clinical examination, and the ability to obtain a highly accurate and faster assessment of treatable injuries from different body segments, are 2 common justifications for this broader WB-CT utilization approach. Multiple studies have shown that WB-CT has sensitivity greater than 95% and a negative predictive value approaching 100% to identify treatable polytrauma injuries.[2,3,11] It can be used to detect unexpected injuries in approximately 22% of patients, and to identify additional traumatic findings that may lead to change in management in up to 34% of patients.[2,3,5–11] There is also questionable evidence demonstrating the beneficial effect on the survival of polytrauma patients evaluated by immediate WB-CT in all such cases,[2,3,6,8,10] and there are data showing shorter time to treatment and length of stay for polytrauma patients who underwent assessment with WB-CT.[2,6,9,10,14]

While WB-CT can provide a rapid and comprehensive diagnosis in polytrauma, some advocate that its routine use is not always justified, and a selective imaging strategy may be more appropriate in certain cases.[4,6,7] Several studies argue that the overutilization of WB-CT on an unselected, commonly young trauma population leads to unnecessary radiation exposure, iodine contrast risk, and elevated costs with a doubtful marginal benefit.[1,4,6,7] In a retrospective cohort on 233 patients, Maghrably and colleagues showed a 20.4% rate of negative WB-CT scans among polytrauma patients, and 31.8% of the positive WB-CT scans had only 1 positive region, supporting the belief that a focused selective CT scan can potentially replace WB-CT in a certain group of polytrauma patients.[4] Understandably, most of the available evidence regarding WB-CT is retrospective. Until more randomized studies are performed to evaluate the mortality impact of routine WB-CT for sub-groups of polytrauma patients, the question of overutilization and suboptimal allocation of health care resources will persist.

WHOLE-BODY COMPUTED TOMOGRAPHY TECHNIQUE

At most trauma centers, blunt polytrauma patients are evaluated with a WB-CT instead of the traditional selective imaging strategy.[12] A non-enhanced brain CT usually precedes the whole-body scan. This scan is followed by an intravenous (IV) contrast injection with variability in the WB-CT protocols used in practice, with some institutions employing a continuous acquisition of the entire body, and others performing a segmented evaluation of the chest and abdomen/pelvis. The most often utilized protocol includes a whole-body scan in 1 sweep in the arterial phase, with a subsequent portal phase of the abdomen and pelvis and selected delayed imaging of the abdominopelvic region in patients with positive findings.

Adding an arterial phase to the standard portal phase of the abdomen and pelvis has been shown to lead to a significant change in the grading of splenic injuries due to increased detection of vascular injuries, resulting in better triage of patients for splenic interventions or conservative management.[15,16] (**Fig. 1**A, B).

Computed tomography angiography (CTA) assessment of the head and neck also has a variable approach with some institutions, including the neck as part of a whole body computed tomography angiography (WB-CTA), which is performed with arms up or abducted, and includes examinations of the neck, chest, abdomen, pelvis, and the entire spine. Others perform dedicated CTA of the neck, timed to optimize head and neck arteries and with arms down or adducted. Sliker and colleagues found similar sensitivities and specificities for dedicated CTA neck versus whole body CT for carotid and vertebral injuries, with digital subtraction angiography (DSA) as the reference standard.[17] However, the topic remains controversial. Dedicated CTA of the neck may be performed in patients with any of the standard risk criteria (eg, most often the Modified Denver criteria) for blunt cerebrovascular injuries (BCVI) and in patients presenting with blunt head or neck trauma who were found to have radiologic findings with potential risk for BCVI on an initial non-enhanced brain

and cervical spine CT. At the author's institution, isolated cranio-cervical trauma necessitating CTA occurs less commonly than multi-system polytrauma. Therefore, WB-CTA is the routine method for screening severe blunt polytrauma patients.[18]

WB-CT is typically performed with modern multi-detector CT (MDCT) scanners with a continuous acquisition, with thin (0.5–0.6 mm) collimation images reconstructed at 1 mm and 3 mm slices for imaging interpretation—the anatomic coverage extending from the head to the symphysis pubis. The authors' institutional protocol involves a biphasic injection of 100 mL of iodinated contrast (350 mg/mL) at 4 cc/s for 15 seconds, then at a rate of 3 cc/s, followed by a 40-cc saline bolus at 4 cc/s. The fixed-time delay method is generally suitable, but issues arise in cases of abnormal anatomy, cardiac function, or severe arterial disease, impacting blood transit time. While bolus tracking is often favored in such scenarios, research shows improved efficiency with a fixed-time empiric delay of 20 or 25 seconds for patients over 55.[19]

Post-processing techniques, including coronal and sagittal multiplanar reformations (MPR) and maximum intensity projections (MIPS) of the torso are also generated and submitted for interpretation. Separate dedicated coronal and sagittal reformations of the neck and thoracolumbar spine in both bone and soft-tissue algorithms are generated, with the liberal use of additional postprocessing techniques by the radiologist.

We perform dedicated neck CTA on 64-slice-multidetector computed tomography (64-MDCT)

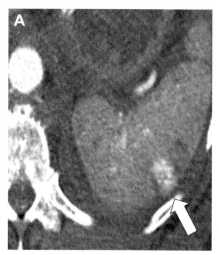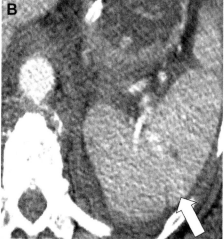

Fig. 1. Splenic pseudoaneurysm: Whole-body computed tomography (WB-CT) arterial phase image through the abdomen (*A*) demonstrates a pseudoaneurysm (*arrow*), which becomes isoattenuating to the splenic parenchyma on portal phase (*B*), consistent with grade IV injury.

scanners with 0.6 mm detector configuration. Our coverage region extends from the aortic arch to the circle of Willis, using an automated triggering device centered in the ascending aorta. The patients receive 50 to 100 mL of iodinated contrast material (350 mg/mL) at 5 mL/s, followed by a 40 mL saline bolus at a similar rate. The images are reconstructed at 0.6 mm and 1.5 mm slices in axial, coronal, and sagittal planes. The radiologist generates 3-dimensional (3-D) reconstructions at the picture archiving and communication system (PACS) workstation using integrated software, as necessary.

Other alternative contrast injection protocols include the split-bolus technique, in which the single pass WB-CT is preceded by 2 or 3 boluses of contrast, given sequentially with a time delay, usually with the larger dose for the first injection, including the portal-venous part. A typical split-bolus protocol comprises a first bolus injection (eg, 80 mL) at a rate of 4 cc/s with an inter-bolus delay of 10 to 30 seconds (eg, 20 seconds), followed by a second bolus of 40 to 70 mL, and a scan delay of 60 to 70 seconds. The split-bolus protocol primarily offers 2 advantages over traditional sequential arterial and venous acquisitions: reduced radiation dose and decreased image overload.[20,21] Regardless of the type of contrast injection technique, a saline chaser should be used at the end of the contrast medium injection.[22]

Ideal patient arm positioning for WB-CT is also a subject of debate and may be limited in the setting of upper extremity injuries. The arms-up position has lower radiation exposure and improves the quality of the torso evaluation with a slight increase in the neck and skull base noise. Crossing the patient's arms over the trunk diminishes beam hardening artifacts. The latter position has also been suggested in the "time optimized" protocol proposed by the European Society of Emergency Radiology in their guidelines on radiological polytrauma imaging for hemodynamically unstable patients.[14]

DUAL-ENERGY COMPUTED TOMOGRAPHY, POST-PROCESSING TECHNIQUES, AND APPLICATIONS IN POLYTRAUMA

It can be challenging to differentiate substances of similar attenuation values on single-phase CT. For instance, a fracture fragment, calcification, or high-density foreign body may mimic areas of hemorrhage and active bleeding. In such scenarios, advanced imaging including dual-energy CT (DE-CT) and post-processing techniques become invaluable tools, allowing for tissue characterization, reduction of artifacts, increased conspicuity of injuries, and quantitative analysis.[23–25]

DE-CT refers to the acquisition of images at 2 different x-ray spectra (low and high kilovolt peak), using dual x-ray source, dual-layer detector, or fast kilovolt (kV)-switching methods, which are then blended to create images that resemble those obtained with conventional CT scanners.[26–28] Low kilo-electron-volt (KeV) images accentuate the iodine content, highlighting the distribution and uptake of contrast material within tissues, which can aid in detecting active bleeding, solid organ, and vascular injuries. High keV images are less susceptible to beam-hardening and metal streak artifacts, improving image quality, particularly in the setting of metallic hardware.[24,29] Material decomposition technique enables the selection of various materials (iodine, urate, bone, water), and assigns them a color, which is then utilized to compose color maps that represent distribution patterns,[29–31] allowing for the assessment of organ perfusion.

Virtual non-contrast images (VNC) are obtained by the subtraction of iodine content from the image, creating a non-contrast phase from a contrast-enhanced data set, reducing radiation dose and exposure time.[23] VNC images are also helpful in differentiating calcium from hemorrhage and evaluating the vasculature, allowing suppression of calcified plaques and improving the diagnostic accuracy of vascular injuries.[28,32–34] With a similar principle, subtracting trabecular bone may help identify areas of marrow edema, detect occult fractures, and differentiate acute from chronic fractures.[32] In summary, DE-CT proves indispensable in the ER trauma setting. It enhances tissue characterization, reduces artifacts, unmasks injuries, and facilitates quantitative analysis, enabling swift and accurate diagnosis.

INJURY SPECTRUM

WB-CT is a non-invasive, dependable, and extremely effective tool allowing for the screening, diagnosis, and timely management of critical injuries. Multi-phasic CT imaging and post-processing techniques enhance diagnostic capability.

CRANIO-CERVICAL INJURIES

Traumatic brain injuries are the most common trauma-related mortality. Intracranial hemorrhage, whether intra-axial or extra-axial, is best appreciated on non-contrast CT. WB-CTA encompassing part of the brain and neck can simultaneously be used to evaluate the presence

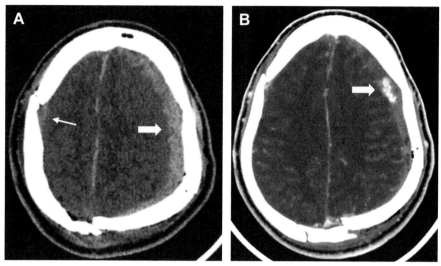

Fig. 2. Bilateral subdural hematomas: Axial unenhanced CT image through the brain (*A*) demonstrates bilateral subdural hematomas greater on the left (*thin arrow* on the *right* and *thick arrow* on the *left*). (*B*) Whole body computed tomography angiography (WB-CTA) demonstrates active bleeding from the left subdural hematoma (*thick arrow*).

and source of active intracranial bleeding and to assess the intracranial and neck vasculature for injury (**Fig. 2**A, B). Biffl and colleagues designed a DSA classification system for BCVI involving the carotid and vertebral arteries, which has been adopted for CTA.[35,36] WB CTA protocols including the head also allow the evaluation of the dural venous sinuses, which may be injured in the setting of an overlying skull fracture and can lead to a venous infarct.

TRAUMATIC AORTIC INJURY

Second to intracranial hemorrhage, traumatic aortic injuries (TAI) are the next most common cause of motor vehicle collision (MVC) deaths, and it is estimated that 80% of patients with aortic injuries die before arriving at the hospital.[37,38] MDCT has been found to be nearly 100% sensitive and specific for the detection of TAIs.[39] Most TAIs occur at the isthmus. Abdominal TAIs are rare, and 25% represent an extension of a thoracic aortic injury.[40] The infrarenal aortic segment is twice as commonly involved as the supra-renal segment.[40] The presence of a vertebral body fracture should prompt the interpreter to closely scrutinize the aorta. Sagittal MPR reconstructions are especially useful in assessing the aorta. Electrocardiography (ECG)-gating techniques that minimize cardiac pulsation artifacts may be used for follow-up CT imaging to re-evaluate areas susceptible to pulsation artifact, including the aortic root, ascending thoracic aorta, heart, and pericardium. The

Society for Vascular Surgery advocates operative management for anything other than a Grade 1 minimal TAI (intimal tear) (**Fig.** 3A–C).[41,42] Some studies have pondered the feasibility of non-operative management for Grade 2 TAIs (intramural hematoma [IMH]). Endovascular Aortic Stent Repair (EVAR) is the primary treatment for most aortic injuries requiring intervention. Open surgical repair with the use of surgical grafts is reserved for injuries that are not amenable to EVAR, such as those involving the distal ascending thoracic aorta, and aortic arch, and when variant vascular anatomy is encountered.[41,42]

DIAPHRAGMATIC INJURIES

Diaphragmatic injuries (DI) may be more common with penetrating injuries but also occur with blunt trauma. The left hemidiaphragm is more often injured in blunt trauma, as the liver is thought to help protect the right hemidiaphragm.[43] DI may occur anywhere along the diaphragm surface but most commonly involves the posterolateral aspect. Identifying a DI is important, because if the defect is large enough initially or expands over time, bowel, solid organs, mesentery, and omentum can herniate into the chest shortly following the trauma, or even years later, predisposing to respiratory compromise, organ ischemia, and bowel obstruction. With MDCT, one can localize and size the DI and identify potential complications.[44] Operative repair is performed for most DIs, particularly those that involve the left hemidiaphragm. Injuries to the

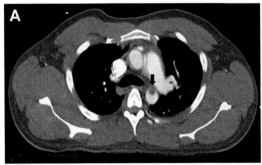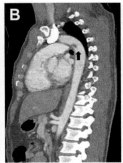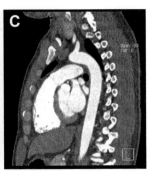

Fig. 3. Traumatic aortic injury: Axial WB-CTA image (*A*) through the thorax demonstrating a Grade 1 blunt traumatic aortic injury (BTAI) (*arrow*). Sagittal multiplanar reformation (MPR) of WB-CTA (*B*) demonstrating a Grade 1 BTAI (*arrow*). Sag MPR of computed tomography angiography (CTA) Chest (*C*) 5 weeks after the trauma after conservative management of the aortic injury demonstrates resolution.

right hemidiaphragm, particularly if the defect is small, may be managed conservatively, as the liver "patches" the diaphragmatic defect.

CARDIAC, PULMONARY TRUNK, AND THORACIC INFERIOR VENA CAVA INJURY

It is rare to identify a cardiac, pulmonary trunk, or inferior vena cava (IVC) injury on CT, as most patients never make it to the hospital. Injuries to these structures may result in massive hemothorax and hemopericardium, predisposing to cardiac tamponade requiring urgent chest tube drainage, pericardial window formation, and cardiorrhaphy.[45] Cardiac injuries on CT may present as some combination of displaced heart, hemopericardium, pneumopericardium, myocardial hematoma, intraluminal thrombus, aneurysm, and contrast extravasation into the pericardium or mediastinum. Clues to the presence of cardiac tamponade include the presence of a large pericardial effusion with associated distension of the superior and IVC, contrast reflux into the IVC or azygous vein, bowing of the intraventricular septum, and compression and deformity of the cardiac chambers.[45]

NON-VASCULAR CHEST INJURY

Lung contusions, lacerations, and rib fractures may lead to respiratory compromise, especially in the elderly. Identifying a flail chest (3 or more consecutive segmental rib fractures) may indicate the need for prolonged mechanical ventilation. Pneumomediastinum may indicate an underlying airway injury, or the rare blunt traumatic esophageal injury.[46] MDCT can also be used to confirm appropriate life support line positioning and radiologically occult pneumothoraces.

BOWEL INJURY

Extraluminal gas, bowel wall discontinuity, mesenteric vessel irregularity, occlusion, or extravasation, and focal bowel wall thickening all have high specificities for bowel injury on CT (**Fig. 4**). Other sources of free air in the setting of blunt trauma may be related to the extension of a pneumothorax or pneumomediastinum, barotrauma from mechanical ventilation, DI, chest tube placement, diagnostic peritoneal lavage (DPL), and intraperitoneal rupture of a recently instrumented bladder. Free fluid on CT, particularly if hyperdense, is the most sensitive finding for a bowel injury (BI), with a 90% to 100% sensitivity, but has only a 15% to 25% specificity.[47] The amount and density of the free fluid are important predictors of injury severity. Free fluid may be unrelated and

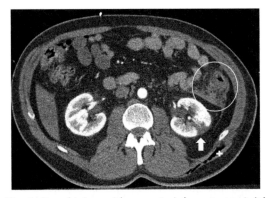

Fig. 4. Bowel injury with mesenteric hematoma: Axial WB-CTA image through the abdomen demonstrates a thickened descending colon with surrounding mesenteric hematoma (*circle*), left renal laceration (*arrow*), and left flank subcutaneous emphysema (*cross*). Contusion and perforation of the descending colon was found on exploratory laparotomy requiring a segmental left colon resection.

pre-exist the trauma but may also suggest the presence of an occult BI. The absence of hemoperitoneum has been shown to have a high negative predictive value for the presence of a BI.[48] The presence of a small amount of free fluid without an identifiable etiology in a stable, alert, and oriented patient without abdominal pain may be managed conservatively, however, with close observation to include serial physical abdominal examinations.[49] A 5 to 8-hour diagnostic delay in the case of a BI can be detrimental. It is important to remember that bowel wall thickening can also be seen with peristalsis, incomplete distension, shock bowel, ascites, infectious or inflammatory bowel disease, portal hypertension, and hypoalbuminemia.[50] Shock bowel in the setting of hypovolemia usually presents on CT as diffuse-long segment submucosal edematous wall thickening and mucosal hyperenhancement.[47,51]

MESENTERIC INJURY

Mesenteric injuries (MIs) may present as an area of fat stranding or induration, as can be seen with contusion and hematoma.[52] The presence of fat stranding alone has been shown to be up to 77% sensitive and 40% to 90% specific on MDCT in suggesting a MI.[48] MIs with IV contrast extravasation increase the likelihood of an adjacent associated BI[47] (see **Fig. 4**; **Fig. 5**A–C). Pre-existing mesenteric panniculitis, granulation tissue, and carcinomatosis can all potentially be misinterpreted as MI.

SOLID ORGAN INJURY (LIVER, SPLEEN, PANCREAS, KIDNEYS, AND ADRENALS)

Solid organ injuries should be graded on CT following the current American Association for the Surgery of Trauma solid organ injury classifications. Solid organ injuries are best detected on the portal venous phase due to optimal organ contrast, however, the arterial phase increases the sensitivity in the detection and characterization of vascular injuries, particularly of contained vascular injuries. Thus, incorporating both phases ensures a more comprehensive assessment of solid organ trauma.[53]

Renal Collecting System and Bladder Injuries: Renal laceration that extends to the collecting system is suspicious for an associated collecting system injury, and delayed CT imaging should be performed to assess for urine contrast extravasation[54] (**Fig. 6**A, B). Bladder and posterior urethral injuries should be suspected in the setting of hematuria, pelvic fracture, or diastasis, and in the presence of a prevesical space hematoma (also known as the space of Retzius) (**Fig. 7**A, B).

Delayed CT imaging alone is not reliable in demonstrating a bladder injury, as the bladder is usually not fully distended. Therefore, a dedicated CT-cystogram should be performed with an attempt for optimal bladder distension.[55] A total of 70% of bladder injuries are extraperitoneal and are associated with pelvic fractures (managed by placing a supra-pubic catheter), and 20% are intraperitoneal (requiring operative repair).

OTHER VASCULAR INJURIES

WB-CTA can adequately demonstrate the presence and severity of a vascular injury and whether it is isolated or associated with a solid organ or hollow viscus injury. Vascular injuries present similarly despite location. Pseudoaneurysms present as a dense non-expanding contained contrast focus that follows aortic attenuation,

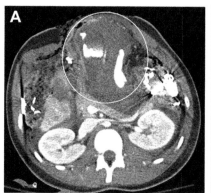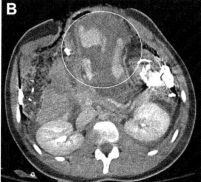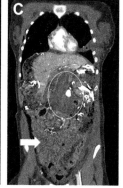

Fig. 5. Mesenteric Injury with large hematoma, active bleed, and shock bowel: (*A*) Axial WB-CT arterial phase image through the upper abdomen demonstrates a large mesenteric hematoma with extensive contrast extravasation (*circle*) that expands on delayed phase imaging (*B*). Coronal MPR WB-CT arterial phase image (*C*) image demonstrating the large mesenteric hematoma with active bleeding (*circle*) and thick-walled and hyperenhancing small intestine compatible with shock bowel (*arrow*).

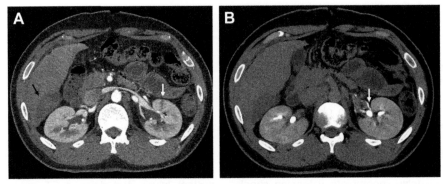

Fig. 6. Grade IV renal laceration: (*A*) Axial WB-CT arterial phase image through the abdomen demonstrates a left renal laceration (*white arrow*) extending to the collecting system. Additionally, subcapsular hepatic hematoma is seen (*black arrow*). (*B*) Axial WB-CT delayed phase image demonstrates urine/collecting system contrast extravasation (*white arrow*) consistent with a Grade IV injury.

decreasing in density and losing its conspicuity on subsequent phases of imaging. Arterial injuries commonly undergo endovascular or surgical repair, whereas venous injuries are often managed conservatively with compression, packing, and the use of hemostatic gauze. Arterial and venous bleeding can be differentiated by the phase of imaging that the bleeding is initially identified and how it changes on subsequent phases of CT imaging. Arterial bleeds present as a dense focus on arterial-phase imaging, which expands and becomes denser on subsequent phases.[56] Venous bleeding, on the other hand, is usually identified on the portal or delayed phases of imaging, is less dense than arterial bleeding, and may also expand[57] (**Fig. 8**A, B).

DIAGNOSTIC PITFALLS

Despite MDCT's high sensitivity and specificity, challenges in interpretation persist, often stemming from inadequate technique or limited image quality. Motion artifacts caused by an increased respiratory rate and poor breath-holding can degrade images, mimicking fractures, contained vascular injuries, fat stranding, and hematomas. The interpreter should refer to lung and bone windows to assess for a background of motion. WB-CT scans, being non-cardiac gated, are prone to pulsation artifacts, which manifest as linear hypodensities resembling aortic dissections in the thorax. Additionally, beam-hardening artifacts from external or indwelling metallic devices may obscure or mimic organ injuries. Arterial-phase contrast bolus timing deficiencies, poor cardiac output, and hypotension can compromise vessel opacification, potentially resulting in a misdiagnosis of an arterial dissection or thrombosis. Meanwhile, a deficient arterial or portal phase resulting in poorly opacified vessels may obscure or resemble solid organ lacerations (**Fig. 9**A, B). Periportal edema may also mimic hepatic lacerations. Pre-existing atherosclerosis may present with intimal irregularities and mural thrombus

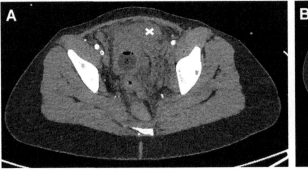
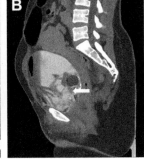

Fig. 7. Extraperitoneal bladder rupture: (*A*) Axial WB-CT arterial phase image through the pelvis demonstrates a space of Retzius hematoma (*X*). (*B*) Sagittal MPR image from CT cystogram demonstrates a defect along the inferior bladder wall with extraperitoneal extravasation of contrast (*arrow*).

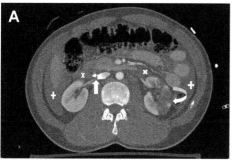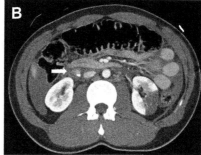

Fig. 8. Inferior vena cava (IVC) injury and traumatic left renal infarcts. (*A*) Axial WB-CT image through the abdomen demonstrates bilateral retroperitoneal hematomas (*X*) related to active bleeding from the IVC (*arrow*) and traumatic left renal infarcts (*curved arrow*). Bilateral upper quadrant hemoperitoneum is noted (*cross*). (*B*) Axial WB-CT portal phase image through the abdomen demonstrates enlarging contrast blush related to IVC injury (*arrow*).

mimicking vascular injuries. These challenges underscore the complexity and importance of optimizing CT techniques for trauma imaging.[58]

Anatomic variants may also potentially mimic traumatic injuries. An aortic ductus diverticulum or aortic spindle may be confused for a pseudoaneurysm (PSA), a remnant patent or calcified ductus arteriosus may be misconstrued for a TAI, thymus may be confused for a mediastinal hematoma, while a splenic cleft or pancreatic lobulation can mimic a laceration. The absence of associated fat stranding or fluid may hint that the finding is non-traumatic.[59–61] Calcifications or foreign bodies may also resemble areas of hemorrhage, which can be differentiated by the area's density and stable appearance in all phases of imaging. Pre-existing abnormalities such as vascular malformations or tumors and even the normal penile bulbar blush may be mistaken for traumatic injuries and active bleeding. Additionally, signs of hypoperfusion syndrome and fluid overload from resuscitation can mimic bowel or mesenteric injuries.[59,60,62] Radiologists should be vigilant of these pitfalls and carefully analyze CT findings to avoid delays in treatment and unnecessary interventions.

INCIDENTAL FINDINGS

One must also consider the screening function of WB-CT as incidental findings result in early detection of disease. Incidental findings of varying importance and relevance are found at rates as high as 54.8%.[63] Studies have shown that incidental findings are more common in women and older patients, with most findings typically located in the abdomen and pelvis.[64] Some abnormalities have distinct characterizing features, but most are non-specific for which the clinical context and patient's history may or may not provide insight. The most common incidental findings include renal cysts of varying complexity, pulmonary nodules, adrenal masses, pulmonary emboli, and thyroid nodules.

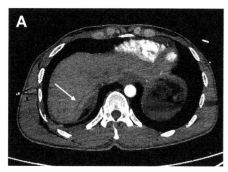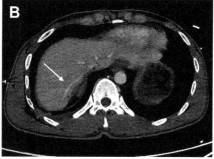

Fig. 9. Unopacified right hepatic vein mimicking a liver laceration. (*A*) Axial WB-CT arterial phase image through the upper abdomen demonstrates an unopacified right hepatic vein resembling a laceration (*arrow*). (*B*) Axial WB-CT venous phase image through the abdomen demonstrates opacification of a normal right hepatic vein (*arrow*).

Some other findings, particularly vascular tumors, may be misinterpreted as acute injuries. The discovery of incidental findings, however, also poses substantial challenges in deciding if the finding warrants further investigation, specialty referral, and treatment, and generate patient anxiety and drive increased health care costs. Many different guidelines are available directing the management of incidental findings. Thus, establishing an efficient feedback mechanism with a reliable referral system is crucial for optimal patient care in the trauma setting.[64-66]

ARTIFICIAL INTELLIGENCE USE IN POLYTRAUMA WHOLE-BODY COMPUTED TOMOGRAPHY

Integrating artificial intelligence (AI) in emergency radiology, particularly in the context of WB-CT scans for polytraumatized patients, represents a substantial advancement in the diagnosis and subsequent management of traumatic injuries. A review of the current literature underscores the promising potential of AI to enhance the accuracy, efficiency, and predictive capabilities of radiological assessments in the emergency and trauma settings. Zhou and colleagues conducted a study on 133 patients comparing the results of rib fracture detection using initial CT and follow-up CT, revealing that AI-assisted diagnosis statistically significantly improved the overall accuracy for the detection of rib fractures.[67]

The development of Total Segmentator by Wasserthal and colleagues represents another milestone in automating tasks for CT analysis. This deep learning segmentation model can automatically segment 104 anatomic structures facilitating the comprehensive analyses of numerous structures, enabling a more detailed and accurate semi-automated assessment.[68] In another study, Polzer and colleagues explored AI-based automated detection and stability analysis of traumatic vertebral body fractures on CT of 257 patients, demonstrating a sensitivity of 88.4% and specificity of 80.3%.[69] The innovative application of AI extends beyond these examples. AI has been employed in the quantitative analysis of traumatic hemoperitoneum,[70] highlighting its ability to aid in diagnosing and managing intra-bdominal bleeding. Seyam and colleagues implemented an AI-based detection tool for intracranial hemorrhage (ICH) and evaluated its diagnostic performance, assessing clinical workflow metrics compared to pre-AI implementation.[71] The study found that the tool demonstrated practical diagnostic performance with an overall accuracy of 93.0%, sensitivity of 87.2%, and a negative predictive value of 97.8%. However, it identified lower detection rates for specific subtypes of ICH, such as 69.2% for subdural hemorrhage and 77.4% for acute subarachnoid hemorrhage. It is important to define a clear framework for clinical integration, recognizing the limitations of AI.

RADIATION EXPOSURE IN WHOLE-BODY COMPUTED TOMOGRAPHY

Excess and, at times, unnecessary radiation exposure comes with the liberal use of WB-CT. It has been estimated that a single-phase WB-CT radiation dose ranges from 10 to 20 mGy correlating with a 0.8% lifetime risk of cancer mortality for a 45-year-old person, although this estimate is controversial and open to substantial debate.[72] On principle alone, the amount of radiation exposure to save a life is worth the theoretic risk, especially in the trauma setting. The organ radiation dose depends on technique and the risk of cancer depends on the patient's age. The theoretic long-term risk of radiation-induced cancer mortality is outweighed by the risk of a traumatic death in older patients.[73] The common younger traumatized patient populations have lower traumatic mortality rates but are more vulnerable to the potential neoplastic risk of radiation.[73] Substantial uncertainty exists in these radiation risk estimates extrapolated from data on atomic bomb survivors exposed to similar doses of radiation. Some believe the cancer risk is significantly exaggerated. Long-term cancer mortality rates are based on a linear no-threshold relationship, suggesting that the risk of cancer is directly proportional to the level of radiation exposure. Despite similar settings, the radiation exposure of different scanner models may differ, and can result in an approximate organ dose differential of up to 35%.[72] Intuitively, the individual estimated radiation doses and subsequent cancer risk will increase for every CT scan obtained, and particularly if occurring during a short-term time interval. Lung cancer is estimated to be the dominant cancer resulting from WBCT radiation exposure.[72] Stengel, and colleagues found that low-dose WBCT protocols maintained diagnostic accuracy with half the standard radiation dose, despite decreased image quality.[74]

Scans should be optimized to decrease radiation exposure while maintaining quality. Modern CT scanners allow less radiation exposure using technical parameters like iterative reconstruction and tube current modulation. Decreasing phases, such as the selective use of delayed images or the split-bolus technique, can also be used to reduce radiation exposure.

STRUCTURED REPORTING

As the workload increases, radiology reports are now the primary form of communication with referring clinicians. The quality of the report is paramount in optimizing patient care. Free form-style reporting has been criticized for its lack of structure, variability, and increased time to generate. While clinicians prefer structured reporting (SR), many radiologists view SR as too rigid, limiting descriptions, especially in determining the clinical significance of uncertain findings and taking away the art of reporting. Some radiologists claim that completing an SR checklist distracts them, potentially leading to missed findings.[75] SR usually consists of templates, with or without picklists, that can provide a further detailed description of the imaging finding. If utilized, it is imperative to tailor SR templates to meet the needs of the referring clinicians.

Implementing SR may improve patient care by decreasing reporting times and subsequently expediting treatment, serving as a guide for the in-depth systematic review of organ systems, increasing the clarity of findings by standardizing language, and decreasing the rate of miscommunication with clinicians.[75,76] Schwartz and colleagues found that both referring clinicians and radiologists felt that using SR allowed for more useful information to be conveyed without compromising the accuracy of the reports.[77] SR also facilitates documenting the reporting of critical findings, comparisons, and data extraction for documentation and research.[78] SR is particularly helpful at the training level as it operates as a checklist of organ systems that should be evaluated; however, it does not improve the satisfaction of search phenomenon.[75] Dendi and colleagues retrospectively evaluated the implementation of a timed interdisciplinary 2-phase checklist SR approach for polytrauma WBCT without the aid of reconstructed images. The first checklist recorded life-threatening injuries, evaluated endotracheal tube position, and had to be completed within 1 minute. The second checklist focused on immediately clinically relevant pathology and had to be completed within 10 minutes. The findings of both checklists were compared to the final radiology report. They found that a shorter reporting time led to a higher diagnostic inaccuracy despite the interpreter's experience.[75]

SUMMARY

The identification of injuries depends on the image quality, diagnostic acumen, and radiologist's experience. It is imperative to be familiar with, quickly recognize, and communicate direct and indirect signs of life-threatening injuries for appropriate and timely management. Even a few hours of a delayed diagnosis may result in a detrimental outcome for the patient. One must utilize all the tools available to enhance the interpretation of images. It is also important to recognize imaging pitfalls and artifacts to avoid unnecessary intervention.

DISCLOSURE

All authors certify they have no competing interests to declare relevant to this manuscript's content.

REFERENCES

1. Munera F, Durso AM. Whole-body CT after motor vehicle crash: when is it necessary? Radiology 2019;292(1):101–2.
2. Dreizin D, Munera F. Blunt polytrauma: evaluation with 64-section whole-body CT angiography. Radiographics 2012;32(3):609–31.
3. Iacobellis F, Romano L, Rengo A, et al. CT protocol optimization in trauma imaging: a review of current evidence. Curr Radiol Rep 2020;8(6):8.
4. Mulas V, Catalano L, Geatti V, et al. Major trauma with only dynamic criteria: is the routine use of whole-body CT as a first level examination justified? Radiol Med 2022;127(1):65–71.
5. Shannon L, Peachey T, Skipper N, et al. Comparison of clinically suspected injuries with injuries detected at whole-body CT in suspected multi-trauma victims. Clin Radiol 2015;70(11):1205–11.
6. Long B, April MD, Summers S, et al. Whole body CT versus selective radiological imaging strategy in trauma: an evidence-based clinical review. Am J Emerg Med 2017;35(9):1356–62.
7. Maghraby NH, Alshaqaq HM, AlQattan AS, et al. Negative whole-body computed tomography scans in polytrauma patients: a retrospective cohort study. Open Access Emerg Med 2020;12:305–13.
8. Yoong S, Kothari R, Brooks A. Assessment of sensitivity of whole body CT for major trauma. Eur J Trauma Emerg Surg 2019;45(3):489–92.
9. Sampson MA, Colquhoun KBM, Hennessy NLM. Computed tomography whole body imaging in multi-trauma: 7 years experience. Clin Radiol 2006;61(4):365–9.
10. Caputo ND, Stahmer C, Lim G, et al. Whole-body computed tomographic scanning leads to better survival as opposed to selective scanning in trauma patients. J Trauma Acute Care Surg 2014;77(4):534–9.
11. Chidambaram S, Goh EL, Khan MA. A meta-analysis of the efficacy of whole-body computed tomography

imaging in the management of trauma and injury. Injury 2017;48(8):1784–93.

12. Sierink JC, Treskes K, Edwards MJR, et al. Immediate total-body CT scanning versus conventional imaging and selective CT scanning in patients with severe trauma (REACT-2): a randomised controlled trial. Lancet 2016;388(10045):673–83.

13. Shyu JY, Khurana B, Soto JA, et al. ACR appropriateness criteria® major blunt trauma. J Am Coll Radiol 2020;17(5):S160–74.

14. Wirth S, Hebebrand J, Basilico R, et al. European society of emergency radiology: guideline on radiological polytrauma imaging and service (short version). Insights Imaging 2020;11(1):135.

15. Hemachandran N, Gamanagatti S, Sharma R, et al. Revised AAST scale for splenic injury (2018): does addition of arterial phase on CT have an impact on the grade? Emerg Radiol 2021;28(1):47–54.

16. Lee JT, Slade E, Uyeda J, et al. American society of emergency radiology multicenter blunt splenic trauma study: CT and clinical findings. Radiology 2021;299(1):122–30.

17. Sliker CW, Shanmuganathan K, Mirvis SE. Diagnosis of blunt cerebrovascular injuries with 16-MDCT: accuracy of whole-body MDCT compared with neck MDCT angiography. Am J Roentgenol 2008;190(3):790–9.

18. Winn A, Durso AM, Lopera CR, et al. Blunt craniocervical trauma. Neuroimaging Clin N Am 2018;28(3):495–507.

19. Adibi A, Shahbazi A. Automatic bolus tracking versus fixed time-delay technique in biphasic multidetector computed tomography of the abdomen. Iran J Radiol 2014;10(4). https://doi.org/10.5812/iranjradiol.4617.

20. Leung V, Sastry A, Woo TD, et al. Implementation of a split-bolus single-pass CT protocol at a UK major trauma centre to reduce excess radiation dose in trauma pan-CT. Clin Radiol 2015;70(10):1110–5.

21. Yaniv G, Portnoy O, Simon D, et al. Revised protocol for whole-body CT for multi-trauma patients applying triphasic injection followed by a single-pass scan on a 64-MDCT. Clin Radiol 2013;68(7):668–75.

22. Jeavons C, Hacking C, Beenen LF, et al. A review of split-bolus single-pass CT in the assessment of trauma patients. Emerg Radiol 2018;25(4):367–74.

23. Hamid S, Nicolaou S, Khosa F, et al. Dual-energy CT: a paradigm shift in acute traumatic abdomen. Canadian association of radiologists. Journal 2020;71(3):371–87.

24. Cester D EMAHEA. Virtual monoenergetic images from dual-energy CT: systematic assessment of task-based image quality performance. Quant Imag Med Surg 2022;1(12):726–41.

25. Cester D, Eberhard M, Alkadhi H, et al. Virtual monoenergetic images from dual-energy CT: systematic assessment of task-based image quality performance. Quant Imag Med Surg 2022;12(1):726–41.

26. Yu L, Primak AN, Liu X, et al. Image quality optimization and evaluation of linearly mixed images in dual-source, dual-energy CT. Med Phys 2009;36(3):1019–24.

27. Marin D, Boll DT, Mileto A, et al. State of the art: dual-energy CT of the abdomen. Radiology 2014;271(2):327–42.

28. Wortman JR, Uyeda JW, Fulwadhva UP, et al. Dual-energy CT for abdominal and pelvic trauma. Radiographics 2018;38(2):586–602.

29. Primak AN, Ramirez Giraldo JC, Liu X, et al. Improved dual-energy material discrimination for dual-source CT by means of additional spectral filtration. Med Phys 2009;36(4):1359–69.

30. Parakh A, Lennartz S, An C, et al. Dual-energy CT images: pearls and pitfalls. Radiographics 2021;41(1):98–119.

31. Chandarana H, Megibow AJ, Cohen BA, et al. Iodine quantification with dual-energy CT: phantom study and preliminary experience with renal masses. Am J Roentgenol 2011;196(6):W693–700.

32. D'Angelo T, Albrecht MH, Caudo D, et al. Virtual non-calcium dual-energy CT: clinical applications. Eur Radiol Exp 2021;5(1):38.

33. Vlahos I, Chung R, Nair A, et al. Dual-Energy CT: vascular applications. Am J Roentgenol 2012;199(5_supplement):S87–97.

34. Wong WD, Mohammed MF, Nicolaou S, et al. Impact of dual-energy CT in the emergency department: increased radiologist confidence, reduced need for follow-up imaging, and projected cost benefit. Am J Roentgenol 2020;215(6):1528–38.

35. Biffl WL, Moore EE, Offner PJ, et al. Blunt carotid arterial injuries: implications of a new grading scale. J Trauma Inj Infect Crit Care 1999;47(5):845.

36. Biffl WL, Moore EE, Offner PJ, et al. Blunt carotid and vertebral arterial injuries. World J Surg 2001;25(8):1036–43.

37. Neschis DG, Scalea TM, Flinn WR, et al. Blunt aortic injury. N Engl J Med 2008;359(16):1708–16.

38. Fox N, Schwartz D, Salazar JH, et al. Evaluation and management of blunt traumatic aortic injury. J Trauma Acute Care Surg 2015;78(1):136–46.

39. Keller SE. Multidetector computed tomography scanning is still the gold standard for diagnosis of acute aortic syndromes. Interact Cardiovasc Thorac Surg 2010;11(3):359.

40. Mellnick VM, McDowell C, Lubner M, et al. CT features of blunt abdominal aortic injury. Emerg Radiol 2012;19(4):301–7.

41. Sandhu HK, Leonard SD, Perlick A, et al. Determinants and outcomes of nonoperative management for blunt traumatic aortic injuries. J Vasc Surg 2018;67(2):389–98.

42. Osgood MJ, Heck JM, Rellinger EJ, et al. Natural history of grade I-II blunt traumatic aortic injury. J Vasc Surg 2014;59(2):334–42.

43. Iochum S, Ludig T, Walter F, et al. Imaging of diaphragmatic injury: a diagnostic challenge? Radiographics 2002;22(suppl_1):S103–16.

44. Desir A, Ghaye B. CT of blunt diaphragmatic rupture. Radiographics 2012;32(2):477–98.

45. Witt CE, Linnau KF, Maier RV, et al. Management of pericardial fluid in blunt trauma. J Trauma Acute Care Surg 2017;82(4):733–41.

46. Spigel Zachary A, Al Fayyadh Mohammed J, Dent Daniel L. Tension pneumomediastinum after blunt chest injury managed with percutaneous mediastinal drain. American College of Surgeons 2020;1(6).

47. Bates DDB, Wasserman M, Malek A, et al. Multidetector CT of surgically proven blunt bowel and mesenteric injury. Radiographics 2017;37(2):613–25.

48. Lansier A, Bourillon C, Cuénod CA, et al. CT-based diagnostic algorithm to identify bowel and/or mesenteric injury in patients with blunt abdominal trauma. Eur Radiol 2022;33(3):1918–27.

49. Kane NM, Francis IR, Burney RE, et al. Traumatic pneumoperitoneum. Implications of computed tomography diagnosis. Invest Radiol 1991;26(6):574–8.

50. Fernandes T, Oliveira MI, Castro R, et al. Bowel wall thickening at CT: simplifying the diagnosis. Insights Imaging 2014;5(2):195–208.

51. Ames JT, Federle MP. CT hypotension complex (shock bowel) is not always due to traumatic hypovolemic shock. Am J Roentgenol 2009;192(5):W230–5.

52. Soto JA, Anderson SW. Multidetector CT of blunt abdominal trauma. Radiology 2012;265(3):678–93.

53. Kawinwongkowit K, Kaewlai R, Kasemassawachanont A, et al. Value of contrast-enhanced arterial phase imaging in addition to portovenous phase in CT evaluation of blunt abdominopelvic trauma. Eur Radiol 2022;33(3):1641–52.

54. Park SJ, Kim JK, Kim KW, et al. MDCT findings of renal trauma. Am J Roentgenol 2006;187(2):541–7.

55. Pao DM, Ellis JH, Cohan RH, et al. Utility of routine trauma CT in the detection of bladder rupture. Acad Radiol 2000;7(5):317–24.

56. Baghdanian AH, Armetta AS, Baghdanian AA, et al. CT of major vascular injury in blunt abdominopelvic trauma. Radiographics 2016;36(3):872–90.

57. Anderson SW, Soto JA, Lucey BC, et al. Blunt trauma: feasibility and clinical utility of pelvic CT angiography performed with 64–detector row CT. Radiology 2008;246(2):410–9.

58. Miller-Thomas MM, West OC, Cohen AM. Diagnosing traumatic arterial injury in the extremities with CT angiography: pearls and pitfalls. Radiographics 2005;25(suppl_1):S133–42.

59. Soto JA. Pitfalls in diagnosis of blunt abdominal trauma, American journal of roentgenology.

60. Patel NR, Dick E, Batrick N, et al. Pearls and pitfalls in imaging of blunt traumatic thoracic aortic injury: a pictorial review. Br J Radiol 2018;16:20180130.

61. Ko JP, Goldstein JM, Latson LA, et al. Chest CT angiography for acute aortic pathologic conditions: pearls and pitfalls. Radiographics 2021;41(2):399–424.

62. Ito K, Hirahara N, Muraoka H, et al. Normal variants of the oral and maxillofacial region: mimics and pitfalls. Radiographics 2022;42(2):506–21.

63. Kolbeinsson HM, Dandamudi S, Gira J, et al. Expecting the unexpected: incidental findings at a level 1 trauma center. Emerg Radiol 2023;30(3):343–9.

64. Paluska TR, Sise MJ, Sack DI, et al. Incidental CT findings in trauma patients: incidence and implications for care of the injured. J Trauma 2007;62(1):157–61.

65. Barrett TW, Schierling M, Zhou C, et al. Prevalence of incidental findings in trauma patients detected by computed tomography imaging. Am J Emerg Med 2009;27(4):428–35.

66. Hanna TN, Shekhani H, Zygmont ME, et al. Incidental findings in emergency imaging: frequency, recommendations, and compliance with consensus guidelines. Emerg Radiol 2016;23(2):169–74.

67. Zhou Q, Qin P, Luo J, et al. Evaluating AI rib fracture detections using follow-up CT scans. Am J Emerg Med 2023;72:34–8.

68. Wasserthal J, Breit HC, Meyer MT, et al. Total segmentator: robust segmentation of 104 anatomic structures in CT images. Radiol Artif Intell 2023;5(5). https://doi.org/10.1148/ryai.230024.

69. Polzer C, Yilmaz E, Meyer C, et al. AI-based automated detection and stability analysis of traumatic vertebral body fractures on computed tomography. Eur J Radiol 2024;173:111364.

70. Dreizin D, Zhou Y, Fu S, et al. A multiscale deep learning method for quantitative visualization of traumatic hemoperitoneum at CT: assessment of feasibility and comparison with subjective categorical estimation. Radiol Artif Intell 2020;2(6):e190220.

71. Seyam M, Weikert T, Sauter A, et al. Utilization of artificial intelligence–based intracranial hemorrhage detection on emergent noncontrast CT images in clinical workflow. Radiol Artif Intell 2022;4(2). https://doi.org/10.1148/ryai.210168.

72. Brenner DJ, Elliston CD. Estimated radiation risks potentially associated with full-body CT screening. Radiology 2004;232(3):735–8.

73. Laack TA, Thompson KM, Kofler JM, et al. Comparison of trauma mortality and estimated cancer mortality from computed tomography during initial evaluation of intermediate-risk trauma patients. J Trauma Inj Infect Crit Care 2011;70(6):1362–5.

74. Stengel D, Mutze S, Güthoff C, et al. Association of low-dose whole-body computed tomography with missed injury diagnoses and radiation exposure in patients with blunt multiple trauma. JAMA Surg 2020;155(3):224.

75. Dendl LM, Pausch AM, Hoffstetter P, et al. Structured reporting of whole-body trauma CT scans using checklists: diagnostic accuracy of reporting radiologists depending on their level of experience. RöFo - Fortschritte auf dem Gebiet der Röntgenstrahlen und der bildgebenden Verfahren 2021; 193(12):1451–60.

76. Jorg T, Heckmann JC, Mildenberger P, et al. Structured reporting of CT scans of patients with trauma leads to faster, more detailed diagnoses: An experimental study. Eur J Radiol 2021;144:109954.

77. Schwartz LH, Panicek DM, Berk AR, et al. Improving communication of diagnostic radiology findings through structured reporting. Radiology 2011; 260(1):174–81.

78. Olthof AW, Leusveld ALM, de Groot JC, et al. Contextual structured reporting in radiology: implementation and long-term evaluation in improving the communication of critical findings. J Med Syst 2020;44(9):148.

UNITED STATES POSTAL SERVICE ®

Statement of Ownership, Management, and Circulation
(All Periodicals Publications Except Requester Publications)

1. Publication Title: RADIOLOGIC CLINICS OF NORTH AMERICA

2. Publication Number: 596 – 510

3. Filing Date: 9/18/2024

4. Issue Frequency: JAN, MAR, MAY, JUL, SEP, NOV

5. Number of Issues Published Annually: 6

6. Annual Subscription Price: $561.00

7. Complete Mailing Address of Known Office of Publication (Not printer) (Street, city, county, state, and ZIP+4®)
ELSEVIER INC.
230 Park Avenue, Suite 800
New York, NY 10169

Contact Person: Malathi Samayan
Telephone (Include area code): 91-44-4299-4507

8. Complete Mailing Address of Headquarters or General Business Office of Publisher (Not printer)
ELSEVIER INC.
230 Park Avenue, Suite 800
New York, NY 10169

9. Full Names and Complete Mailing Addresses of Publisher, Editor, and Managing Editor (Do not leave blank)

Publisher (Name and complete mailing address)
DOLORES MELONI, ELSEVIER INC.
1600 JOHN F KENNEDY BLVD. SUITE 1800
PHILADELPHIA, PA 19103-2899

Editor (Name and complete mailing address)
JOHN VASSALLO, ELSEVIER INC.
1600 JOHN F KENNEDY BLVD. SUITE 1800
PHILADELPHIA, PA 19103-2899

Managing Editor (Name and complete mailing address)
PATRICK MANLEY, ELSEVIER INC.
1600 JOHN F KENNEDY BLVD. SUITE 1800
PHILADELPHIA, PA 19103-2899

10. Owner (Do not leave blank. If the publication is owned by a corporation, give the name and address of the corporation immediately followed by the names and addresses of all stockholders owning or holding 1 percent or more of the total amount of stock. If not owned by a corporation, give the names and addresses of the individual owners. If owned by a partnership or other unincorporated firm, give its name and address as well as those of each individual owner. If the publication is published by a nonprofit organization, give its name and address.)

Full Name	Complete Mailing Address
WHOLLY OWNED SUBSIDIARY OF REED/ELSEVIER, US HOLDINGS	1600 JOHN F KENNEDY BLVD. SUITE 1800 PHILADELPHIA, PA 19103-2899

11. Known Bondholders, Mortgagees, and Other Security Holders Owning or Holding 1 Percent or More of Total Amount of Bonds, Mortgages, or Other Securities. If none, check box ► ☐ None

Full Name	Complete Mailing Address
N/A	

12. Tax Status (For completion by nonprofit organizations authorized to mail at nonprofit rates) (Check one)
The purpose, function, and nonprofit status of this organization and the exempt status for federal income tax purposes:
☒ Has Not Changed During Preceding 12 Months
☐ Has Changed During Preceding 12 Months (Publisher must submit explanation of change with this statement)

PS Form **3526**, July 2014 (Page 1 of 4) (see instructions page 4)] PSN: 7530-01-000-9931   PRIVACY NOTICE: See our privacy policy on www.usps.com.

---

13. Publication Title: RADIOLOGIC CLINICS OF NORTH AMERICA

14. Issue Date for Circulation Data Below: JULY 2024

15. Extent and Nature of Circulation

	Average No. Copies Each Issue During Preceding 12 Months	No. Copies of Single Issue Published Nearest to Filing Date
a. Total Number of Copies (Net press run)	847	766
b.(1) Mailed Outside-County Paid Subscriptions Stated on PS Form 3541 (Include paid distribution above nominal rate, advertiser's proof copies, and exchange copies)	592	548
b. Paid Circulation (By Mail and Outside the Mail) (2) Mailed In-County Paid Subscriptions Stated on PS Form 3541 (Include paid distribution above nominal rate, advertiser's proof copies, and exchange copies)	0	0
(3) Paid Distribution Outside the Mails Including Sales Through Dealers and Carriers, Street Vendors, Counter Sales, and Other Paid Distribution Outside USPS®	198	179
(4) Paid Distribution by Other Classes of Mail Through the USPS (e.g. First-Class Mail®)	0	0
c. Total Paid Distribution (Sum of 15b (1), (2), (3), and (4))	790	727
d.(1) Free or Nominal Rate Outside-County Copies included on PS Form 3541	40	25
d. Free or Nominal Rate Distribution (By Mail and Outside the Mail) (2) Free or Nominal Rate In-County Copies Included on PS Form 3541	0	0
(3) Free or Nominal Rate Copies Mailed at Other Classes Through the USPS (e.g. First-Class Mail)	0	0
(4) Free or Nominal Rate Distribution Outside the Mail (Carriers or other means)	40	25
e. Total Free or Nominal Rate Distribution (Sum of 15d (1), (2), (3) and (4))	40	25
f. Total Distribution (Sum of 15c and 15e)	830	752
g. Copies not Distributed (See Instructions to Publishers #4 (page #3))	17	14
h. Total (Sum of 15f and g)	847	766
i. Percent Paid (15c divided by 15f times 100)	95.18%	96.67%

* If you are claiming electronic copies, go to line 16 on page 3. If you are not claiming electronic copies, skip to line 17 on page 3.

16. Electronic Copy Circulation

	Average No. Copies Each Issue During Preceding 12 Months	No. Copies of Single Issue Published Nearest to Filing Date
a. Paid Electronic Copies ►		
b. Total Paid Print Copies (Line 15c) + Paid Electronic Copies (Line 16a) ►		
c. Total Print Distribution (Line 15f) + Paid Electronic Copies (Line 16a) ►		
d. Percent Paid (Both Print & Electronic Copies) (16b divided by 16c × 100) ►		

☒ I certify that 50% of all my distributed copies (electronic and print) are paid above a nominal price.

17. Publication of Statement of Ownership
☒ If the publication is a general publication, publication of this statement is required. Will be printed in the NOVEMBER 2024 issue of this publication.   ☐ Publication not required.

18. Signature and Title of Editor, Publisher, Business Manager, or Owner

Malathi Samayan - Distribution Controller

Malathi Samayan   **Date** 9/18/2024

I certify that all information furnished on this form is true and complete. I understand that anyone who furnishes false or misleading information on this form or who omits material or information requested on the form may be subject to criminal sanctions (including fines and imprisonment) and/or civil sanctions (including civil penalties).

PS Form **3526**, July 2014 (Page 2 of 3)   PRIVACY NOTICE: See our privacy policy on www.usps.com

Moving?

Make sure your subscription moves with you!

To notify us of your new address, find your **Clinics Account Number** (located on your mailing label above your name), and contact customer service at:

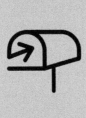

Email: journalscustomerservice-usa@elsevier.com

800-654-2452 (subscribers in the U.S. & Canada)
314-447-8871 (subscribers outside of the U.S. & Canada)

Fax number: 314-447-8029

Elsevier Health Sciences Division
Subscription Customer Service
3251 Riverport Lane
Maryland Heights, MO 63043

*To ensure uninterrupted delivery of your subscription, please notify us at least 4 weeks in advance of move.

Printed and bound by CPI Group (UK) Ltd, Croydon, CR0 4YY

08/05/2025

01864750-0018